UNDERGRADUATE
SURGERY SIMPLIFIED

Disclaimer

Whilst the advice and information in this book is believed to be true and accurate at the time of going to press, neither the author nor the publishers can accept any legal responsibility or liability for any errors or omissions that have been made. Readers are advised to confirm the information contained in this book with other sources and are advised to check the current product information sheet provided by the manufacturer for any drug they plan to administer to be certain that the recommended dose, method, duration of administration and contraindications contained in this publication are accurate. It is the responsibility of the doctor/practitioner to determine the best treatment and drug dosage for each individual patient. Neither the author nor the publisher can assume any liability for injury and/or damage to persons arising from the content of this publication. Note that normal values of investigations vary between laboratories and from country to country.

Every attempt has been made to trace and acknowledge copyright of material used in this publication. The publisher apologizes for any accidental infringements and would welcome any information to redress the situation.

This book has been produced for the purposes of medical education only.

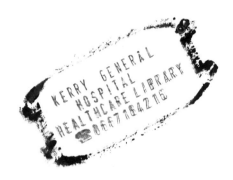

UNDERGRADUATE SURGERY SIMPLIFIED

A Directed Self-Learning Course for Undergraduate Surgical Students

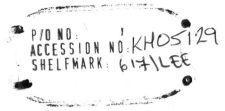
Peter Lee

MD FRCS FRCS [Edin] FRCSI [Hon]
Formerly, Professor and Head
Department of Surgery
Penang Medical College
Penang, Malaysia

Consultant General and Colorectal Surgeon
Hull and East Yorkshire Hospitals, UK

Foreword
Professor Sir Norman Williams

MS FRCS FMed Sci FRCP FRCP [Edin]
FRCA FDS [Hon] FACS [Hon] FRCSI [Hon] FRCSEd [Hon]
Past President, Royal College of Surgeons of England

Illustrations
Stephen Hill
MBBS MRCP MRCGP

![JAYPEE] *The Health Sciences Publisher*

New Delhi | London | Philadelphia | Panama

Jaypee Brothers Medical Publishers (P) Ltd.

Headquarters

Jaypee Brothers Medical Publishers (P) Ltd.
4838/24, Ansari Road, Daryaganj
New Delhi 110 002, India
Phone: +91-11-43574357
Fax: +91-11-43574314
E-mail: jaypee@jaypeebrothers.com

Overseas Offices

J.P. Medical Ltd.
83, Victoria Street, London
SW1H 0HW (UK)
Phone: +44 20 3170 8910
Fax: +44 (0) 20 3008 6180
E-mail: info@jpmedpub.com

Jaypee-Highlights Medical Publishers Inc.
City of Knowledge, Building 235, 2nd Floor
Panama City, Panama
Phone: +1 507-301-0496
Fax: +1 507-301-0499
E-mail: cservice@jphmedical.com

Jaypee Medical Inc.
325, Chestnut Street
Suite 412, Philadelphia, PA 19106, USA
Phone: +1 267-519-9789
E-mail: support@jpmedus.com

Jaypee Brothers Medical Publishers (P) Ltd.
17/1-B, Babar Road, Block-B, Shaymali
Mohammadpur, Dhaka-1207
Bangladesh
Mobile: +08801912003485
E-mail: jaypeedhaka@gmail.com

Jaypee Brothers Medical Publishers (P) Ltd.
Bhotahity, Kathmandu, Nepal
Phone: +977-9741283608
E-mail: kathmandu@jaypeebrothers.com

Website: www.jaypeebrothers.com
Website: www.jaypeedigital.com

© 2017, Jaypee Brothers Medical Publishers

Inquiries for bulk sales may be solicited at: jaypee@jaypeebrothers.com

Undergraduate Surgery Simplified: A Directed Self-Learning Course for Undergraduate Surgical Students

First Edition : **2017**

ISBN : 978-93-5152-894-4

Printed at Sanat Printers

Dedicated to

Sam and Ben
Perhaps some day, they will read it—I hope so

FOREWORD

It is a pleasure to write this foreword to Peter Lee's superb undergraduate textbook. I have known Peter for many years, ever since he and I were trainees at Leeds General Infirmary in the 1970s. He was always an inspirational teacher for both undergraduates and postgraduates. His teaching sessions were full of common sense and practical tips delivered clearly and always with a sense of humor that appealed to students and colleagues. His enthusiasm for all things surgical shone through and was infectious. But in addition, this gift for imparting knowledge was overlain by a deep humanity which is such an important part of medicine. His love of teaching has clearly led him to think deeply about improving education methods. As he says, the undergraduate curriculum has become more overloaded with less and less time for students to spend in surgical placements. Yet 'surgical' diseases still make up a significant proportion of the conditions that present to the doctors in the community. Students therefore need to be cognizant of such disorders and understand the principles of management. However, patients do not present with a disease, they present with a symptom that needs unraveling and that is why problem-based learning is so important. This is a discipline, which is also essential to impart gradually for a future career in medicine. One cannot rely on being "spoon fed". Medicine moves at such a pace that if a doctor cannot think for himself and know how to access and importantly utilize new information, he/she will soon become de-skilled. This book helps inculcate these skills as well as providing knowledge of surgery, which will I be sure benefit the student no matter what discipline, he/she wishes to pursue. It is a gem of a book, and I warmly recommend it to you.

Professor Sir Norman Williams
MS FRCS FMed Sci FRCP FRCP [Edin]
FRCA FDS [Hon] FACS [Hon] FRCSI [Hon] FRCSEd [Hon]
Past President
Royal College of Surgeons of England

PREFACE

Modern medical students have too much to learn in too little time. This book is designed to simplify and enhance the learning process of the students by involving the students in acquiring their own surgical knowledge through the use of directed or modified problem-based learning.

Undergraduate Surgery Simplified is a series of case-based tutorials in a question and answer format. The book covers the most common problems, which the students will meet during their general surgical clinical training. Each tutorial is centered on a presenting clinical symptom or sign—exactly as the student will encounter them in hospital or general practice. Using the question and answer format, the tutorials encourage the student to search out and source further surgical knowledge; thus, promoting deeper and longer-lasting learning. This is in contrast to most standard surgical textbooks where the surgical curriculum is artificially divided into 'disease' categories and centered on the less efficient model of didactic or 'rote' learning.

The book is arranged into three modules. The first module is centered on history taking and physical examination, the second deals with differential diagnosis and investigation and the final module with patient management and house officer/intern tasks. Many of the same case scenarios (or patients) spiral into all three modules so that the student gradually builds up knowledge of their overall presentation and management. The content of the book is designed to allow the students to use the tutorials from the first day of their clinical course, when their clinical knowledge and experience is minimal, to their last; hopefully making their transition from final year student to house officer, a seamless and non-traumatic experience. With this in mind, emphasis is placed on basic science, ethics, communication skills and on the practical tasks they will be expected to perform in their house officer/intern years.

Although primarily intended for the undergraduate surgical students, the book may also appeal to surgical house officers and interns, Foundation year 1 and 2 doctors in the United Kingdom and Surgical Course Curriculum Directors looking to update and standardize their surgical undergraduate curriculum.

The question and answer format of this book is similar to the Modified Essay Question (MEQ) widely used in modern day undergraduate and postgraduate examinations. This allows the readers to use the content as an important revision tool before summative examinations, regardless of whether or not they have previously used the book.

Undergraduate Surgery Simplified is a directed self-learning course based on modern day teaching methods. Whether used as a stand-alone course carried out at the student's individual rate, as an adjunct to their own medical school curriculum or as a revision tool, the book will enable the student to acquire the surgical knowledge and skills in a graded and enjoyable manner—promoting deeper and longer-lasting knowledge.

This book is based on the Directed Self-Learning Course developed over several years at Penang Medical College, Malaysia (affiliated to the Royal College of Surgeons in Ireland and University College, Dublin) where I was Professor of Surgery for 9 years. The content was an integral component of the Surgical Curriculum used alongside didactic lectures, tutorials and hospital experience. It was universally praised by both students and tutors alike, with feedback suggesting it as enjoyable, relevant and leading to more easily assimilated and retained knowledge.

Peter Lee

ACKNOWLEDGMENTS

The Urology and Head Injury tutorials were written, in the main, by Dr Ban Eng Lau (Consultant Urologist at The Loh Guan Lye Specialist Medical Center, Penang, Malaysia)

The Inflammatory Bowel Disease tutorials were written by Dr Tom Lee (Consultant Gastroenterologist, Newcastle, UK)

My colleagues in the Department of Surgery, Penang Medical College: Professor Premnath, Professor Kevin Moissinac and the teaching staff at Penang General Hospital, especially, my good friend Mr Manjit Singh, contributed greatly as the tutorials were developed and used in the teaching program.

The book could not have been produced without the radiological illustrations contributed by Dr Dennis Tan Gan Pin (Department of Radiology, Penang General Hospital), Dr Mohammed Ali (Chief, Nuclear Medicine Department, Penang General Hospital), Dr Risha Ratnalingam and Dr Annette Richardson, Leeds, UK and Dr James Cast, Department of Radiology, Hull Hospitals, UK.

Several of the clinical illustrations are reproduced with the permission of The Royal College of Surgeons in Ireland (special thanks to Professor Sean Tierney) and Mr BJ Wilken, formerly Consultant Surgeon in Scunthorpe, UK. Other individual contributions and publishers have been acknowledged where appropriate in the text. May I also thank James McCaslin, Professor Nick Stafford, Riz Farouk and Jawaid Akhbar for illustrations.

Tutorial content checking and editing have been carried out by Mr John Hartley (Hull, UK), Mr Bert Wilken (Norfolk, UK) Professor John MacFie (Scarborough, UK) and in Penang by Manjit Singh, Ban Eng Lau, Professor Liam Kirwan, Miss Lim Lay Hooi and Mr Yoong Meow Foong. Samir Pathak, Specialist Registrar in Surgery, read through and criticized the whole manuscript.

My former PA Paulina Bany carried out a lot of retyping and Trudy Lim retyped and edited the whole document—what a task. Kenneth Acharia photographed many of the X-rays, and Tim White in Beverley, Jon and Aidon in Leeds, UK and Richard in Aintree, UK helped with image difficulties.

The editorial team at M/s Jaypee Brothers Medical Publishers (P) Ltd, New Delhi, India turned the mass of words and pictures into a book, I hope we can be proud of.

I must also acknowledge the many hundreds of medical students who passed through the Department of Surgery at Penang Medical College between 2003 and 2011, the course was written for them and changed and evolved with their inspiration and feedback. Two in particular: Ronstan Lobo and Dhir "Trinidad" Bhattacharya require special mention for their help.

Finally, and perhaps most importantly, I should like to thank Dr Stephen Hill, the medical illustrator, who without complaint spent hundreds of hours on the drawings as well as many hours as a sounding block for my ideas and my moans.

In a book like this, so many people made contributions—if I have omitted anyone, my sincere apologies.

By Case Scenario

M = Module number

T = Tutorial number

CONTENTS 2

Module 3 Management and House Officer/Intern Tasks				
Tutorial	Symptoms/Signs/Topic	System/organ	Page no.	
			Questions	Answers
M3.1	Lump in neck: Solitary thyroid swelling Lump in neck: Multinodular goiter Lump in neck: Parotid tumor, submandibular swelling patient consent: Thyroidectomy	Endocrine	197	249
M3.2	Lump in breast: Cancer Lump in breast: advanced and recurrent breast cancer how to record clinical findings of a breast lump patient consent: mastectomy	Endocrine	200	250
M3.3	Difficulty in swallowing: Cancer esophagus Indigestion: Duodenal ulcer Acute abdominal pain: Perforated duodenal ulcer patient consent: upper G/I endoscopy consent for emergency laparotomy writing a prescription for drugs reading CVP manometer	Upper gastrointestinal	203	252
M3.4	Jaundice and gallstones: Cholecystectomy jaundice, fever and rigors: Cholangitis	Hepatobiliary	207	257
M3.5	Jaundice and weight loss: Cancer of pancreas Chronic abdominal pain: Chronic pancreatitis Acute abdominal pain: Acute pancreatitis	Panceas	207	259
M3.6	Rectal bleeding: Colorectal cancer Postoperative fever: Anastomotic leak Pain on defecation: Fissure in ano Perianal pain: Anal abscess Perianal soreness: Fistula in ano and pruritus ani Stoma complications Anal cancer; Rectal prolapse; Pilonidal sinus prescribing preoperative drug prophylaxis; marking a stoma	Lower gastrointestinal Minor anorectal	210	261
M3.7	Calf pain: Claudication Acutely painful leg: PVD; Arterial embolus Communication skills: Explanation of PVD and consequences	Vascular	216	265
M3.8	Acute RUQ abdominal pain: Cholecystitis Acute LLQ abdominal pain: Diverticulitis Colicky abdominal pain: Small bowel obstruction	Gastrointestinal	219	268
M3.9	Varicose veins Leg ulcer: Varicose ulcer Swollen leg; Lymphedema obtaining consent: vv operation	Vascular	223	272
M3.10	Acute loin pain: Renal stones drug prescription for pain	Urology	225	276
M3.11	Painful scrotum: Epididymitis; Scrotal gangrene Enlarged testis: Testicular tumor Difficulty with intercourse: Phimosis Scrotal ache: Varicocele Absent testis (infant) communication skills: explaining testicular cancer to patient communication skills: explaining retractile testis to a mother	Urology	227	278

HOW TO USE THIS BOOK?

Essential Information for the Reader

The content of this book can be used in one of four ways:

1. As a 'standalone' course for the clinical section of the students' undergraduate surgical training—performed in their own time and at their own pace
2. As a supplement (or adjunct) to the student's own medical school clinical surgical curriculum
3. To 'dip in and out of' when wanting to explore a particular symptom or sign which has been encountered on the ward or in the clinic
4. For revision purposes before examinations—particularly, those of the Modified Essay Question (MEQ) type.

Unless the book is used for revision, the reader will obtain maximum learning benefit by adopting the Directed Self-Learning approach on which the book is based. This can only be achieved by a *Disciplined Approach* to the tutorials, as described here.

Each tutorial will present a patient or patients with specific symptoms and signs. You will be asked to answer questions related to the patient, based on the sequence of history taking, physical examination, differential diagnosis, investigation and management. This is the way the patient will, in real life, present to the general practitioner's surgery, the outpatient clinic or on the ward. This attempt to simulate the situations you will face as a house officer or intern and qualified doctor is called *Case Based* learning and will be performed using *Directed Self Learning (DSL)*—a technique which is explained here.

When using the text please note:

The *Question numbers* are highlighted in red and the *Questions* themselves follow in non-bold type.

The *Initial History* of the Case Scenario is highlighted in an orange box with the ongoing history, examination findings, investigations and results following in bold type.

Any comments or instructions, out with the details of the 'ongoing' case scenario are given in non-bold type.

Note also that the relevant *Answers* are provided at the end of each module. They have been deliberately placed remote from the questions to discourage the learner from looking at the answer without first formulating their own.

It is suggested that you approach each tutorial in the *identical* way:

1. First read the appropriate chapter of your standard surgical textbook*, lecture or tutorial notes
2. Work through the DSL questions and answer as many as you can *without* the textbook or notes
3. List those questions or points you cannot answer or do not understand
4. Look up the answers or explanations in your surgical textbook, lecture notes, in journals or the net
5. Re-do the questions and answers with your new knowledge
6. Only then should you check your own answers with the tutorial answer section
7. Make a note of any further explanations to ask at your tutorials or directly to your teachers.

Print out the tutorial or use the computer with appropriate spaces for the answers. Condense and summarize the answers as appropriate (another textbook of surgery is not necessary!): This makes one think, as well as making the questions and answers ideal for revision or correction purposes.

Resist the temptation to 'cheat': If the answer section of the tutorial is used before you work out and record your own answer, much of the self-learning value will be lost.

All of this takes a lot of *time, thought* and *effort,* but if done conscientiously throughout the three modules, *as you go along*, a lot of knowledge will be assimilated, hopefully as deeper rather than superficial, crammed knowledge.

---

*Each medical school and student will have their own favored standard surgical textbook.

MODULE 1 will concentrate on *history taking and physical examination*; however, there will be some questions on diagnosis, investigation and management. The first reason for this is so that from the beginning, some idea of the overall management of the patient is obtained. Each case scenario hopefully then becomes more meaningful. The second reason is that the whole of the appropriate chapters in your standard surgical textbook should have been read before answering the case-based questions. Do not just read the section on symptoms and signs but also the relevant differential diagnosis and management. Clearly, all of this may not be understood to start with but the more times you look at a chapter or section of the book, the more familiar the content will become. If you do not have a protocol for taking a general surgical history and the relevant surgical examinations, please look at the Appendix 1 before starting Module 1—all these protocols will come into the text as you go along.

MODULE 2 will concentrate on differential diagnosis and investigation.

MODULE 3 will concentrate on management and house officer/intern tasks. On many occasions, the same 'patients' appear in all three modules (called *spiralling in* or vertical and horizontal integration by medical educationalists), but in practice means the reader will have experienced the complete sequence of a patient's care.

Note from the Author: The format of the first four tutorials is slightly different from the rest of the book, really just to provide some stimulus and guidance in the difficult first week or two when you have not taken clinical histories or sat face-to-face with real-life patients! Do not worry, the more interesting and stimulating standard case-based format starts in Tutorial 5! No apology is made for repeating the directed self-learning instructions at times throughout the tutorials—*resist the temptation to skip directly to the answers*. It will be worth it in the end—as will be attested to by the hundreds of medical students who used the course at Penang Medical College (and did not have access to the answer section!).

Good luck.

Addendum

Medicine and Surgery constantly change. The reader's attention is brought to some recent developments. These do not materially change the content or purpose of this book; rather they emphasize the importance of the Self-Directed Learning on which the text is based. The theme and content of the developments will have relevance to the appropriate section of the modules.

1. The increasing use of Minimally Invasive Surgery ("keyhole surgery"), particularly in the abdominal and thoracic cavities as well as in the repair of hernias and many urological procedures. Review at *www.patient.info/doctor/minimally-invasive-surgeryneeds*—plus accompanying references.

2. The availability of CT scanning for the initial assessment of the Acute Abdomen (reducing the use of plain abdominal X-rays) Review at *www.pubs.rsna.org/doi/full/10.1148/radiol.2531090302*

3. Bariatric (obesity) surgery Review: *www.patient.info/doctor/bariatric-surgery*

4. The use of Endovascular Aneurysm Repair (EVAR) in the management of elective and emergency Abdominal Aortic Aneurysm Repair. Review at *interventions.onlinejacc.org/article.aspx?articled=1378838* and Endovascular open repair for ruptured abdominal aortic aneurysm: *BMJ 2014;348doi:http://dx.doi.org/10.1136/bmj.f7661.*

ABBREVIATIONS

AAA	Abdominal Aortic Aneurysm		CA 19-9	Cancer Antigen 19-9 (tumor marker)
ABCDE	Airway/Breathing/Circulation/Disability/Exposure (in Primary Survey)		CNS	Central Nervous System
AAFB	Acid and Alcohol Fast Bacilli (Tuberculosis)		CT	Computerized Tomography imaging scan also called CAT scan
ABGs	Arterial Blood Gases		COPD	Chronic Obstructive Pulmonary Disease
ABO	Blood Group System		CVP	Central Venous Pressure
ABPI	Ankle Brachial Pressure Index		CVS	Cardiovascular System
A and E	Accident and Emergency (Department)		CXR	Chest X-ray
AF	Atrial Fibrillation		DD	Differential Diagnosis
AFP	Alpha-Fetoproteins		DOB	Date of Birth
ALT	Alanine Aminotransferase (liver function test)		DRE	Digital Rectal Examination
ALP	Alkaline Phosphatase (Alk. Phos) (liver function test)		DSL	Directed Self-Learning
AP	Anteroposterior (X-ray)		DU	Duodenal Ulcer
APER	Abdominoperineal Resection of Rectum		DVT	Deep Vein Thrombosis
AR exam.	Anorectal examination		ECG	Electrocardiogram
ASP	Aspartate Aminotransferase (liver function test)		ERCP	Endoscopic Retrograde Cholangiopancreatography
ARDS	Acute Respiratory Distress Syndrome		ESWL	Extracorporeal Shock Wave Lithotripsy
AR	Anterior Restorative Resection of the Rectum		ETA	Expected Time of Arrival
ASA	American Society of Anesthesiology Physical Classification System		Ex	On examination (clinical)
BEDDS	Mnemonic for examination of ulcer (see Appendix 1)		FAP	Familial Adenomatous Polyposis
			FH	Family History
Bioprofile:	Blood chemistry – Urea/electrolytes/LFTs		FBC	Full Blood Count
BMT	Best Medical Therapy		FNAC	Fine Needle Aspiration Cytology
BP	Blood Pressure		GA	General Anesthesia
BPH	Benign Prostatic Hypertrophy		GCS	Glasgow Coma Score (Scale)
BS	Blood Sugar (Blood glucose)		GERD	Gastroesophageal Reflux Disease
BUSE	Blood Urea and Serum Electrolytes		GI	Gastrointestinal (system)
Ca	Calcium		GN	Glomerulonephritis
CA	Cancer		GP	General Practitioner/Family Doctor
CBD	Common Bile Duct (UK) Continuous Bladder Drainage (Asian Abbreviation –not used in this book)		GTN	Glyceryl Trinitrate
			GTT	Glucose Tolerance Test
CEA	Carcinogenic Embryonic Antigen level		GU(S)	Genitourinary (System)

GU	Gastric Ulcer
H2 receptor	Histamine 2 receptor
Hb	Hemoglobin concentration
HCC	Hepatocellular Carcinoma
hCG	Human Chorionic Gonadotropin
HDU	High Dependency Unit
HI	Head Injury
HIV	Human Immunodeficiency Virus
HNPCC	Hereditary Nonpolyposis Colon Cancer
HO	House Officer (UK terminology) as in Intern or Foundation 1 (F1) doctor
HP	*Helicobacter pylori* also *H. pylori*
Hx	History – as in patient history and examination
Hx PC	History of Presenting Complaint
IBD	Inflammatory Bowel Disease
ICU	Intensive Care Unit
ICP	Intracranial Pressure
IHD	Ischemic Heart Disease
INR	International Normalized Ratio –measure of blood coagulation based on prothrombin time
I+D	Incision and Drainage (of abscess)
IV	Intravenous
IVC	Inferior Vena Cava
JVP	Jugular Venous Pressure
KUB	Plain X-ray abdomen to show area including Kidneys/Ureters and Bladder
L	Left side (as opposed to Right)
L	Liter as in mm/L
LDH	Lactate Dehydrogenase
LFTs	Liver Function Tests
LHRH	Luteinizing-Hormone Releasing Hormone
LMWH	Low Molecular Weight Heparin
LNMP	Last Normal Menstrual Period
LUQ	Left Upper Quadrant of abdomen

MB ChB	Bachelor of Medicine, Bachelor of Surgery (Medical qualification)
MCH	Mean Corpuscular Hemoglobin (as in Full Blood Count)
MCHC	Mean Corpuscular Hemoglobin Concentration (as in Full Blood Count)
MCV	Mean Corpuscular Volume (as in Full Blood Count)
MDT	Multidisciplinary Team meeting
METs	Metastases
MI	Myocardial Infarction
Micro C+S	Microscopy, Culture and Sensitivity (bacteriology examination of urine)
MNG	Multinodular Goiter
MRI	Magnetic Resonance Imaging
MR angio	Magnetic Resonance Angiogram
MRICP	Magnetic Resonance Imaging Cholangiopancreatography
MSU	Mid-Stream Urine
MS	Musculoskeletal
MVA	Motor Vehicle Accident
NAD	Nothing Abnormal Detected
NBM	Nil by Mouth
NG/ng	Nasogastric tube
O/E	On Examination
OCP	Oral Contraceptive Pill
EGD	Esophagogastric Duodenoscopy –as in Upper Gastrointestinal Endoscopy
OK	Expression of agreement or acceptance
OPD	Out-Patient Department
O_2 Sat	Oxygen saturation in arterial blood
OT	Operating Theater (Room)
P	Pulse Rate
PaO_2	Partial pressure of oxygen dissolved in arterial blood
PA	Posteroanterior (X-ray)
PCV	Packed Cell Volume (as in Full Blood Count)
PCA	Patient Controlled Analgesia

PE	Pulmonary Embolism		SH	Social History
PEEP	Positive End- Expiratory Pressure		SRN	State Registered Nurse
PMH	Past Medical History		SOB	Shortness of Breath
POD	Pouch of Douglas		STD	Sexually Transmitted Diseases
POSSUM score	Physiological + Operative Severity Score for the enUmeration of Morbidity and Mortality		T/L	Thoracic/Lumbar (as in vertebrae)
			T3	Triiodothyronine (as in thyroid function studies)
PPF	Plasma Protein Fraction		T4	Thyroxine (as in thyroid function studies)
PR	Digital examination of rectum		Tb/TB	Tuberculosis
p.r.n	pro re nata : means 'as needed' or 'as the situation arises'		TBI	Traumatic Brain Injury
			TCC	Transitional Cell Carcinoma of bladder
PSA	Prostate Specific Antigen (tumor marker)		TED stockings	ThromboEmbolism Deterrent stockings (compression stockings)
PV	Vaginal examination			
PVD	Peripheral Vascular Disease		T, N and M	Tumor, Nodes and Metastases
q	each or every, e.g. q 2hours means: every 2 hours		TME	Total Mesorectal Excision (in operation for rectal cancer)
R	Right side (as opposed to L –Left side)			
RCC	Renal Cell Carcinoma		TRH	Thyroid Releasing Hormone
Rh fever	Rheumatic fever		TSH	Thyroid Stimulating Hormone
Rh(D)	Rhesus Blood Group D		TV	Television
RIF	Right Iliac Fossa (of abdomen)		U+Es	Serum Urea and Electrolytes
ROS	Review of Systems –as in patient history Cardiovascular System, etc.		UK	United Kingdom
			US	Ultrasound
RR	Respiratory Rate		UTI	Urinary Tract Infection
RS	Respiratory System		V/Q scan	Ventilation/Perfusion Scan of lungs
RUQ	Right Upper Quadrant of abdomen		WCC	White Cell Count
SSS, etc	Mnemonic for examination of lump (see Appendix 1)		WHO	World Health Organization

History and Examination

TUTORIAL 1: Symptoms and Signs of Gastrointestinal (GI) Diseases

Question 1: Make a list of the basic questions you would ask in the history of a patient presenting with:

1.1 Difficulty in swallowing

1.2 Vomiting

1.3 Heartburn

1.4 Abdominal pain

Use a mnemonic to start with if you need to. Try to avoid writing it on the history sheet. Remember—pain is a very important symptom of many diseases. We are going to list the bare minimum of questions, in many cases, these will have to be expanded (if you get the chance, read Tim de Dombal's *'Diagnosis of Acute Abdominal Pain' (Churchill Livingstone, 1980)*—short and immensely valuable).

1.5 Indigestion

We will be dealing with indigestion in a later tutorial. Remember different people mean different things by this symptom and your questions must elucidate this.

1.6 Change in bowel habit

First list the general questions you would ask.

Then the specific questions relating to:

Diarrhea

Constipation

1.7 Change of appetite

1.8 Weight loss.

Question 2: Make a simple list of the common physical signs of gastrointestinal tract disease.

Use the headings face/eyes/mouth/hands/arms/legs/neck/axilla/chest/abdomen/anorectal exam.

Question 3: Case scenario

> A 60-year-old man presents as an emergency with abdominal pain, vomiting and has not had his bowels open for 48 hours.

Question 3.1: What questions would you ask him regarding these symptoms under the headings: Pain, vomiting, bowels

The pain started 3 days ago. It came on suddenly. He has never had it before. The pain started around the umbilicus but now it seems to be over his whole abdomen.

He says it is colicky in nature; it started off mildly and then became severe coming in waves every few minutes. When the pain was bad, he sometimes bent over or walked about but most of the time, he lay flat. He says he felt sick as soon as the pain started and he first vomited after about 2 hours. The vomit was initially mucusy with some green bile but now was brownish and smelled a little. He vomits every few hours and feels a little better after he had vomited. He has not noticed any blood in the vomit.

He has not had his bowels move for 2 days but thinks he has passed some flatus. His normal bowel habit is once per day.

Question 3.2: On examination, what features would you be looking for? Both in general examination and examination of the abdomen.

On examination:

He is alert, conscious and orientated. He is in obvious pain. He is pale but his mucous membranes are injected. He is not clinically jaundiced or cachexic.

He is dehydrated. His lips are not cyanosed, his tongue is dry and his dentition is good.

His hands are cold. He has no nail or palmar abnormalities. His pulse is 100 beats per minute, BP 110/60, temp 38.4/RR 20.

His abdomen is moving normally with respiration and is distended. There are no scars.

He is obese and no peristalsis is visible. There are no masses to see and his umbilicus is normal and inverted.

On palpation, he is slightly tender over the whole abdomen but with no guarding or rebound. There are no masses to feel and no organomegaly. He has no demonstrable ascites. He has high pitched bowel sounds coming in waves.

He has no groin hernias and rectal examination shows an empty rectum.

Question 3.3: What is your diagnosis?

Question 3.4: What might be the causes?

TUTORIAL 2: Symptoms and Signs of Urological Diseases

Question 1: Make a list of the basic questions you would ask in the history if a patient presented with:
- 1.1 Blood in the urine (hematuria)
- 1.2 Difficulty in passing urine
- 1.3 Pain when he passes urine (dysuria)
- 1.4 Dribbling of urine
- 1.5 Passing bubbles in urine (pneumaturia)

Question 2: Case scenarios

A 70-year-old man presents with difficulty in starting to pass urine, poor stream and dribbling over a period of some months.

Question 2.1: What basic group of symptoms is he describing?

A 35-year-old lady comes complaining of burning pain on passing urine together with daytime frequency.

Question 2.2: What basic group of symptoms is she describing?

A 30-year-old man who has just visited Bangkok comes complaining of a severe painful urge to pass urine. When he urinates, it is a small amount and he says it burns along his penis.

Question 2.3: What symptom is he describing and what is its significance?

The problem of how to lead into the question of sexually transmitted diseases is always difficult, especially when you are an inexperienced 'historian'.

Here are some suggestions:
1. Only ask the STD questions if you have a reason for doing so, i.e. the patient presents with STD symptoms.
2. Only ask questions to a patient at potential risk, i.e. do not start asking older, unmarried ladies or men unless you have a good reason for doing so.

Question 2.4: List the symptoms of a sexually transmitted disease.

Question 2.5: How will you lead into the necessary questions?

Question 3: Case scenario

A 30-year-old man presents with colicky right-sided abdominal pain and blood in his urine.

Question 3.1: What questions will you ask him?

The patient says he has never had the pain before, it came on suddenly 24 hours ago and he has had 3 attacks since then with a few hours of relief between. It is the worst pain he has ever had. It comes in waves. The pain is in the right side of his abdomen and moves into his groin and right testis. The blood is in the middle of his 'stream'— bright red and in small amounts. He has not noticed any clots. He has taken some nurofen tablets which helped a little. He is not on any other medications.

Question 3.2: What is the significance of the blood being in the middle of his stream?

Question 3.3: In this patient, what physical signs will you look for on general examination and examination of his abdomen and genitalia?

On general examination, he is not in obvious pain, he is flushed and has a low grade pyrexia. On abdominal examination, he is slightly tender in his R loin with no other signs. His groins and external genitalia are normal.

Question 3.4: What is your diagnosis?

Question 4: Make out your own table of the types of renal/ureteric stones, their frequency and how you would recognize them.

TUTORIAL 3: Symptoms and Signs of Vascular Diseases

Question 1: Make a list of the basic questions you would ask in the history if a patient presented with:
- 1.1 Pain in his calf on walking
- 1.2 Pain in his foot at night
- 1.3 An ulcer on his lower leg
- 1.4 Transient loss of vision

Question 2: Case scenario

A 50-year-old man presents to the A and E department with pain in his right calf. This came on while he was hurrying to catch an airline flight and went away when he sat down.

Question 2.1: What questions will you ask the patient when taking his history.

> Think—what might this be: Claudication/DVT/injury/ neurological. So questions will be based around this (history taking is dynamic (not a static list of facts)) and starts immediately with you *thinking* what might be wrong.

Question 2.2: Describe how you will examine this patient, under the headings: General and Specific—in this case CVS/ RS/abdomen/lower limbs including appropriate neurological examination where indicated.

TUTORIAL 4: Symptoms and Signs of Endocrine Diseases

Question 1: Make a list of the basic questions you would ask in the history if a patient presented with:
  1.1 Lump in the breast (female)
  1.2 Pain in the breast at period time
  1.3 A lump in the neck

Question 2: Case scenario

> A 54-year-old lady presents with a 2 cm diameter swelling in her right breast.

Question 2.1: What questions will you ask this lady?

The patient says she noticed the lump while showering 4 weeks ago and thinks it may have become bigger. She says that this is the first lump she has felt in her breasts for years. She used to have lumpy breasts at period times. This swelling is not painful and does not change in size. She had the menopause at age 50. She has not noticed any nipple discharge. She has 3 children, all of whom were breast-fed, the first one was born when she was 19. She had the menarche at 13 years and, as has been said, the menopause at 50. She was on the contraceptive pill for years. She is not taking hormones now.

Question 2.2: What are the features on clinical examination which may make you think this lump is malignant?

Question 2.3: What are the features on clinical examination which may make you think the lump is benign? List under LOOK, FEEL, MOVE.

Question 3: Case scenario

> A 50-year-old lady present with a diffuse enlargement of her thyroid gland.

Question 3.1: What questions will you ask her? Include the symptoms and signs of hyperthyroidism.

Question 3.2: List below the findings you would expect on examining the patient if she had Graves' Disease.

These should be listed under GENERAL and SPECIFIC (Neck):

Finally, one or two questions to help with your examination procedures:

Question 4: What is the difference between lid lag and lid retraction?

Question 5: Make a simple drawing of the relation of the IRIS to the eyelids in the normal state and in lid retraction and exophthalmos. This will really help you to remember them.

TUTORIAL 5: Difficulty in Swallowing and Heartburn

INSTRUCTIONS

It is suggested that you approach each tutorial in the identical way, that is, in a directed self-learning manner:
1. Read the appropriate chapter of your standard, recommended surgical textbook and use any appropriate lecture or tutorial notes you may have.
2. Work through the DSL questions and answer as many as you can without the textbook or your notes.
3. List those questions or points you cannot answer or do not understand.
4. Look up the answers or explanations in your surgical text book, lecture notes, in journals or the net.
5. Redo the questions and answers with your new knowledge.
6. Only then should the answer section of the tutorial be viewed.
7. Make a note of any further explanation you may need to ask your teachers directly or raise at the appropriate tutorial.

Print out the DSL or use your computer with appropriate spaces for the answers. Condense and summarize the answers appropriately. This makes your questions and answers ideal for revision and also easier to correct.

Resist the temptation to 'cheat'—if the answers are viewed without your own written answer attempt or the appropriate knowledge search, a lot of the self-learning value will be lost.

Question 1: Case scenario

Mr T is a 73-year-old retired laborer who presents with an 8-week history of difficulty in swallowing.

Question 1.1: What system are we dealing with?

Question 1.2: What questions will you ask him about his difficulty in swallowing?

Question 1.3: What other questions will you ask him next?

The patient says he started to be sick (vomiting) on and off 4 weeks ago.

Question 1.4: What will you ask about the vomiting?

He says the vomit now contains both liquids and food which he has just eaten. It is getting so bad now he can only keep a bit of porridge down. There is no blood that he can see. He has lost 10 kg in weight in the last 2 months and is never hungry. His bowels have become very constipated. He has not passed any blood or dark stools.

Question 1.5: What will you ask him about the constipation?

Question 1.6: How will you explain 'mucus'?

You have now obtained the details of his 'presenting complaint'.

Question 1.7: What will you do next?

Question 1.8: Write out the history taking protocol in full.

Back to the Case Scenario

Mr T has not had any serious illness, hospital admissions or surgery.

He has never had an anesthetic. He has not had diabetes/jaundice/chest pain/high blood pressure, a stroke/Rh fever or Tb.

His mother and father died of old age in their 70s. He has 2 brothers and a sister who are alive and well. There are no family illnesses. He is married and his wife is alive and well. He has 3 children who are all well and working.

He owns his own home and is financially able to support himself. He drinks 3 bottles of beer in a day. He has smoked 40 cigarettes per day since he was young. He has never traveled abroad and ate a diet of meat, rice and vegetables until his problem started.

In the review of systems under the respiratory system he says he has started to bring up dirty sputum when he is in bed at night—only in the last week or two. He has had chest infections in the past and his doctor told him to stop smoking.

In endocrine symptoms, he mentions that he has noticed a hoarseness of his voice in the last month and his wife has commented on it (Please note we will be going into the relevance of the sputum and hoarseness in Module 2 but think about what they might mean).

You have now completed his history. Look back over the details you have obtained and prepare a summary of them. Please note that the **summary should contain:**

1. The patient's name, age and occupation.
2. Any serious comorbidity.
3. The presenting complaint and its duration.
4. The 'lead' points of the history which are making you think about the differential diagnosis (do not worry too much about this at the moment, it will become easier as you gain experience and core knowledge of the symptoms of common surgical diseases).
5. It should be only a few lines maximum and is not a repeat of all the history you have just taken.

Remember the history and summary should be in the patient's words and not your interpretation into medical terms, i.e. difficulty in swallowing not dysphagia.

Question 1.9: Write your summary of this patient's history.

When you have gained more experience, even at this stage in the patient's assessment, you will be thinking of a differential diagnosis, this will lead you into what to look for when you examine him.

Question 1.10: What do you think is wrong with him?

We will now move onto examination of the patient:

Just as you have a routine protocol for history taking, you should develop a routine for your physical examination. This will be the same format whatever the presenting complaints.

Question 1.11: List the four headings which will form the basis of your routine examination.

Many physicians tell you to start with general appearance of the face, then the hands and then go back to the face for conjunctival pallor, etc. This seems illogical. When you examine the patient what do you look at first? The face—so deal with all this first. However, it does not really matter as long as you perform the same process every time and do not miss anything out.

Now we are going to consider the examination of this patient in detail, this will form the basis of your own physical examination protocol. Remember, when you are more experienced you will already have some idea of what is wrong with the patient, so you will be looking for specific signs. However, to start with you must rely on your routine (and you must include this, anyway, no matter how experienced you are. Do not cut corners!!).

Question 1.12: What will you look for on general examination?

List under the following headings:
Face, hands, arms, legs.

Question 1.13: What vital signs will you list?

In this case, we will examine his neck and chest before we proceed to abdominal examination (this is a convenient progression).

Question 1.14: What will you be looking for in neck and chest?

Then we come on to the specfic system—The abdomen:

Question 1.15: Write the headings of the abdominal examination protocol and under each heading, which features you would comment on or examine for:

Question 1.16: What will the rest of the routine examination consist of?

Now, we think this patient has a malignant lesion of his esophagus (probably a carcinoma of the esophagus).

Question 1.17: Based on your examination protocol, list the physical signs you might expect to find in a patient with an esophageal cancer. Think about this, then look it up in the relevant section in your surgical textbook and then write your answer.

In other words what physical signs might you expect to find in a patient with a carcinoma of the esophagus that you will be particularly looking for when you carry out your routine examination?

When the house officer examined Mr T, he listed the following:

Mr T is alert, conscious and orientated. He looks thin and cachexic. He is not in any obvious pain. He does not appear obviously dehydrated. He is pale and his mucous membranes are pale. He is not obviously jaundiced and his sclera are white. Inspecting his mouth, the mucous membranes are moist, his tongue is furred. There are no obvious ulcers to see or feel. His dentition is poor.

Inspection of his hands shows pale palmar creases. There are no signs of liver failure. His finger nails are normal.

His pulse is 72 and BP 120/80. He is apyrexial, respiration rate 15 (part of this comes from checking his charts).

There are no masses to feel in his neck and in particular no glands in the supraclavicular area.

There are no obvious abnormalities to see on his chest.

Inspection of his abdomen shows evidence of weight loss. The abdomen is not distended and moves normally with respiration. There are no scars present, no masses to see, no abnormalities of the skin and no distended veins or pulsations. His umbilicus is inverted and normal.

Palpation: There is no tenderness on superficial or deep palpation. His liver is palpable 2 cm below the right costal margin and has an irregular border which is very firm. It has a normal span. Spleen is not palpable and the kidneys are not ballotable.

Percussion: Liver edge is dull. There is no shifting dullness or percussion tap thrill.

Auscultation: Normal bowel sounds and no bruit.

Inspection of the groins and genitalia are normal.

Digital rectal exam from the house officer's notes is normal (as student you would not be expected to perform a routine rectal examination unless specifically asked to do so by a senior staff member and supervised by him). This does not mean you should not acquire the information from the notes if available.

His legs are normal with no edema.

The CVS and RS are examined: The base of his left lung is dull to percussion with reduced air entry and multiple crepitations.

Question 1.18: What do you think may be the significance of the following findings?
a. His cachexia?
b. His pale appearance and pale mucous membranes?
c. The findings on liver examination?
d. The findings on examination of his chest?
e. The history of voice change?

Question 2: Case scenario

Miss Q is a 40-year-old obese lady who presents with a 3-month history of a burning sensation in her chest, especially when she lies down at night.

Question 2.1: What questions would you ask her in taking your routine history?

The patient says she has had problems for about 3 months. Before that she cannot remember having any problems. When the burning sensation started, it was always at night and was intermittent. Now she gets it every night. She also has episodes in the day time after she has eaten. She has a lot of belching which is sometimes accompanied by acid in her mouth. She has noticed it

be worse with chocolate and coffee. She has also noticed she gets burning in her chest when she has a hot drink or drinks whiskey. She has never had any indigestion pain or abdominal discomfort after eating. She has put on a lot of weight recently and thinks this has made her symptoms worse.

Note: You must complete the rest of the protocol questions for the gastrointestinal system and PMH/FH/SH/ROS

Question 2.2: What is the likely cause of Miss Q's symptoms?

Question 2.3: Write a brief note about the pathophysiology of gastroesophageal reflux including the risk factors (basic science).

Question 2.4: What does the Figure 5.1 show and how was it obtained?

Question 2.5: What type of X-ray is shown in Figure 5.2 and what abnormalities does it show?

Question 2.6: What is achalasia of the cardia?

Question 2.7: How does the history of achalasia differ from that of say CA esophagus?

Question 2.8: How common is achalasia?

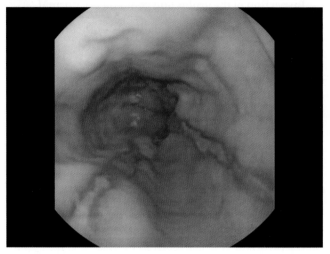

Fig. 5.1

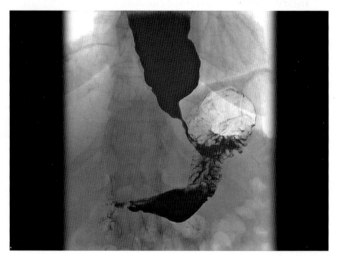

Fig. 5.2

TUTORIAL 6: Dyspepsia

Question 1: What is the difference between indigestion and dyspepsia?

Question 2: Case scenario

Mr F, aged 46, is referred to the OPD clinic with a history of upper abdominal discomfort for 2 years.

Question 2.1: What questions will you ask him?

Mr F says he has had the symptoms for 2 years. They were infrequent to start with but now occur every day. When asked to show where the discomfort is, he points to his epigastrium. He says it comes on when he is hungry and is relieved by eating food and by the antacid tablets he buys from the pharmacy. He also has a lot of belching and bloating.

Sometimes the discomfort wakes him at night and he gets up and takes a glass of milk.

His bowels are regular, he has not passed any blood, his appetite is good and, if anything, he has put on a few kilos in weight. He does not take any medications other than the antacids.

Question 2.2: What would be your diagnosis at this stage?

Because this is the likely diagnosis (and you should already be thinking of this), there are a few more specific questions you should ask him, mainly related to ulcer etiology and complications.

Question 2.3: What are these questions?

Question 2.4: What do you understand by the term hematemesis. How do you recognize it and how do you quantitate the amount?

Question 2.5: What do you understand by the term 'melena'?

What question do you ask the patient to try and establish that he has actually passed melena (this is very important as a lot of patients say they have passed dark bowel motions, which is not melena).

Question 2.6: You are now going to examine Mr F. You will be using your routine examination protocol for the gastro-intestinal tract. Write down below under the headings general and specific system what physical signs you would be specifically looking for in Mr F and why.

On examination, the patient looks well, is not clinically anemic or jaundiced. He is well-hydrated, well-nourished, his lips and oral cavity are normal and his teeth are in good condition.

His hands are normal and vital signs are within normal limits. Neck examination and chest inspection are normal.

Abdomen:

Inspection: Moving normally with respiration, no distension, no mass, no scars, no skin changes, no dilated veins or pulsations, umbilicus normal.

Palpation: Slightly tender in the epigastrium, no guarding, no organomegaly.

Auscultation: Normal bowel sounds.

Percussion: No ascites.

Groins: Normal.

PR: Negative.

Question 2.7: What is your diagnosis now?

The patient's hemoglobin comes back as 13 g/dL.

An upper GI endoscopy is carried out—the findings in the duodenum are shown below (Fig. 6.1).

Question 2.8: What does this show?

Question 2.9: What other investigation would you carry out with the endoscopy, i.e. what 'status' would you need to know?

The patient is diagnosed as having a duodenal ulcer and is found to be HP +ve. He is treated with triple therapy but does not come back for follow-up. Eighteen months later he is admitted to the general hospital as an emergency. For a year, he has been free of his indigestion but it started to recur three weeks ago. He now complains of sudden onset of severe epigastric pain (for 6 hours) which has spread over his whole abdomen. He has vomited twice and says he feels very ill and shaky.

Question 2.10: What is the likely diagnosis and what physical signs would you expect to find on examination (i.e. the signs of ----------).

On examination he looks ill and in pain. He is pale, has sunken eyes, a dry tongue and his pulse is 100 and his BP 100/60. His peripheries are cold. His abdomen does not move with respiration and shows diffuse board-like rigidity and guarding. He has no bowel sounds.

Question 2.11: What term would you use to describe his circulatory status and give a definition of this term.

Question 2.12: What term would you apply to the condition of his abdomen and what does this mean?

Question 2.13: What is the difference between tenderness, guarding and rebound tenderness and how would you elicit these signs?

The patient's erect chest X-ray is shown below (Fig. 6.2).

Question 2.14: What abnormality does it show?

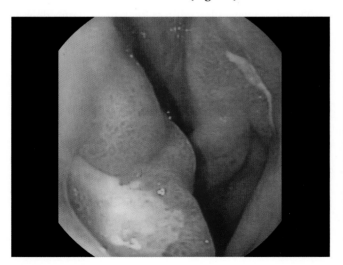

Fig. 6.1 Endoscopic view of duodenum

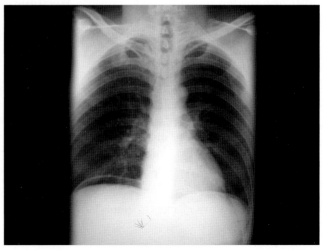

Fig. 6.2 Erect chest X-ray

Question 2.15: What will be the likely management? (Answer in one word only)

These are the findings at his operation (Fig. 6.3):

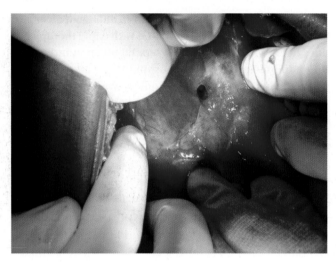

Fig. 6.3

Question 2.16: What is shown?

Question 2.17: In a few words what operative procedure will likely be performed (not greater than 8 words).

Question 3: Case scenario

Mr M is a 70-year-old man who is referred to the surgical clinic with weight loss, loss of appetite and what he calls indigestion.

Question 3.1: What questions will you ask him?

Mr M says he has had indigestion for the last year and has lost 6 kg. He says this is because he no longer feels like eating. In addition, in the last 2 months, he feels full after a small meal and has vomited on two occasions. When asked he says the vomit is the food he ate two hours before.

When asked to say what he means by 'indigestion' he says a feeling of discomfort and fullness in his upper abdomen. He has also been belching a lot.

On direct questioning he says for the last year he has felt tired and unwell.

Question 3.2: What do you think might be the differential diagnosis?

Question 3.3: List the classical history of cancer of the stomach.

Question 3.4: List the risk factors of stomach cancer.

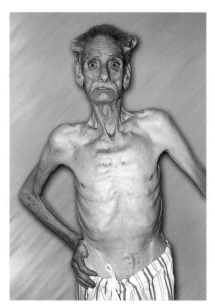

Fig. 6.4 From Bailey and Love, A Short Practice of Surgery, Ed. Williams N. Hodder, 2008. Reproduced by permission of Taylor and Francis Books, UK (*Courtesy:* Hodder Education with permission)

Question 3.5: This is a picture of Mr M (Fig. 6.4) Looking at him what physical signs do you see?

Question 3.6: What physical signs in the face indicate loss of weight?

On examination Mr M looks unwell. He has clearly lost weight and looks pale. His conjunctivae are pale but he is not jaundiced. He has a palpable gland in the left supraclavicular fossa. His abdomen is thin with evidence of weight loss. He has a vague mass in the epigastrium. His liver is not palpable. On rectal exam, he has a hard mass in the pouch of Douglas.

Question 3.7: What is the significance of:
a. The supraclavicular node (plus whose name does it carry)?
b. What is the significance of the mass in Pouch of Douglas (POD)?

Finally a little basic science:

Question 3.8: In outline only:

Where does cancer of the stomach spread to?

Question 3.9: Therefore, how do you stage cancer of the stomach?

You do not need to know the details of this, but remember the important prognostic factors are the depth of invasion of the stomach wall and the level of lymph nodes involvement.

TUTORIAL 7: Obstructive Jaundice

Question 1: Case scenario

A 35-year-old lady is admitted to the ward with upper abdominal pain, nausea and vomiting.

Question 1.1: What questions will you ask?

Question 1.2: List your parameters of pain.

The patient states this episode of pain started 2 days ago. The pain came on suddenly in the upper part of her abdomen and has been present ever since. She describes it as severe.

It radiates to her back. She has felt sick ever since it started and has vomited on 2 occasions. It is better when she lies still and takes paracetamol. Nothing makes it worse.

Question 1.3: List the other routine questions for the GI tract (from your protocol).

Examination of this patient shows the following:

General inspection:
The patient is alert, conscious and orientated. She is in pain and looks flushed. She is not clinically anemic or jaundiced but appears dehydrated. No abnormality of the lips or mouth. Dry tongue, good dentition.
Hands: Nothing abnormal detected (NAD)
She has a temperature of 38°C and a pulse of 90 beats per minute; BP = 120/70; RR = 20.

Question 1.4: What are the clinical signs of dehydration?

Abdominal examination:
On inspection, her abdomen is not distended and is moving normally with respiration. There are no abdominal scars, no masses to see, no dilated veins or pulsations. The skin shows no abnormalities and the umbilicus is normal and inverted. On palpation, she is tender in the right upper quadrant (RUQ) with a positive Murphy's sign. Liver is not palpable.

Question 1.5: What is Murphy's sign and how do you elicit it?

Question 1.6: What is your diagnosis in this patient and why?
The house surgeon arranges the relevant investigations:

Her white cell count (WCC) is raised and her liver function tests (LFTs) are normal. Plain X-ray of abdomen shows calcified opacities in RUQ and ultrasound shows gallstones in a thick walled gallbladder. The imaging investigations are shown (Figs 7.1 and 7.2).

You will note shortened 'abbreviations' have been used for some of the parameters. Medicine is now bedeviled with

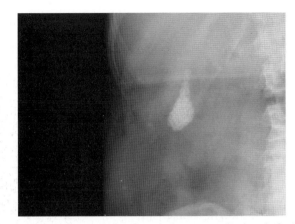

Fig. 7.1 Plain X-ray of abdomen showing multiple calcified opacities in right upper quadrant

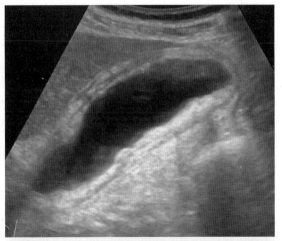

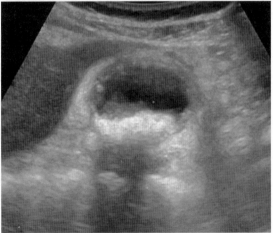

Fig. 7.2 Ultrasound scan of abdomen showing thickened gallbladder wall and multiple gallstones (Permission of Dr Taco Geertsma)

these abbreviations. Use only the very common ones and then only sparingly, remember they can cause confusion and may lead to errors.

For example, in the Western world, CBD is used to mean common bile duct but in Asia, CBD means continuous bladder drainage.

The consultant decides to treat the patient conservatively. She is put on nil by mouth, an IV infusion started and given antibiotics.

On day 3 in hospital, she says she does not feel well. She has developed shivering, a high temperature and now looks clinically jaundiced. Her pulse rate has risen but her abdominal signs have not changed.

Question 1.7: What do you think has happened? What clinical state has she now developed?

Question 1.8: Draw a simple diagram of the biliary tree and name the anatomical components.

Question 1.9: What routine questions will you ask every patient who presents with jaundice?

Question 1.10: What clinical examination features will help you to say the patient has obstructive jaundice?

Question 2: Case scenario

A 73-year-old woman presents with jaundice which has been present for several months. To start with, she had no abdominal pain but now she has a dull ache in her upper abdomen.

Question 2.1: What questions will you ask?

On examination she looks cachexic and has clearly lost weight. She is clinically jaundiced and has a mass in the right upper quadrant of her abdomen.

Question 2.2: What do you think may be wrong with her?

Question 2.3: What does Courvoisier's law state?

Question 2.4: Write down the classical history of carcinoma of the head of the pancreas.

Question 2.5: What is the outcome for this disease?

We will be dealing with the investigation of jaundice in more detail in Module 2, but as an introduction you should study the radiographs below.

Question 2.6: What investigation is shown in Figure 7.4 and what abnormalities does it show?

Question 2.7: What type of investigation is shown in Figure 7.5 and what abnormalities are seen?

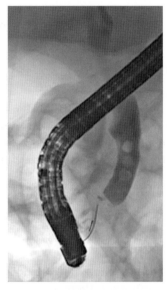

Fig. 7.4

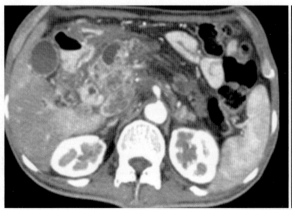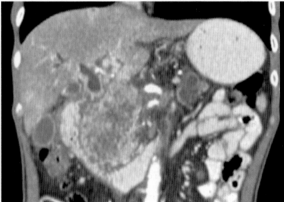

Fig. 7.5

TUTORIAL 8: Abdominal Pain (The Pancreas)

Question 1: Case scenario

A 40-year-old lady presents as an emergency with abdominal pain. The history the house officer (intern) obtains is as follows:

Over the past 3 years, the patient has complained of infrequent bouts of upper abdominal discomfort brought on by eating fatty foods. These have never been severe enough for her to visit her doctor. Eight hours prior to admission, she had the sudden onset of severe pain in her upper abdomen. This made her vomit (bile-stained fluid). Since then the pain has remained present the whole time and after 2 hours spread over the whole abdomen. She has vomited twice more, does not feel like eating and cannot hold down any liquids.

On direct questioning she has had no difficulty in swallowing, she has had heartburn and flatulence for 3 years. No change in bowel habit, no blood PR and no weight loss.

No PMH of note and she is a nondrinker and smoker.

On examination she looks unwell, she is pale, possibly slightly jaundiced and she is clinically dehydrated. Her pulse is 100/min, BP 120/70. Her abdomen shows diffuse tenderness and guarding with no bowel sounds heard. Rectal examination is negative.

Question 1.1: How do you elicit rebound tenderness?

Question 1.2: What does the absence of bowel sounds indicate?

Question 1.3: List your differential diagnosis for this patient. Write alongside each diagnosis the classical history and examination findings of each disease you list and then see if you can still justify including that diagnosis.

You might say that it is too early to be asked to make a differential diagnosis. However, the purpose of the reading you do in Module 1 (in addition to any lectures you are attending) is to start the development of your knowledge of the core symptoms and signs of the common surgical diseases.

In this tutorial we are also considering some basic aspects of investigation and management. This is to emphasis that although we are concentrating on history and examination, you must read up the disease entities as a whole.

It helps to use the same basic surgical textbook all the time—familiarity helps memory.

Question 1.4: What investigations will you (the house officer/intern) arrange and why?

Question 1.5: The patient's serum amylase comes back as >2000 IU. What is the diagnosis?

Question 1.6: What clinical sign is shown in Figure 8.1 below?

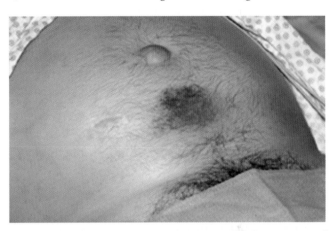

Fig. 8.1 CC (Creative Commons) Fred H. van Dijk H, Images of memorable cases: Case 21 (connections website), 2008. Available at http://cnx.org/contents/m/4942/1.3/

Question 1.7: What clinical sign is shown in Figure 8.2 below?

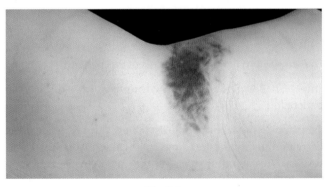

Fig. 8.2

Question 1.8: How is acute pancreatitis classified clinically?

Question 1.9: What do you understand by Ranson's criteria and the Glasgow Prognostic Score? How are they used?

Question 1.10: What are the causes of acute pancreatitis?

Question 2: Case scenario

A 50-year-old man presents with severe epigastric pain which radiates to the back and is relieved by sitting forwards. He has had bouts of similar pain on and off for 2 years and has noticed they are made worse by eating and drinking alcohol.

Question 2.1: What questions will you ask about his alcohol consumption?

He says that he drinks 4 big bottles of beer every day and has at least 3 small glasses of whiskey a day. He has done this for years.

Question 2.2: How will you quantitate his alcohol intake?

He says he has diarrhea, and has lost a lot of weight.

Question 2.3: What questions will you ask about his diarrhea?

He says his bowels work 5 times a day and that the stools are difficult to flush away and stink!

Question 2.4: What do you think this means? What condition may he have developed?

He also complains of being thirsty all the time and passing urine 20 times a day.

Question 2.5: What may this indicate?

On examination he is very thin and looks unwell. His abdomen is tender in the epigastrium and there are brownish red marks over the center of his abdomen.

Question 2.6: What is the physical sign shown in Figure 8.3 called and how is it caused?

The patient's plain abdominal X-ray is shown in Figure 8.4.

Question 2.7: What does it show?

Question 2.8: What is the diagnosis of this patient?

Question 2.9: Describe the pathophysiology of chronic pancreatitis.

Question 2.10: Make a simple list of how chronic pancreatitis is treated, using the headings medical (conservative) and surgical. This is your first real venture into management, look it up and try to understand the principles rather than the details at this stage.

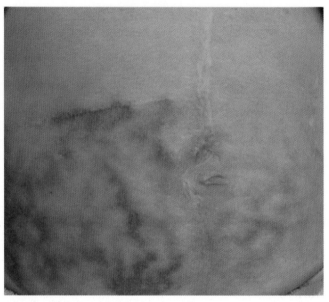

Fig. 8.3 (*Courtesy:* Heilman J. Available at http://Wikipedia.org/wiki/file; Hotbottlerash.JPG)

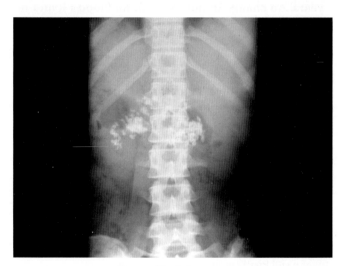

Fig 8.4

TUTORIAL 9: Rectal Bleeding 1

Question 1: Case scenario

A 65-year-old man presents to his general practitioner (GP) with bright red rectal bleeding of 3 months' duration.

Question 1.1: What questions should the GP ask the patient about the bleeding?

Question 1.2: What other questions related to the GI tract will be very important in this case?

The patient says the blood is bright red, he sees it mixed with the bowel motion every time he goes to the toilet. It is small in amount. He has never had this before. He has also noticed a definite change in his bowel habit, his normal bowel habit was once per day. In the last three months, he has been going 4 times a day. He has no pain either in the anus or his abdomen. His appetite is good and he has not lost any weight.

Question 1.3: What is the significance of the color of the blood?

Question 1.4: What is the significance of the change in bowel habit?

Question 1.5: Why must you always enquire about the patient's normal bowel habit?

Question 1.6: Why do we ask about pain in the anal area?

Question 1.7: Would the GP ask about family history and, if so, why?

Question 1.8: Write down below what you understand by the terms:
a. Adenomatous polyp of large bowel.
b. Familial adenomatous polyposis (FAP).
c. Hereditary nonpolyposis colorectal cancer (HNPCC).

NB: If you do not know the answers, look them up, you will be coming across these terms again as we go along.

Question 1.9: In this patient with rectal bleeding, what examination should the general practitioner carry out once he has obtained the full history?

The GP's findings are as follows:

On examination, the patient is not clinically anemic or jaundiced and has no physical signs in his abdomen.

Anal inspection and digital rectal examinations are normal.

Question 1.10: Should the GP refer this patient to the hospital? Justify your answer.

Question 1.11: If you think he should be referred, to whom and with what urgency?

The patient is referred urgently to the local colorectal surgeon. He repeats the history and carries out a full anorectal examination.

Question 1.12: What will this examination consist of?

Anorectal examination is negative apart from a trace of bright blood in the feces—found on rigid sigmoidoscopy.

Question 1.13: What other investigations will the surgeon arrange?

Colonoscopy shows the following lesion (Fig. 9.1) at about 18 cm from the anal verge. This is the classical appearance of an ulcerating cancer.

Question 1.14: Describe the macroscopic types and microscopic appearance of cancer of the large bowel.

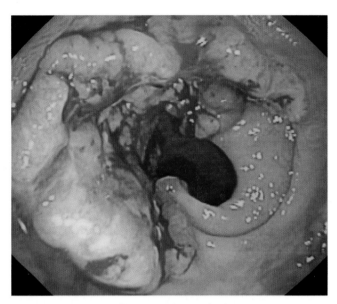

Fig. 9.1 Colonoscopic view of colon cancer

Question 1.15: Draw a diagram showing the percentage anatomical site distribution of large bowel cancers.

The site incidence statistics are important from the point of view of screening for bowel cancer.

Question 1.16: Does a right-sided cancer present in a different manner to a left-sided one? Give the right versus left features.

Question 1.17: Where does large bowel cancer spread to?

Question 1.18: What does the term 'staging' of a tumor mean?

Question 1.19: How does knowing the basic pathology of the disease help you in staging?

Question 1.20: What investigations are required to stage colon and rectal cancer?

Question 1.21: Draw a diagram of the operation that would be performed for a cancer of the cecum.

Question 1.22: Draw a diagram of the operation that would be performed for a cancer of the splenic flexure.

Question 1.23: There are 2 main operations used for cancer of the rectum. What are they?

Question 1.24: Draw a simple line drawing of each of these operations.

Question 1.25: Which main factor decides which of these operations would be performed and why?

TUTORIAL 10: Rectal Bleeding/Anal Pain 2—Minor Anorectal Disorders

Question 1: Case scenario

A 40-year-old man, Mr Smith, presents with rectal bleeding.

Question 1.1: What features in the history will suggest this is hemorrhoidal bleeding?

He states that he has had the bleeding on and off for about 3 years. The blood is bright red in color, usually small in amount and seen on the bowel motion or the toilet paper. Occasionally, the bleeding is more severe and drips into the toilet bowl at the end of defecation. He has noticed a lot of itching around the anus and also some perianal swellings recently which he cannot reduce. His bowel habit is normal. He eats a good diet.

Question 1.2: What is the significance of 'pain' in a history suggestive of hemorrhoidal bleeding?

Question 1.3: What is the significance of his bowel habit in this case?

Question 1.4: What is the significance of the 'good diet'?

Question 1.5: What is the pathophysiology of hemorrhoids (basic science)?

Question 1.6: How do you classify hemorrhoids?

Question 1.7: Of what value is this classification?

Mr Smith, the patient undergoes a full anorectal examination.

Question 1.8: What does this consist of?

On examination: Inspection shows skin tags and cushions. Digital exam is normal. Rigid sigmoidoscopy to 16 cm is normal. Proctoscopy shows hemorrhoids which come down on straining and only go back with manual pressure.

Question 1.9: Classify these hemorrhoids.

Question 1.10: What are the significance of the skin cushions seen around the prolapsed hemorrhoids in the Figure 10.1.

Question 1.11: List the appropriate treatment for the 4 degrees of hemorrhoids in a table.

Question 1.12: What is a proctoscope?

Question 1.13: What is a sigmoidoscope?

Question 1.14: Make a simple line drawing of the anatomy of the rectum and anal canal.

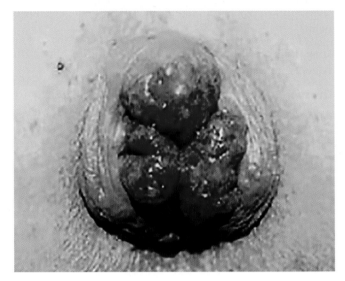

Fig. 10.1 Prolapsed hemhorroids. Reprinted from Surgery (Oxford), 21, 7, Hemorrhoids, Acheson AG, Scholefield J. 2003. pp. 165-7 with permission from Elsevier

Question 1.15: Which part of the rectum is examined by the proctoscope and sigmoidoscope?

Question 2: Case scenario

A 22-year-old girl, Miss Jones, comes to the rectal clinic with a history of pain in her bottom end (anus).

Question 2.1: What questions will you ask her about:
a. The anal pain?
b. Associated symptoms?

Miss Jones says the pain has been present for 4 weeks and occurs every time she has her bowels open. It first started after an episode of diarrhea after eating some bad prawns. The pain is severe and lasts for 2 hours. She describes it as like 'passing glass'. She has also noticed some bleeding.

Question 2.2: What would you expect her to say about bleeding?

Question 2.3: This is a classical history of what?

Question 2.4: What would you expect to find on examination? Make a simple line drawing.

Question 2.5: Answer the following: *(Try without the book first and then check your answers).*

a. At which anatomical positions do fissures occur in the anal canal?
b. What diseases are fissures associated with?
c. What are the clinical features, on examination, of an ideopathic fissure in ano?
d. What are the clinical features, on examination, of a fissure associated with Crohn's disease?

Figure 10.6 shows a classic posterior idiopathic fissure in ano with the white fibers of the internal sphincter clearly seen in its base and a large skin tag at the anal verge. The hypertrophied apical polyp is not seen in the picture.

Question 2.6: How is idiopathic fissure in ano treated? Make a simple list.

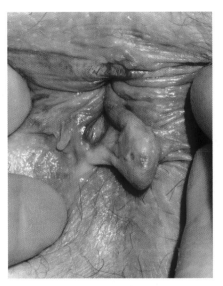

Fig. 10.6 Idiopathic fissure in ano

TUTORIAL 11: Lump in Breast

Question 1: Case scenario

A 45-year-old lady, Mrs Cox, presents with a lump in the left breast.

Question 1.1: List the questions you will ask her about the lump.

Question 1.2: List the risk factors for breast cancer (Enquiry about these must always be included in the history of a patient with breast symptoms).

Question 1.3: Write below your routine for breast examination—do this first without looking at any protocol and then check it with the one you have been advised to use.

Below is shown a picture of Mrs Cox's left breast (Fig 11.1).

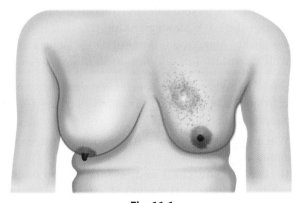

Fig. 11.1

Question 1.4: Describe what you see on inspection.

Question 1.5: List the findings on examination which suggest a breast lump is malignant.

In this case, the lump is 3 cm in diameter and lies in the upper inner quadrant of the breast. It is firm and irregular and fixed to the skin but not deeply. There are no nodes in the axilla. There are no supraclavicular nodes, no enlarged liver, no ascites and the other breast and axilla are normal.

Question 1.6: Basic sciences:

List the microscopic pathology of breast cancer—with the percentages of each type—this should be a simple list—no more than a few lines.

Question 1.7: Where does breast cancer spread to? Remember the following guideline:

In any solid malignancy: Make the differential diagnosis from the hx and ex; make the diagnosis with help of appropriate investigations; confirm it with tissue biopsy and then stage the tumor.

Question 1.8: How will we make the diagnosis and confirm it in this case? Clue: The answer consists of only two words and is the process to which every breast lump must be subjected.

Question 1.9: What does the triple assessment of a breast lump consist of?

Question 1.10: How do we stage breast cancer?

Question 1.11: What is the purpose of staging?

Question 2: Case scenario

A 17-year-old girl presents with a solitary mobile swelling in her left breast.

Question 2.1: What is the likely diagnosis?

Question 2.2: What is the pathophysiology of a fibroadenoma? How would you treat it?

Question 2.3: What would you say to this patient?

Question 3: Case scenario

A 33-year-old premenopausal lady comes complaining of pain in her breasts.

Question 3.1: What questions would you ask?

She says she has had the pain on and off for 2 years but it is getting worse. It is worst just before her periods and goes away when her periods finish. Her breasts have become very lumpy. She is worried because her mother had breast cancer. There are no other risk factors and she is otherwise fit and healthy.

Question 3.2: What is your likely diagnosis?

On examination, her breasts are generally soft but with marked areas of thickening in both upper outer quadrants, which are both very tender.

On the right side there is a discrete, smooth, non-mobile swelling at the 10 o'clock position. There are no palpable glands in the axilla.

Question 3.3: Write a brief summary of the pathophysiology of cyclical mastalgia.

Question 3.4: How would you manage this lady?

Question 3.5: What would you say to the patient?

TUTORIAL 12: Blood in the Urine (Urology 1)

Question 1: Case scenario

Mr M is 50 years of age and presents to the urology clinic with a 3-week history of passing red colored urine which he thinks is due to blood.

Question 1.1: What will you ask about his 'red urine'?

Remember that taking a history is an active, thinking process not a static one (the protocol is just there to guide you to start with). As soon as the patient describes red urine you call to mind the causes of red urine and hematuria and your questions are then designed to elicit the necessary information to make a diagnosis or differential diagnosis.

So with this in mind, ask further questions.

Question 1.2: What are the common causes of blood in the urine (hematuria)?

Question 1.3: Apart from blood, what else might make the urine red?

Back to the patient:

Mr M says that he first noticed the red urine about 3 months ago and has never had it before. He has seen it almost every day since then. He thinks it is blood because it is bright red and he occasionally sees clots in it. The blood is throughout his urinary stream. He has no dysuria, or other urinary tract symptoms. However, he says that he has had intermittent loin pain and night sweats for the last 2 months. His appetite is moderate and he thinks he has lost a few pounds in weight. He is diabetic and has ischemic heart disease (IHD). He is not on any drugs other than his cardiac medications and has not been eating beetroot.

Question 1.4: What can the time relationship of the hematuria during the urinary stream (i.e. initial stream, whole stream or terminal stream) tell you about the probable site of bleeding within the urinary tract?

Question 1.5: What further questions concerning his loin pain will you ask?

Question 1.6: What are the causes of "night sweats"?

Question 1.7: What is your differential diagnosis in this patient at this stage (based on the above history)? Do not worry if you have problems here, read the appropriate chapter and work out which 'core histories' may fit with Mr M's symptoms.

Question 1.8: What are the specific physical signs you are going to look for in your physical examination based on each of your differential diagnoses?

When Mr M is examined the house officer/intern notes the following:

He is alert, conscious and orientated and does not appear in any distress. He looks pale. He is well hydrated, not cachexic, not jaundiced and there are no physical signs in his lips or mouth.

He has no signs in his hands.

His vital signs are normal.

He has no neck abnormalities and his chest is normal on inspection/palpation/percussion and auscultation.

Examination of back: No abnormality.

Question 1.9: What are the clinical features (signs and symptoms) of anemia? List these.

Question 1.10: What signs may lead you to think the patient is uremic?

Abdominal examination of Mr M is as follows:

Inspection shows normal movements with respiration, no skin color changes and fullness on the left side of the abdomen.

There is no abdominal distension, no distended veins or pulsations and his umbilicus looks normal.

Palpation: There is no guarding or tenderness. There is a mass over the left upper quadrant of the abdomen. Renal punch sign is negative. His liver, spleen and right kidney are not palpable.

Auscultation: Bowel sounds are normal.

Percussion: There is no evidence of ascites.

His groins and genitalia are normal except for a soft swelling in his left scrotum above the testicle.

Digital rectal examination is normal. Legs: No abnormality.

Question 1.11: What is the significance of a positive renal punch sign?

Question 1.12: Enlargement of which organs can give you a mass in the left upper quadrant of the abdomen?

Question 1.13: What are the clinical features of a palpable kidney mass?

Question 1.14: How do you distinguish an enlarged kidney from:
a. An enlarged spleen on the left side?
b. An enlarged liver or gallbladder on the right side?

Question 1.15: Make out a table for the signs which differentiate between an enlarged kidney, spleen, liver and gallbladder, using the following headings:
Shape/ability to get above/movement on inspiration/ballotable/others.

When Mr M's abdomen is examined, the clinical feature of the left upper quadrant (LUQ) mass suggests it is enlarged kidney.

Question 1.16: What are the causes of an enlarged kidney and what do you think is the most likely diagnosis in this case?

Finally: A soft swelling has been noted in Mr M's left scrotum. When he is asked to stand up, it is much easier to feel and feels like 'a bag of worms'.

Question 1.17: What is this swelling and what is the pathophysiology in this case likely to be?

TUTORIAL 13: Loin Pain (Urology 2)

Question 1: Case scenario

A 37-year-old lady presents with a sudden onset of pain on her right side. When asked to show exactly where it is, she puts her hand on her right loin area.

Question 1.1: What questions will you ask about the right loin pain?

As in the previous case, as soon as the patient describes loin pain you should be thinking of the causes of pain in this area and moderating your history questions to try and establish which of the known causes is likely in this case. (History taking is active not static).

Question 1.2: What are the possible causes of right loin pain? Remember pain in this area can come from other systems outside the renal tract.

The patient points to her renal angle as the site of pain. She says it started as a dull ache and then became severe and constant and radiated to her right lower abdomen. She has never had it before. The pain goes away a little when she takes some painkillers (tablets she had previously taken for backache). She feels nauseated but has not vomited.

Question 1.3: What systems may be involved here?

Question 1.4: What other questions will you now ask her?

The patient says she has no other urinary tract symptoms. She feels feverish and unwell. Her periods are regular and have not changed recently. She has 2 children who are fit and well. She does not think she is pregnant. She has no other GI symptoms, in particular her bowels are regular and she has not passed any blood or slime. Her appetite is poor since the pain started but she has not lost any weight recently. She has had back pain on and off for 3 years when she works hard. She takes some painkillers from the chemist and has never been to the doctors with the back symptoms. She has no other joint problems.

We will now proceed to examine the patient.

Question 1.5: You will be using a protocoled examination of her GU/GI and M/S systems but list below what physical signs you will be looking for under general and specific.

On physical examination:

The patient appears in pain. She is pale, well-nourished and not jaundiced. She is flushed but not obviously dehydrated. There are no abnormalities in her lips or mouth.

Her hands are warm and moist.

Her pulse is 100/min, BP 140/90, temperature is 37°C, and RR rate normal.

On abdominal examination, inspection is normal. She is tender in the right renal angle and has a positive 'renal punch' test. She is tender in the RIF but has no guarding or rebound.

Liver and spleen are not palpable. Left kidney is not ballotable.

Her groins and external genitalia are normal.

M/S: Examination of back and legs is negative.

Question 1.6a: What is the difference between the lumbar region and the renal angle and the loin and the flank? This question is asked because even experienced physicians are confused by these terms.

Question 1.6b: How do you perform a renal punch test and what is its significance?

Question 1.6c: What is the anatomical position of the kidneys?

Question 1.6d: Describe how you would ballot a kidney.

Question 1.7: Are you going to perform a rectal examination in this patient, and if so, why?

Question 1.8: Are you going to perform a vaginal examination in this patient, and if so, why?

Finally:

Question 1.9: What is your differential diagnosis in this patient at this stage?

Question 1.10a: What is pyelonephritis?

Question 1.10b: What is pyonephrosis?

Question 1.10c: What is hydronephrosis?

We are now going to concentrate on the history and particularly the examination of scrotal swellings.

Question 2: Case scenario

A 58-year-old man presents at the clinic saying that he has noticed that his scrotum is getting bigger

Question 2.1: What further questions will you ask him?

Question 2.2: What differential diagnosis is going through your mind in a 58-year-old man with a scrotal swelling?

Question 2.3: The differential diagnosis should include hydrocele, hernia and tumor. With these diagnoses in mind what other questions will you ask him?

The patient says he first noticed the swelling about a year ago although it may have been longer. The swelling has gradually become bigger and seems to only affect the left side. It sometimes aches a bit but there is no bad pain. He says he has come to hospital because it is starting to get in the way when he rides his bicycle. The swelling never goes away and he cannot push it away. He has had to get up at night to pass urine in the last year which he did not do before. There is no history of trauma. His appetite is good and he has not lost any weight. He continues his work as a gardener and has had no serious illnesses or operations.

The rest of his PMH, SH, FH and review of systems is noncontributory.

We are now going to examine him:

Question 2.4: What systems will you be concentrating on?

You may not have been given a protocol for the examination of the scrotum.

Question 2.5: Make out your own protocol, it must be concise and easy to remember.

Question 2.6: Here is a picture of the gentleman's scrotum (Fig. 13.3). Describe what you see.

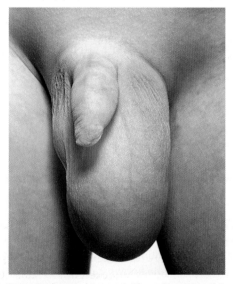

Fig. 13.3 From Bailey and Love, A Short Practice of Surgery, Ed. Williams N. Hodder, 2008. Reproduced by permission of Taylor and Francis Books, UK

In this gentleman, on palpation, it is possible to get above the swelling and define a normal spermatic chord above the swelling.

The swelling measures 12×12 cm and is smooth. It is tense and not fluctuant. It is nontender. The testis is not palpable. The swelling transilluminates.

The overlying skin feels a little warm, and on closer inspection, is slightly reddened.

The R scrotum is normal with a normal testis and chord. There is no evidence of a hernia on either side and no palpable lymph nodes.

Question 2.7: What do you think this swelling is?
(Please note that this patient will be revisited in Module 2).

TUTORIAL 14: Vascular Disease (Arterial): Calf Pain of Chronic Onset and Leg Pain of Sudden Onset

Question 1: Case scenario

Mr P is a 68-year-old man who presents to his general practitioner with pain in his right leg on walking.

Question 1.1: What questions will the general practitioner ask Mr P?

Mr P says he has had the pain nearly everyday for 3 months now. He says it is in the back of the calf in the right leg. It comes on after he walks 100 meters to collect his newspaper in the morning. He stops, lights up a cigarette and the pain goes away after a few minutes. It has not got better or worse. He does not have any pain in his other leg.

He has not injured his leg recently, has no abdominal or back pain and is otherwise fit and well.

Question 1.2: What symptom, even at this early stage in his assessment, do you think he is describing?

He is describing the symptoms of intermittent claudication.

He is referred by his GP to the vascular clinic at the hospital.

You are the house officer/intern and the consultant asks you to take Mr P's history and examine him.

Question 1.3: What other questions will you now ask him in the history of the presenting complaint?

Mr P says he has no chest pain and has not had a heart attack. His GP has told him he has high blood pressure and has treated him for this for 3 years now with tablets. He always takes these. He was asked to go to the surgery every 3 months to have his BP checked but he does not bother because he feels OK. He has not had any problems with his vision, has not had any blackouts, or weakness of his arms or legs and has never had a stroke.

He has put on weight recently because he does not get much exercise. He used to play golf but cannot do this now because of his leg. He eats a lot of fatty things because he likes them. He has never had his cholesterol checked because he does not believe in 'tests'! He is not diabetic but his father died young of a heart attack. He has 2 brothers, both older, and they both have trouble with their hearts.

You then work through the rest of your history taking protocol.

Question 1.4: What will you be interested in when you ask about his social history?

Mr P says he lives alone in a 3 storey house since his wife died 3 years ago. It has a lot of stairs. His 2 daughters come and see him a lot and cook for him. He retired as an accountant 3 years ago and has plenty of money. He smokes 40 cigarettes a day and has done so for 30 years. He drinks about 4 pints of beer a week and has a large whisky every night. (30 units per week)

Question 1.5: What is the relevance of these questions?

Question 1.6: What questions will you ask in the cardiovascular system (CVS) enquiry?

Question 1.7: What questions will you ask in the central nervous system (CNS) enquiry?

Why are the CVS and CNS questions particularly important?

Mr P's review of systems does not give any further positive information except that he is taking his BP tablets which he has read on the packet are beta-blockers and he takes an aspirin each day because his golfing buddies told him to do this.

Question 1.8: Why is he on these medications?

Question 1.9: Make a brief summary of his history. Remember this should contain only the most relevant aspects of the history which you think fit in with the diagnosis(es) you are thinking of (It should not be a repeat of the whole history!).

Now before we move on to his examination—a little basic science revision.

Question 1.10: Write a short paragraph on the pathophysiology of atherosclerosis.

Question 1.11: Draw in outline a simple diagram of the main arteries of the lower limb starting with the aorta and moving down.

Question 1.12: On a second diagram, put in the common sites where atherosclerotic changes occur in the lower limbs.

Next you are going to examine Mr P from the point of view of assessing his arterial vascular system including the CVS.

In the Module 1 Tutorial 3, we have already looked at the examination of the arterial vascular system, revise your answer before you move on to the next question.

Question 1.13: Now make out a protocol for examination of the arterial vascular system which you will then use routinely for the rest of your career!!

We now go back to the case scenario 1: Mr P

The findings on examination of Mr P are as follows:

General:

He is alert, conscious and orientated and not in any distress.

He is well-nourished and well-hydrated

He is not pale, his mucous membranes are well injected and his sclera are normal.

He is not cyanosed.

He has arcus senalis but no xanthelasma.

Mouth and dentition are normal.

Hands:

No palmar pallor. No palmar erythma. Palms are dry.

No finger clubbing or other nail changes.

Vital signs:

Pulse 80/min, regular good volume

BP: 160/100.

RR: 15.

Temperature: Normal, peripheries well-perfused.

CVS:

Radial pulses equal and normal. No collapsing pulse.

Brachial pulses equal and normal.

Carotid pulses present. No bruits.

JVP normal.

Apex beat 5th intercostals space.

Heart sounds normal. No murmurs.

RS:

No abnormality on Inspection: Percussion, Palpation.

Abdomen:

No visible pulsation.

No dilated veins.

No mass on palpation.

No bruits on ausculatation.

Legs:

Look:

Both legs look of equal size.

They do not look pale or blue.

There are no ankle swelling and no varicose veins.

There are no ulcers, including inspecting the toe web spaces and ventral surface of the feet.

On the right side the skin is shiny and hairless on the toes and the toe nails are thickened and irregular.

There is no muscle wasting or obvious deformity.

Feel:

The right leg feels a little cooler than the left.

Examination of the peripheral pulses is as shown below (Fig. 14.3).

There is no sensory loss in either leg to light touch.

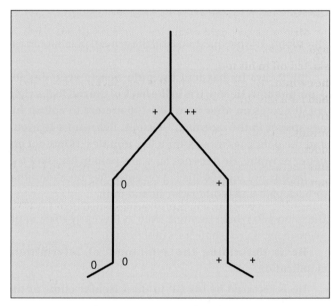

Fig. 14.3 Mr P's peripheral pulses

Move:

Normal power and tone of all lower limb muscle groups. No fixed deformity.

Auscultation:

No bruits.

Question 1.14: What do you think is wrong with Mr P?

Question 1.15: At what level do you think the atherosclerotic block is occurring?

Draw the 'block' on a diagram similar to that in Answer 1.11.

To finish with answer the following relevant questions:

Question 1.16: What do you understand by the term 'dystrophic'?

Question 1.17: What is the anatomical location of:

a. Femoral pulse
b. Popliteal pulse
c. Posterior tibial pulse
d. Dorsalis pedis pulse

Question 1.18: Make a table of the risk factors for atherosclerosis and opposite each factor list the general medical management of that factor.

Question 2: Case scenario

> Mr S is 70 years old and is brought into A and E complaining of the sudden onset of severe pain in his right leg. You are the house surgeon/intern on call and are asked to come and see him urgently.

Question 2.1: What questions will you ask him?

Mr S says the pain came on suddenly about 2 hours ago. He was watching the television at the time. The pain started off in his foot and now the whole leg is painful and he cannot move it much now. It is very severe. He has never had pain like this before. For about 3 years he has had pain in his right calf when he walks which goes away in a few minutes when he rests. He has hypertension. He says the doctor told him he has an irregular heart beat but nothing has been done about it. He is otherwise fit and well. He is not diabetic and is not taking any medications.

Question 2.2: What do you think has happened here, i.e. what is your working differential diagnosis at this stage?

Question 2.3: What physical signs will you be looking for when you examine the patient?

Use the arterial vascular protocol you have developed in the earlier case. Write this out in full.

Back to the Case Scenario

Mr S is alert, conscious and orientated but looks pale, restless and in a lot of pain. He has a tachypnea and is sweating.

His pulse is 100 beats per minute and is irregular. His BP is 100/90. His respiration rate is 20/min. His temperature is normal. His hands are pale and cold.

Abdominal examination is negative, in particular there is no pulsatile mass.

Legs:

Look:

Right leg bigger than left.
Right leg pale compared to left.
No visible mottling or bruising.
No obvious ulceration or gangrene (right).
Toe nails thick and mis-shapen (right).
Skin of toes hairless and shiny (right).

Feel:

Right leg cool compared to left.
Capillary refill time very slow, femoral pulse palpable on right (and irregular) but no pulses palpable below this.
All pulses palpable on left.
Right side has tenderness on squeezing calf muscle.
Sensation diminished on right leg.

Move:

Cannot lift right leg or flex knee.

Question 2.4: What is your diagnosis? And why?

Question 2.5: Write down the 6 'P's of acute limb ischemia. Are these reliable?

Question 2.6: An acutely ischemic limb undergoes a series of color changes as the ischemia progresses. What are these and how are they related to whether or not the limb is salvageable? What is the significance of the calf muscle tenderness?

TUTORIAL 15: Vascular Disease 2: Leg Ulcers and Diabetic Foot

Question 1: Case scenario

> Mrs N is a 60-year-old lady who has had varicose veins for many years. Three months ago, she developed an ulcer on her leg and has come to the hospital because she is worried about it.

You are the house officer/intern who sees her in the clinic.

Question 1.1: What questions will you ask her about the ulcer?

Mrs N replies that the ulcer is on the inside of her left leg. You ask her to show you where at this stage, because it may help with the history). *See* **Figure 15.1.**

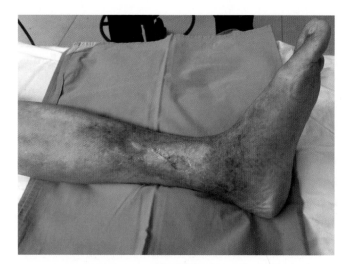

Fig. 15.1

Mrs N says she first noticed it about 3 months ago and thinks the cause is due to her varicose veins. It has started to get bigger. It has never healed over since she first noticed it. She does not remember injuring her leg and the ulcer has not been painful. It has been discharging some sticky fluid and she has taken to putting a bandage over it. She has not noticed any ulcers anywhere else. She has had bad varicose veins for years, worse on the left side. She thinks these came on after she was admitted to hospital with a swollen leg after the birth of her first child. The skin on the left leg has been getting darker and thicker over the last few years. The rest of her PMH/FH/SH and ROS is negative. She is not on any medications.

Question 1.2: Describe the ulcer which you see in the above picture. Before you do this look back at the protocol for describing an ulcer you have been given in the history and examination protocols (Appendix 1) or in Norman Browse's book: An introduction to the Symptoms and Signs of Surgical disease, Third edition. Arnold, London. p. 34.

You then proceed to palpate both Mrs N's legs. The right leg is normal apart from minor below knee varicose veins. On the left side, the leg is of normal temperature and the same temperature as the other leg. All the peripheral pulses are present in both legs. The skin surrounding the ulcer is thickened, hard, discolored and slightly tender. She has multiple varicose veins both above and below the knee along the distribution of the long saphenous vein.

You assess sensation over the lower limbs using 'light touch' with a piece of cotton wool, this is normal in both legs.

Movement, tone and power of both lower limbs are normal.

Question 1.3: What type of ulcer do you think this is?

Question 1.4: What other types of ulcer occur on the lower limb?

Question 1.5: The edge of an ulcer is very important in deciding its likely cause. Draw the 5 types of edge which help to differentiate the cause of the ulcer and name them appropriately.

Question 2: Case scenario

Mr O is 69-year-old and lives alone in the housing estate. He has been diabetic for 20 years and takes insulin. He is a very poor attendee at the GP diabetic clinic and does not test his sugar level regularly. Since his wife died 3 years ago, he has neglected himself. The general practice nurse goes to visit him at home because he has rung the surgery to say his leg is infected and he is having problems walking. The nurse is very worried about his leg and his diabetic control and brings him to A and E, where you are the medical officer on duty.

He shows you his right foot, a picture of which is shown below as Figure 15.3.

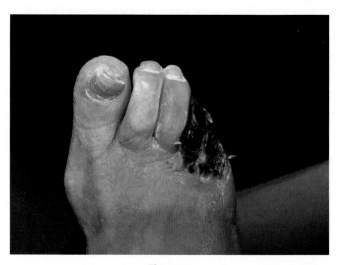

Fig. 15.3

Question 2.1: What term will be applied to Mr O's 4th and 5th toes?

Question 2.2: What initial questions will you ask Mr O?

Mr O says about 4 weeks ago he knocked his toes against a chair in his flat. He noticed that some sores developed, so he cleaned them with some TCP (antiseptic) and put a plaster on. It seemed to be OK at first but then they became red and inflamed. In the last week, they have changed color and started to smell. He did not go to the doctor because he lives alone and has no transport. He has been a diabetic for 20 years and gives himself his insulin. He does not measure his blood sugar level very often and usually takes the same dose night and morning. He has been told by the clinic in the past to be careful with his feet, but since his wife died he has lost a lot of interest in his life. He rarely goes out and when he does, in the last 6 months, he has noticed pain in his right calf on walking and has to keep stopping. He does not feel well at the moment and does not feel like eating. He does not think he has a fever.

You take the rest of his routine, protocoled history and then start to examine him.

Question 2.3: Describe the changes you see in the picture of his foot (Fig. 15.3).

Question 2.4: Before we go on to examine his foot further, write below a short description of the pathophysiology of the diabetic foot in bullet point form.

Question 2.5: Describe a Charcot's joint.

Question 2.6: What are the pressure points of the foot and why are they important in the diabetic foot?

Helped by the above basic clinical science you are now going to examine Mr O's legs.

Question 2.7: Based on the look/feel/move protocol you have developed in the previous arterial cases, describe what examinations you will be performing.

Question 2.8: We are going to look at some more pictures of the ischemic/diabetic foot. For each picture describe what you SEE and say what you think has happened.

a. Figure 15.4:

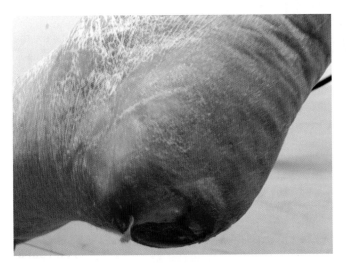

Fig. 15.4

b. Figure 15.5:

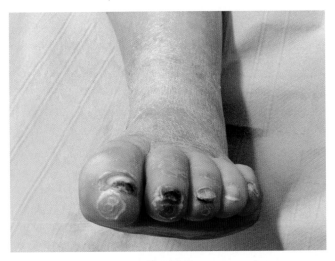

Fig. 15.5

c. Figure 15.6:

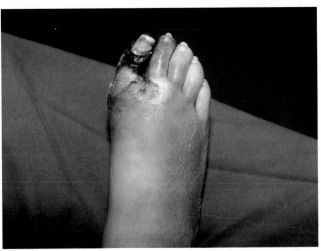

Fig. 15.6

Finally

Question 2.9: When you have completed your examination of Mr O's feet and legs and you proceed to complete his general examination, what will you be examining for as evidence of both atherosclerotic and diabetic pathology in the rest of his examination?

TUTORIAL 16: Head Injuries

Reread your lecture notes and textbook chapter on head injuries. Then try and answer as much of the DSL without the book and notes as possible. Finally check all your answers with the book/notes, altering the answers and adding to them where necessary. This is how you should be doing all the tutorials, you will be amazed at how much more you retain if you take the time and trouble to do this.

Question 1: Case scenario: A patient with a head injury

Patient presentation

> Mr S is a 26-year-old student. He is a front-seat passenger in a car and is not wearing his seat belt. The car collides with another vehicle and he is thrown against the windscreen. On arrival at A and E, he has a bleeding scalp laceration over the right frontal area and is confused.

Question 1.1: Before assessing his head injury what basic protocol would you go through?

Question 1.2: How will you assess his level of consciousness?

The primary survey does not reveal any signs of injury other than his head injury. His airway is patent; he is breathing normally and is peripherally well perfused. His pulse is 90 per minute and his BP is 120/80, RR 12. He is oozing from his scalp laceration but with no obvious arterial pulsation.

You arrange for a neck support, put up an IV line and send off his baseline blood investigations.

Question 1.3: How do you assess his conscious level—make out a table for this but underneath describe exactly how you would make the assessments.

The table is in all the books but often they do not actually tell you what to do!

The patient opens his eyes spontaneously, is confused when asked about his name, age, address and where he is. However, he obeys commands and localizes his pain to the area of his laceration.

Question 1.4: What is his Glasgow Coma Score (GCS)?

Question 1.5: How do you classify head injuries? (Traumatic Brain Injury (TBI))

Question 1.6: What is the role of the GCS in head injuries?

Question 1.7: Apart from the GCS, what other neurological examinations do you need to carry out in an unconscious, traumatized patient?

Question 1.8: Describe how you will carry out a full pupillary examination and what you will include in the neurological examination.

Question 2: Case scenario

> A 10-year-old boy falls out of a tree and strikes his head. His friends say he was knocked unconscious for a few seconds. He goes home and appears well–he is talking and laughing. After 8 hours, he becomes confused, complains of a headache and vomits once. His parents rush him to A and E.

Question 2.1: What is the likely diagnosis?

Question 2.2: What is an extradural hematoma and what are the mechanisms of injury? Include a small diagram to make you understand the basic anatomy of the skull, the meninges and the associated spaces, and simple diagrams to show an extradural and subdural hematoma schematically.

Question 2.3: List the clinical symptoms and signs of an extradural hematoma.

Question 3: Case scenario

> An 83-year-old lady fell in her house. Her neighbors said she was shaken but appeared otherwise unharmed. Four weeks later her daughter sees that she is becoming confused and at times is very drowsy in the daytime. She brings her to see the GP.

Question 3.1: What is the likely diagnosis?

Question 3.2: What is a subdural hematoma and what are the mechanisms of injury and clinical signs and symptoms?

Question 3.3: Now a bit of practice on Glasgow Coma Scores. Please make sure you have learned the GCS and then answer these questions without your notes:
a. A patient is brought into A and E after a head-on car collision. The patient does not open his eyes to painful stimuli, does not make any sound and withdraws from painful stimuli. What is his GCS?
b. A young girl is brought to A and E having crashed into a tree while riding her bike. When seen in A and E, she opens her eyes spontaneously, responds to questions in a confused manner and wrongly and moves all 4 extremities to command. What is her GCS?

Question 4: Now, without reading the books or your notes, summarize in note form the way you would assess a head injury and the principles of management of head injuries.

TUTORIAL 17: Preoperative Assessment and Postoperative Complications

PART 1: PREOPERATIVE ASSESSMENT

The history and examination taken by the house officer admitting a patient for either elective or emergency surgery is one of the most important events in the care of the patient. On it, the optimal care of the patient preoperatively, intra-operatively and postoperatively may depend (Table 17.1).

The history and examination is better protocoled and must be complete and problem orientated.

An example of a standard surgical, protocoled history has already been given to you in Module 1, Tutorial 5, but is appended below for revision purposes.

You must not miss out any of the suggested questions. If you do, this could have serious consequences for the patient, the surgeon and for you! (That is not to say you cannot ask additional relevant questions).

In addition to a protocoled history, you should, by this stage, understand the meaning of a problem-orientated history and should be starting to practice this routinely:

A PROBLEM-ORIENTATED HISTORY AND EXAMINATION

Obviously the purpose of the history is to establish the diagnosis and this is usually the number one entry in your list of problems. However, especially in the surgical patient, the house officer/intern must identify any other 'problems' the patient might have, which will impact on their surgical management. These should be listed at the end of the history and examination.

The house officer should then write alongside what action is proposed and make sure these are done.

For example, you might write:

Diagnosis: Probable small bowel obstruction.

Table 17.1 History taking protocol
Surgical history: Suggested protocol
Name: Age: Occupation:
Presenting complaint(s): Duration of each
History of presenting complaints:
Past medical history: Serious illnesses/operations/ever been in hospital/had anesthetic, if so, any problems—diabetes/jaundice/heart attack/high BP/stroke/Rh Fever/TB
Family history: Mother died of, Father died of? Brothers/sisters? Any family illness
Social history: Married? Children? Smoke, drink, home/financial circumstances diet, travel

Review of systems:

CVS:	Chest pain	**RS:**	SOB/asthma
	SOB		Cough
	Palpitations		Sputum +/– blood
	Ankle swelling		Fever/night cough
Abd:	Difficulty in swallowing	**GUS:**	Frequency
	Nausea/vomiting +/– blood		Dysuria
	Heartburn/acid reflux		Nocturia
	Indigestion/abd pain/abd distention		Hematuria
	Change in bowel habit +/– blood		Periods/pregnancies
	Appetite		Postmenopausal bleeding
	Weight loss		(+ if indicated: Hx of sexual contact)
CNS:	Headaches	**MS:**	Painful/stiff/swollen joints
	Fits/blackouts/dizziness		Neck/back pain
	Weakness/numbness/tingling		Fingers white/blue in cold
	Stroke/sleep well/depressed		
Hemo:	Bruise easily	**Endocrine:**	Swelling in neck
	Difficulty stopping bleeding		Hands tremble
	Lumps under arms, in neck, groins		Prefer hot/cold weather
	Clots in legs/lungs: DVT/PE		Increased sweating/fatigue
			Change in appearance/voice
DRUGS and MEDICATIONS		**ALLERGIES**	

Abbreviations: BP, blood pressure; Rh fever, rheumatic fever; TB, tuberculosis; SOB, shortness of breath; MS, musculoskeletal system, Abd, abdominal; CNS, central nervous system; GUS, genitourinary system; CVS, cardiovascular system; RS, respiratory system; Hemo, hematological system; DVT/PE, deep vein thrombosis/pulmonary embolism

Problems:	Action:
1. Confirm diagnosis	CXR, erect and supine abdominal X-rays
2. Known hypertension	Monitor blood pressure, medications
3. COPD	Chest X-ray review, respiratory function tests, physiotherapy, (?) antibiotics.

The purpose of this tutorial is to get you to think about these concepts and understand why they are so important.

In the past medical history you will ask a series of designated questions.

Let us look at the justification for some of these:

Question 1.1: Why do you ask if he has had any serious illnesses?

Question 1.2: Why do you ask if he has had any previous operations?

Question 1.3: Why do you ask if the patient has had any previous anesthetics?

You then ask the patient a series of direct questions— has he had diabetes, jaundice, chest pain, high blood pressure, stroke, TB, rheumatic fever? These 7 disease entities in particular are chosen because they are very relevant to surgical care.

Let us examine two of them in more detail to illustrate this.

Lets say the patient replies he was jaundiced when he was a teenager:

Question 2: Write down what questions you would then ask about his jaundice.

Question 3: Explain below the relevance of the past history of jaundice to his surgical management—lets say this patient is in for a right hemicolectomy for cancer.

Question 4: The history is problem-orientated, so what tests would you order in this patient who has a past history of jaundice?

Question 5: The patient's serology shows him to be a hepatitis B carrier. What precautions would this lead to when he is on the ward and having his right hemicolectomy?

On direct enquiry, the patient also states he has had chest pain in the past.

Question 6: What questions will you ask about this?

The patient says he has had a heart attack in the past and still gets angina. This is clearly a problem in a man who is about to undergo a right hemicolectomy.

Question 7: What tests will you order on him?

Question 8: What practical steps will you take with the information about his cardiac status, remembering he is about to undergo major surgery.

The other routine diseases asked about are diabetes, hypertension, stroke, rheumatic fever and tuberculosis.

Question 9: If the patient we have been discussing above were to answer in the positive for any of these conditions (he is having a right hemicolectomy) write down below how this may affect his surgery and what steps you as the house officer/intern would take.

PART 2: POSTOPERATIVE COMPLICATIONS

You will remember from your lecture course or textbook that there are several ways of classifying postoperative complications. The commonly used ones are shown in Table 17.2.

Table 17.2 Classifications of postoperative complications
Classification
General—to all operations
Specific—to certain operations
Early, intermediate or late complications
Anesthetic/surgical complications
Specific symptoms or signs

In this tutorial and the next we are going to use the specific symptoms or signs classification, because this is how they will be presented to you as the house officer/intern. For instance, a nurse will not ring up the house officer and say Mrs X has developed 'an early postoperative complication'; she will say Mrs X is complaining of pain and vomiting. This method of classification will be more useful in practical terms.

The postoperative complications we are going to consider are:
1. Pyrexia.
2. Postoperative pain.
3. Wound discharge.
4. Nausea and vomiting.
5. Constipation.
6. Breathlessness.
7. Confusion/agitation.
8. Low urine output: oliguria/anuria.
9. We will start with postoperative pyrexia.

Question 10: Make a list of the common causes of postoperative pyrexia you may encounter on the ward.

It is worth remembering that these complications occur more commonly at certain times during the patient's

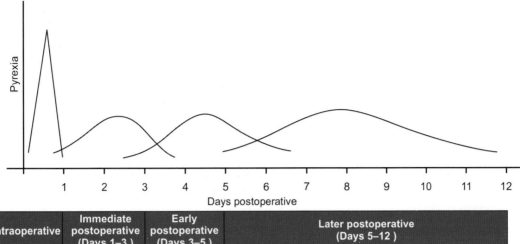

Intraoperative	Immediate postoperative (Days 1–3)	Early postoperative (Days 3–5)	Later postoperative (Days 5–12)
Drugs Blood transfusion	Inflammatory mediators Atelectasis Specific infections* Hematoma	Broncho- pneumonia Sepsis Wound infection Canula sepsis DVT	Anastomotic leak Abscess formation Wound infection and breakdown DVT and pulmonary emboli Distal sites of infection, e.g. UTI

*e.g. Biliary infection postbiliary surgery
Urinary tract infection posturinary tract surgery

Fig. 17.1 Relationship of postoperative complications to time after operation
Abbreviations: DVT deep vein thrombosis; UTI, urinary tract infection

Table 17.3 Postoperative complications					
Patient complaint	*Cause*	*Etiopathology*	*Presentation*	*Diagnosis investigation*	*Management*

postoperative course (perhaps best illustrated by the simple drawing—Figure 17.1) but this is by no means a hard and fast rule.

We are going to work through the possible causes of postoperative pyrexia—identify the presenting features and etiopathology of each cause, decide what investigations you would arrange to confirm your diagnosis and make a very brief outline of the appropriate management you would introduce.

Prepare your answers so that they can be inserted in a simple table for the complication with the following headings shown above (Table 17.3). This will make you extract only the essential core knowledge. Later in the tutorial, you will be asked to prepare similar tables for each of the main groups of postoperative complications. This will involve a lot of time,

thought and effort, but will be well worthwhile when you become the house officer/intern who actually has to deal with these problems.

Let us first consider postoperative atelectasis/bronchopneumonia as a cause of pyrexia under each of the headings.

Question 11: What is the etiopathology of postoperative pulmonary atelectasis or bronchopneumonia?

Question 12: What is the clinical presentation of this complication?

Question 13: How do you make the diagnosis including investigations?

Question 14: What is the management?

Let us now consider wound infection as a cause of postoperative pyrexia under the same headings.

Question 15: What is the etiopathology of postoperative wound infection?

Question 16: What is the clinical presentation of a wound infection?

Question 17: How do you make the diagnosis and what investigations are necessary?

Question 18: What is the management?

The next cause of postoperative pyrexia to consider is intra-abdominal sepsis or abscess.

Question 19: Following abdominal surgery, where are the main sites of associated abscess formation and sepsis?

Let us consider each of these in turn under our headings:
Pelvic Abscess:

Question 20: What is the etiopathology?

Question 21: How do you make the diagnosis?

Question 22: What is the management?

'Abdominal sepsis': By this is meant interloop and sub-visceral collections of pus in the general abdominal cavity.

Question 23: What is the etiopathology?

Question 24: What is the clinical presentation?

Question 25: How is diagnosis made?

Question 26: What is the management?
Subphrenic:

Question 27: What is the likely etiopathology in the postoperative period?

Question 28: What is the clinical presentation?

Question 29: How do you make the diagnosis?

Question 30: What is the management?

Liver abscess (pyogenic)—Just considering the post-operative situation:

Question 31: What is the etiology?

Question 32: What is the presentation?

Question 33: How is diagnosis made?

Question 34: What is the management?

Now let us look at urinary tract infection (UTI) as a cause of postoperative pyrexia:

Question 35: What is the etiology of the UTI?

Question 36: What is the clinical presentation and how is diagnosis confirmed?

Question 37: What is the management?

Now let us look at the inflamed IV site as a cause of pyrexia. Remember also that infection of a central line can also cause pyrexia. CVP lines will be discussed in a later tutorial.

Question 38: What is the etiopathology?

Question 39: What is the presentation?

Question 40: What is the management?

Now lest us consider thromboembolism (*Deep Venous Thrombosis*) which may present with a small spike of temperature.

Question 41: What is the etiopathology?

Question 42: What is the clinical presentation?

Question 43: How is the diagnosis made?

Question 44: What is the management?

Because it is very important for the house officer/intern, let us consider under the same headings the complication of pulmonary embolism coming from the DVT.

Question 45: What is the etiopathology of pulmonary embolism as a postoperative complication?

Question 46: What is the presentation?

Question 47: How is the diagnosis made and what investigations will help?

Question 48: What is the management?

Now let us look at blood transfusion problems as a cause of postoperative pyrexia.

Question 49: What is the etiopathology of transfusion reactions?

Question 50: What is the clinical presentation?

Question 51: What is the management?

Finally for pyrexia, let us look at septicemia:

Question 52: What is the etiopathology in the postoperative situation?

Table 17.4 Complications					
Patient complaint	Cause	Etiopathology	Presentation	Diagnosis investigation	Management

Question 53: What is the clinical presentation?

Question 54: How is diagnosis made and what are the investigations?

Question 55: Outline the management.

Question 56: Now transfer all the answers to the above questions on pyrexia into a simple table (as outlined above in Table 17.4) with the headings:

- Patient complaint.
- Cause.
- Etiopathology.
- Clinical presentation.
- Diagnosis and investigation.
- Management.

TUTORIAL 18: Postoperative Complications (2)

In this tutorial, we are going to consider the rest of the postoperative complications which we listed in Tutorial 17. Most of these will be studied by constructing a table as we have done for pyrexia.

This will involve a lot of work, if however, you do it fully and in the format chosen, then:

1. You will acquire knowledge by deeper learning.
2. By using the 'tables' you will be condensing this to 'core knowledge'.
3. You will have an excellent revision 'tool' for the future.
4. You will acquire practical knowledge.
   We will next consider:
   - Postoperative pain
   - This will be divided into:
     – Wound pain
     – Chest pain
     – Abdominal pain
     – Leg pain.

Question 1: Imagine you are the houseman and the patient complains of wound pain. List the presenting features of the causes of wound pain, what you would look for and what you would do about it in the way of investigations and treatment and enter these answers into the same type of table we have used for pyrexia.

Question 2: Make out a table for chest pain under the following causes:
- Cardiac
- Pulmonary
- Gastric/esophageal
- Musculoskeletal.

Question 3: Make out a table for abdominal pain with the following causes: Anastomotic leak, intestinal obstruction, postoperative hemorrhage, perforated viscus, pancreatitis/cholecystitis, intestinal ischemia, intra-abdominal abscess/sepsis.

Question 4: Make out a table for leg pain with the following causes:
- DVT, trauma and lumbar disc prolapse.
- Let us now consider the patient whose complaint is:
  Discharge from his wound

Question 5: Construct the same table using the same headings with the following causes:
  Bleeding, wound infection, wound breakdown, fistula.
  Now we will consider postoperative, nausea and vomiting:

Question 6: Make out the table using the following cause of postoperative nausea and vomiting:
- The anesthetic
- Related to the surgery

- Medications
- Electrolyte disturbance
- Pseudo-obstruction.

Now we will consider postoperative constipation:

Question 7: Make out a table for the patient complaint of constipation.

Now let us consider the patient complaint or sign of postoperative breathlessness:

Question 8: Make out the table with the following causes for the breathlessness:

- Respiratory
- Cardiac
- Wound pain
- Blood loss
- Sepsis.

We will now consider the complication of postoperative confusion/agitation.

This is an important and common complication especially amongst the elderly. You may be rung in the middle of the night by the nurses to say that Mrs Jones who is day 4 following her bowel surgery has become confused and agitated. She is trying to climb out of bed and has pulled her IV line out.

Inexperienced house officers find it a difficult situation to deal with but provided you have thought about the causes, the management becomes easier.

Question 9: What are the risk factors for postoperative confusion?

Question 10: Make a list of the underlying causes of postoperative confusion, i.e. the etiopathology.

Question 11: What will be your management when you are called to see the confused patient in the night?

Finally we are going to look at the common postoperative complaint of low urine output (oliguria) or no urine output (anuria).

Question 12: What are the causes of oliguria or anuria in the postoperative patient. Do this on a general, easy to remember basis rather than just a list.

Question 13: Make a simple list of the steps in management you will carry out as a house officer/intern to prevent postoperative renal failure.

Question 14: You are the house officer on call and the nurse rings you to say Mr M who is 24 hours postoperative anterior resection has dropped his urine output over the last 2 hours. Make a bullet point list of exactly the initial practical steps you will undertake.

TUTORIAL 19: Blood Transfusion

Read the appropriate chapter in your surgical textbook and then answer the following questions:

Question 1: Case scenario

Mr P, a 48-year-old businessman presents with the history of passing of melena stools for one week. He has no significant past medical history. Clinical examination shows that he is pale. His pulse is 92/min and BP 130/80 mm Hg. His hemoglobin level is 9.5 g/dL. Upper GI endoscopy shows a chronic duodenal ulcer with no stigmata of recent hemorrhage.

Question 1.1: Does this patient need a blood transfusion at this stage? Justify your answer.

Question 1.2: What do you understand by the term "transfusion trigger" or "trigger level for transfusion"?

The patient's condition and his hemoglobin level remain stable and he is discharged home after 2 days and advised to take the histamine H2 receptor antagonist **cimetidine. One week later he again presents with passing fresh melena. He is hemodynamically stable. This time his hemoglobin is 5.3 g/dL. EGD shows fresh blood clot over the duodenal ulcer.**

Question 1.3a: Does Mr P need a blood transfusion now and, if so, why?

Question 1.3b: If you decide to transfuse him, which blood component are you going to use?

Question 1.3c: List the components that can be prepared from a single donated blood unit.

Question 1.3d: What is the difference between 'type and screen', group and hold and full cross matching?

Question 1.4: What procedures should be taken to prevent transfusion errors before blood is given to a patient?

Back to the patient scenario:

Mr P is worried about the possible adverse effects of blood transfusion.

Question 1.5: How are you going to counsel him regarding the possible adverse effects of blood transfusion?

Mr P has read in the newspaper about autologous blood transfusion. He wants to know more about this.

Question 1.6: What is an autologous transfusion? Would Mr P be suitable to have autologous blood transfusion?

Under what circumstances is autologous transfusion indicated?

Question 2: Case scenario

Mr Q is a victim of a motor vehicle accident and suffers multiple injuries to his thorax, abdomen and pelvis. His pulse is 124/min and BP is 70/40 mm Hg when he arrives at the A and E department. He is given 2 liters of normal saline and 2 bottles of colloid expander but remains tachycardic and hypotensive. His hemoglobin taken on arrival at hospital is 4.4 g/dL.

Question 2.1: Mr Q needs urgent blood transfusion. Which type of blood can you give him while waiting for cross-matching and why?

Question 2.2: What does the term "massive transfusion" mean?

Question 2.3: What are the likely complications of massive transfusion?

We are now going to give you a practical patient scenario. Make sure you have read the chapter in the surgical textbook and then try and answer the scenario without 'help'. When you have finished, check your answers with the textbook and correct your own answers where necessary or discuss the problems with your tutor. You might like to look at "Blood transfusion—a clinician's reference:" *www. transfusionguidelines.org.uk/transfusion-handbook*

Question 3: Case scenario

Mr W has undergone a partial gastrectomy. On the ward round four days after the operation the consultant is told by the house officer that Mr W's postoperative hemoglobin is only 7.2 g/dL. They decide that he would benefit from transfusion and the HO is asked to recross match him and give him the packed cells from 3 pints.

Question 3.1: In order to fill out the request form you will need to know certain information. Write down the information you will need to fill out the form.

The patient information in this case is as follows:
Name: Arthur W   Admission date: 31/05/07
DOB: 12/6/43
Gender: Male

Pt identification number: PG 192345
Place: Ward 9   Surgeon: Mr L
Require packed cells from 3 pints
Date of request: 6/6/07
Date required: 7/6/07
Blood group at preoperative X-match A Rh +ve
Transfused packed cells from 2 pints on 2/6/07
Diagnosis: Neoplasm stomach postsurgery
Reason for transfusion : Postoperative Hb = 7.2

Question 3.2: Fill out the form below marked Table 19.1 (University Hospital blood transfusion request form) Do this by scanning and printing it or if digital by downloading and printing.

When the blood arrives, the nurse on the ward says she has never started a transfusion herself before and sister and the other nurses are busy. Sister asks that the house officer/intern helps the nurse to start the transfusion.

Question 3.3: What would you check before putting up the blood?

The nurse says she is not sure what readings (charts) the patient should be on.

Question 3.4: What readings will you tell the nurse to put the patient on?

The transfusion is started. The first packet of packed cells is to be run in over 2 hours. Towards the end of the first packet the nurse rings you (the house officer) and says the patient's temperature is 38°C and that he has developed a rash. He otherwise is well.

Question 3.5: What do you think has happened?

You go and see the patient and the situation is as the nurse says. Pulse is 80/min, BP 120/80. Very fine rash on chest. The patient says he is fine and does not know what the fuss is about.

Question 3.6: What would you do as the HO?

Now, let's just say that with the same patient, the nurse calls you and asks you to come urgently. A few minutes after starting the transfusion the patient has become breathless and complains of pain in his abdomen. He has a tachycardia, his temperature is 40 degrees C and he has a diffuse rash on his back chest and arms.

Question 3.7: What are the possible causes for this change in his condition?

Question 3.8: What will you do when you arrive on the scene?

The patient improves. His pulse is down to 80, BP at 110/80.

Question 3.9: What will you watch for over the next few hours? What readings will the patient be on?

Table 19.1 Cross match, blood and blood products request form

UNIVERSITY HOSPITAL

Name   : ....   Admission date :. ....   Room no. :. ....

RN   : ....   Doctor   : ....

Unit No. : ....   Request date : ....   Time :. ....

DOB   : ....   Sex: M/F   Time received : ....

CROSS MATCH, BLOOD AND BLOOD PRODUCTS REQUEST FORM

TEST REQUESTED PLEASE MARK ☑ APPROPRIATE BOX(ES)

Diagnosis	Reason for transfustion	Blood group	
		Hb	Patient

Any previous transfusion? Yes/No	If yes, state date of last transfusion	Complication?

Transfusion required	Blood given immediately without crossmatch (to save life)

Transfusion required

☐ (a) Urgent

☐ (b) Date. .... time. .... am/pm

☐ (c) Reserve for 46 hours

☐ Blood given immediately without crossmatch (to save life)

☐ Whole blood. .... ☐ Platelet concentrate. ....

☐ Packed cells. .... ☐ Cryoprecipitate. ....

☐ Fresh frozen plasma. ....

☐ Group screen and hold

Signature. ....

Chop and name of
consultant ....

TUTORIAL 20: Acute Abdomen: Abdominal Pain and Vomiting (Intestinal Obstruction)

Question 1: Case scenario

A 40-year-old lady is admitted to the surgical ward with abdominal pain.

Question 1.1: What questions will you ask about the pain?

The patient says the pain started 48 hours before admission. It came on suddenly and has been present on and off ever since. She describes it as colicky in nature, coming in waves. She may be free of pain for a few minutes between the waves. The pain is situated around her umbilicus and radiates over her whole abdomen. There is nothing that makes it worse or better. She has never had it before. She says she has just started to vomit.

Question 1.2: What are the features of visceral pain and what causes it? Which part of the gut do you think this ladies' pain is from and why?

Question 1.3: What other questions are you going to ask this lady in the history of the presenting complaint?

She says she started to vomit a few hours after the pain first started. She has been sick 3 times. The vomit was like water to start with then greenish colored. The last time she was sick, the vomit was brownish and smell bad.

Question 1.4: What is the significance of the facts she has told you about the vomiting?

The patient says her bowels have not opened since the pain started and she has not passed any flatus. She is otherwise fit and well. Her appetite was good until the pain started and she has not lost any weight recently. She has no symptoms of difficulty in swallowing, acid reflux, indigestion and has not noticed her abdomen swelling. Her bowel habit has not changed recently and she has not passed any blood or slime.

In her PMH, she says that she had her gallbladder removed 2 years ago. She had no problems with the operation or the anesthetic but thinks the scar on her abdomen is ugly.

Question 1.5: What do you think is the likely diagnosis?

Question 1.6: When you go to examine her what will you be looking for?

On examination, she is clinically dehydrated. Her pulse is 100 and BP 100/70. Her abdomen looks slightly distended and there is a suggestion of visible peristalsis. There is a well-healed upper midline scar. On palpation, she is very slightly tender over the whole abdomen. There are no masses to feel and no organomegaly. There is no demonstrable ascites and her bowel sounds are high pitched and come in runs. No hernia is identified in the groin. When asked to cough and lift her legs no incisional hernia is identified. Rectal examination is negative.

Question 1.7: What is your differential diagnosis? List below your reasons for each.

Question 1.8: What investigations will you, as the house officer/intern, order for this lady and why?

When her electrolytes come back she has a urea of 13 and a potassium of 3.0 mmol/L.

Question 1.9: What are the normal values of the routine electrolytes, urea and creatinine?

Question 1.10: Why is her urea raised? Why is her potassium low?

Question 1.11: List the clinical signs of dehydration.

Question 1.12: What fluids would you give this lady and why?

The patient's plain abdominal X-rays are shown in Figures 20.1 and 20.2).

Question 1.13: What positions are these X-rays taken in?

Question 1.14: What is the diagnosis from these X-rays? Identify the radiological abnormalities shown.

Question 1.15: What are the two most common causes of small bowel obstruction?

Question 1.16: Describe very briefly how you could manage this lady.

Question 1.17: What are the indications for operating on her? In two sentences!

These are the findings at her laparotomy (Fig. 20.3):

Question 1.18: What does this operative picture show?

At this stage in your lecture series, reading, tutorials and clinical exposure, you will start to realize how important the "acute abdomen" is in general surgery. You should also be starting to become familiar with the presenting symptoms and signs of the common acute abdominal conditions.

Question 1.19: Make out a table with little boxes for all the common abdominal emergencies—their symptoms, signs and diagnostic tests, each box should contain only a few lines and represents the core knowledge (see Table 20.1).

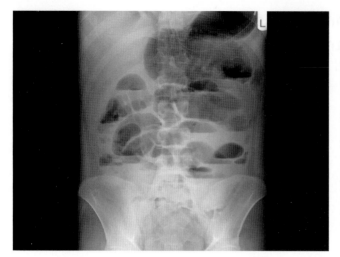

Fig. 20.1 Plain X-ray of patient's abdomen

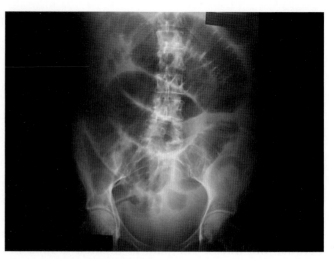

Fig. 20.2 Plain X-ray of patient's abdomen

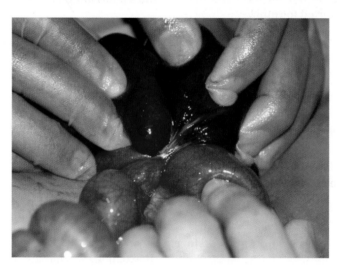

Fig. 20.3 Findings at laparotomy

Do this for the following acute abdominal conditions:

Appendicitis

Cholecystitis

Pancreatitis

Intestinal obstruction

Diverticulitis

Ureteric colic

Ruptured ectopic pregnancy

Dissecting abdominal aortic aneurism

The table should take the following form:

Condition	Pain				Other symptoms	Physical signs	Diagnosis test
	Localization	Character	Aggravating factors	Relieving factors			

Table 20.1 Common abdominal emergencies

Spend some time preparing this table and then learning it. The contents will form the basis of much of your work as a houseman and perhaps afterwards. When you have learned it perfectly, work with a fellow student asking each other the 'boxes' until they become second nature!

Question 1.20: Now without looking at your table write out the presenting features of:
1. Acute appendicitis
2. Ruptured abdominal aortic aneurism
3. Ectopic pregnancy
4. Perforated DU
5. Acute cholecystitis/biliary colic
6. Intestinal obstruction
7. Ureteric colic
8. Acute diverticulitis.

TUTORIAL 21: Swellings in the Neck

Question 1: Case scenario

A 30-year-old lady presents with a 3-month history of a swelling in the front of her neck in the region of the thyroid gland.

Question 1.1: List below the questions you will ask her about the swelling.

The patient says she has had the swelling for about 6 years. She did not bother about it until recently when her husband told her it was getting bigger. It is not painful. She thinks it has grown slowly over the last year.

Question 1.2: List below the other questions you will now directly ask her.

The patient says she is otherwise very fit and well. Her appetite is good but she has put on 4 kg in the last 2 years. She has no difficulty in swallowing and has not noticed any change in her voice. She does not have a cough. Her bowel habit is regular and has not changed recently. Her periods are regular and have not changed recently. She does not prefer either hot or cold weather.

Question 1.3: List the symptoms of:
a. Thyrotoxicosis:
b. Hypothyroidism or myxedema

Question 1.4: Do you think this lady is hyper, hypo or euthyroid from her symptoms?

Question 1.5: What is a goiter?

Question 1.6: How do you confirm the swelling is in the thyroid gland by clinical examination?

Question 1.7: How do you tell by clinical examination if the swelling involves either the whole of the gland or only part of it?

Question 1.8: You are now going to examine the patient. In this case, we are going to start with the neck first. List below the physical signs you will be looking for:
a. On inspection
b. On palpation (*look, feel, move*)
c. On percussion
d. On auscultation
e. Pemberton's sign.

Question 1.9: What are the significance of the following signs in relation to a thyroid swelling?
a. There are multiple discrete swellings in both lobes.
b. There is one discrete swelling in one lobe.
c. The whole of the gland is uniformly enlarged and non-tender.
d. The whole of the gland is enlarged and tender.
e. The whole of the gland is very hard and irregular and seems fixed to the underlying structures (old person).
f. The whole of the gland is soft, enlarged and there is a bruit present on auscultation.
g. The gland is enlarged and nodular but you cannot define a lower edge and there is an area of dullness with dullness to percussion over the sternum.
h. Pemberton's sign is positive.

When this lady is examined, you note she has a visible swelling in the R anterior triangle. It appears to be about 2 cm in diameter. There are no scars, no changes in the skin and no distended veins or pulsations. The swelling moves up when she swallows and does not move when she sticks out her tongue. On palpation, the swelling is 2 cm in diameter, firm, nonfluctuant and has a discrete edge. It moves up on swallowing. It is nontender, not warm and does not pulsate. It is not fixed to the skin or deep tissues. There are no neck glands palpable. Both carotid pulses

are present. The trachea is central; there is no dullness to percussion over the sternum and no bruit. Pemberton's test is negative.

Question 1.10: What is your differential diagnosis?

Question 1.11: How do you clinically (i.e. on examination) assess a patients' thyroid status, i.e. how do you tell clinically whether the condition is hyperthyroid, euthyroid or hypothyroid?

Back to this patient:

She has no exophthalmos, lid lag or lid retraction, divergence or diplopia. There is no chemosis. Her hands are dry; there is no clubbing and no tremor. Her pulse is 80 per min and regular. She has no proximal muscle weakness. She has no skin changes on her legs and her ankle reflexes are normal.

Question 1.12: What is her clinical thyroid status?

Just to prepare you for Module 2 and to make sure you have read the whole chapter in your book:

Question 1.13: What investigations will you order for this lady?

To finish off anatomy/basic science revision questions:

Question 1.14:
a. Write below the anatomical borders of the anterior and posterior triangles.
b. Why does the thyroid move on swallowing?
c. What is the difference between proptosis and exophthalmos?
d. What is the pathophysiology of exophthalmos?
e. What does pretibial myxedema look like? How common is it?

TUTORIAL 22: Swelling in Groin

Question 1: Case scenario

A 40-year-old man comes to the surgical outpatient clinic. He has with him a referral letter from his GP which is as below:

Dear Mr Cox
Please see this man who noticed a swelling in his groin after doing some heavy lifting at work last week. I think he has a hernia and the patient wants to have something done about it.

Yours sincerely,
Dr Joe Mancini
MB ChB

You are the house officer in the clinic and Mr Cox, the consultant, asks you to assess the patient.

Question 1.1: What questions will you ask the patient about the swelling? Your answer should include general questions about the swelling and also specific questions related to the possibility that the swelling is a hernia. With the 'specific' questions please state your reason for asking the question.

Question 1.2: Assuming that the answers to the above questions indicate that the swelling is likely to be a hernia; what other questions are important that you should ask the patient-specifically to help you decide:
a. What treatment he needs?
b. With what urgency is that management required?

Below is the history which the patient gives:

The patient is a 40-year-old factory worker who lifts heavy bales of rope. While lifting one of the bales 10 days ago, he felt a sudden pain in his right groin. This was severe enough for him to sit down. He called the supervisor and asked to be allowed to go home. He did not notice a swelling at that stage.

When he got home he lay down on the couch and watched the TV and the pain gradually went away after 4 hours. When he had a shower that night he noticed a swelling in his groin, this went away when he went to bed but came back when he stood up in the morning. He went to see his GP the next day who told him he had a hernia and told him he would refer him to the hospital and not to go back to work.

He says he has never felt a swelling in his groin before that day at work. He has always had a heavy manual job. The pain he felt when the swelling came on has not come back again but now he sometimes feels a dull ache in the groin when he is walking around. The swelling in his groin is present when he is on his feet and always goes away when he goes to bed.

He has not had any abdominal pain or vomiting. His appetite is good and he has not lost any weight. His bowels work regularly. He has not passed any blood and he has no urinary tract symptoms. He has had no serious illnesses apart from the fact that he is diabetic. He has never been in hospital before except to get his diabetes controlled.

He has had no operations. On systems review, he has no CVS symptoms and no RS symptoms, in particular, he has no cough. He takes tablets for his diabetes which he says is well-controlled.

Question 1.3: Before going onto the examination, please write out in bullet form the protocol which you would use for hernia examination, and in a way that you can remember; try and do this without looking at any protocol you have been given previously.

Now for a bit of basic anatomy:

Question 1.4: Define a hernia and describe its components.

Question 1.5: Make a simple line drawing of the anatomy of the inguinal and femoral canals—do this first without looking in the books and then check it.

Question 1.6a: What are the bony landmarks of the inguinal ligament?

Question 1.6b: How do you locate them?

Question 1.6c: What is the anatomical location of the deep ring?

Going back now to the original patient: When you examine him you find he has an easily reducible R indirect inguinal hernia.

Question 1.7: Draw a simple diagram below to show that you understand the anatomical relationship of an indirect inguinal hernia to a direct one.

Question 1.8: The following questions are designed to make sure that you understand the 'specific' terms which are often applied to hernia in the clinical situation—often incorrectly!! What do you understand by the following terms?
a. An irreducible hernia?
b. An incarcerated hernia?
c. An obstructed hernia?
d. A strangulated hernia?
e. An infant hernia?
f. An inguinoscrotal hernia?

Question 1.9: List the factors which decide whether a patient is advised to have surgery for his/her inguinal hernia.

Question 1.10: In the adult, what are the 2 components of an inguinal hernia operation?

Question 1.11: What types of herniorraphy or hernioplasty are used today?

Question 1.12: What do you understand by the terms 'open' and 'laparoscopic' repair of an inguinal hernia?

Question 1.13: You are the house surgeon and your consultant has asked you to consent his patient for an open right inguinal hernia repair. What will you say?

This is the sort of duty you may well be called upon to perform when you become a house officer. It requires that you have a basic understanding of the anatomy of an inguinal hernia, how the surgeon will perform the operation and the ability to convert this knowledge into a form that the patient will understand (communication skills).

You will probably find this 'task' difficult at this stage in your knowledge and experience but the earlier you think about the knowledge and skills involved, the better you will become. If you have no idea how to start, then the following are recommended:

Go to the ward on the operation day and ask if you can listen while the HO or registrar consents the patient.

Go on the internet and download a 'patient information' leaflet for hernia repair.

Look up how an open hernia repair is done (in the textbook) and try and translate this into terms a patient will understand.

Try 'consenting' one of your fellow students—practice makes perfect.

Answers

TUTORIAL 1: Symptoms and Signs of Gastrointestinal (GI) Diseases

Answer 1.1:
- How long have you had the problem?
- Describe what it is like?
- Have you had it before?
- Did it come on gradually or suddenly?
- Is it becoming worse?
- Do you have difficulty with solids and/or liquids?
- Which came first?
- Does the food seem to stick. Show me where?
- Have you been vomiting, what, etc. (see below)?
- How is your appetite?
- Have you lost weight?
- Plus, all the other GI protocol questions (see end of tutorial).
- Plus, do you feel anything else wrong with you at present.

Answer 1.2:
- When did the vomiting start?
- What do you vomit?
- Is it food/water/bile/greeny stuff/acid/blood?
- If food, is it food you have just eaten or old food?
- If it is blood, how do you know? Amount, color, clots, coffee grounds.
- How often do you vomit?
- Do you feel sick (nauseated) all the time?
- Does anything bring the vomiting on (worse)?
- Does anything make it better?
- Does it shoot out with great force (projectile)?
- Any coughing or choking?

Answer 1.3:
- Describe it to me.
- How long have you had it?
- Have you had it before this episode?
- Did it come on gradually or suddenly?
- Is it becoming worse?
- What makes it worse (e.g. lying down in bed, bending over, certain types of food and drink—spicy food/alcohol/coffee)?
- What makes it better (sleeping, sitting up, avoiding certain drinks or food, medications)?

- Do you get any acid reflux—acid or water coming into your mouth, describe this please (distinguish acid reflux and water-brash).
- Do you have any difficulty swallowing? Describe.
- Do you have any pain behind the chest bone? Describe.
- Do you vomit?
- Do you have indigestion?
- Have you put on weight recently?

Answer 1.4:
- When did the pain start?
- Where is it, show me?
- Have you ever had it before?
- Did it come on suddenly or gradually?
- Does it go anywhere else? Show me.
- How bad is it, worst you have ever had, severe, very severe, mild, moderate, just an ache (do not use x/10 unless you define 10!!!!)?
- Is it the same all the time?
- Have you had time completely free of pain since it started?
- Is it constant or comes in waves?
- Is it getting worse?
- What makes it better, e.g. lying still/painkillers?
- What makes it worse, e.g. moving about?
- Have you got any other symptoms with it, give examples, e.g. vomiting/fever?

Answer 1.5:
- Do you have any indigestion, if says 'yes'?
- Ask what do you mean by this, if says 'no', ask: do you have any discomfort or pain in your tummy after eating?
- Where is the discomfort, show me (pointing sign of DU)?
- When do you get it—before meals/after meals?
- Does it wake you at night (DU), what do you do about it, e.g. get up have some milk and a biscuit (DU)?
- How often do you get it, e.g. every day?
- Have you had it before?
- Have you seen your GP about it or been investigated in hospital (e.g. endoscopy)?
- What did they say was wrong with you?
- What makes the indigestion worse/better?
- Have you been vomiting any blood?
- How is your appetite; have you lost weight?

- Do you take any medications for it (define)?
- Are you taking aspirin/NSAIDs/steroids/herbal medications?

Answer 1.6:

Bowel Habit
- Has your bowel habit changed recently?
- If patient does not appear to understand—Explain.
- Have you developed diarrhea or constipation recently (means different things to different people)?
- Define their normal bowel habit.
- Define what it has changed to, e.g. normal is × 1 per day now is × 3 per day.
- If has diarrhea—define content, color, offensive, blood/floats (see set of questions below).
- If has constipation—is it constipation or incomplete evacuation? or even tenesmus (see below set of questions)?
- Have you passed any blood or slime? Define both.
- Have you had any abdominal pain or weight loss?
- On any drugs (e.g. antibiotic)?

Diarrhea
- Frequency of defecation (>x3 = abnormal).
- Recent or present for long time.
- Solid/liquid/mixed. Bulky may be steatorrhea.
- Color: Black (melena), red (blood), pale (steatorrhea, obstructive jaundice), silver (because of mixture of melena and fatty stool in tropical sprue, carcinoma (Ca) of ampulla of Vater).
- Pus or mucus.
- Smell—very offensive, may be infective/melena.
- Floats/difficult to flush away, may be steatorrhea.
- Any other symptoms, e.g. vomiting.
- Been abroad recently.
- Anyone else in family with it (gastroenteritis).
- NB: Some gastroenterologists divide by physiological cause into secretory, osmotic, exudative, malabsorption (not very useful in practice).
- (If you want to explore the 'physiological' types further look at Talley and O'Connor: Clinical Examination, Churchill Livingstone, 5th Ed, 2006. pp. 130).

Constipation
- What do you mean by constipation—infrequent bowel action or very hard motion or difficulty in evacuation?
- Is this a new symptom or long standing?
- If recent, define 'change': Normal bowel habit versus old bowel habit.
- Any blood or mucus?
- Incomplete emptying—have to go again—is a symptom of pelvic floor descent or rectal cancer.

- Painful almost continuous urge to defecate is tenesmus (rectal equivalent of urinary strangury) indicates inflammation or tumor involving anal sphincters.
- Other GI symptoms, e.g. abdominal pain/distension.
- On any drugs, e.g. codeine.
- Alternating diarrhea + constipation, some say symptom of tumor but more likely irritable bowel syndrome (large bowel tumor is more often change from normal to more frequent).
- Any incontinence—overflow or otherwise?

Answer 1.7:
- When did this happen, did it start same time as other GI symptoms?
- Loss of appetite (anorexia) + weight loss = Suspicious of malignancy.
- Increase in appetite, may suggest hypermetabolic state, e.g. thyrotoxicosis.

Answer 1.8:
- When did it start?
- How much (in kg over weeks) if patient not sure, ask about loose clothes?
- Why do you think lost weight—may say on diet!
- Are there other symptoms—may need full review of systems, e.g. fever/thirst?

Answer 2:

Face:	Jaundice
	Lemon yellow (uremia, CA cecum, pernicious anemia)
	Weight loss
	(temporalis muscles, cheeks)—cachexia
	Dehydration
	Distress (pain)
	Pale (anemia/pain)
	Flushed (temperature)
Eyes:	Yellow sclera
	Pale mucous membranes
	Kayser-Fleischer rings (Wilson's disease)
Mouth:	Angular stomatitis (B_{12} deficiency, Fe deficiency)
	Pigmentation (Peutz-Jeghers syndrome)
	Ulcers (Crohn's disease)
Hands:	Finger nails leukonychia (low protein)
	Koilonychia (Fe deficiency)
	Clubbing (UC/cirrhosis)
	Palms Pale creases (anemia)
	Palmar erythema (liver failure)
	Liver flap (liver failure)
Arms:	Scratch marks (obstructive jaundice)
Legs:	Superficial thrombophlebitis (pancreatic CA)
Neck:	Enlarged lymph nodes (supraclavicular—CA stomach)

Axilla: Acanthosis nigricans (CA stomach)

Chest: Spider nevi (liver failure)

Gynecomastia (liver failure)

Abdomen: Inspect: No movement with respiration (peritonitis)

Jaundiced

Distended (obstruction, ascites)

Weight loss (malignancy)

Scars (previous surgery)

Fistula (Crohn's)

Everted umbilicus (ascites)

Mass (tumor, abscess)

Visible peristalsis (intestinal obstruction)

Enlarged veins + caput medusa (liver disease)

Cullen's/Grey Turner's sign (pancreatitis)

Erythema ab igne (pain/hot water bottle use)

Sister Joseph's nodule (transcelomic spread of tumor)

Cellulitis (abscess—diverticular disease/tumor)

Palpate: Tenderness/guarding/rebound (inflammation)

Mass (tumor)

Organomegaly: Liver (primary CA/metastases)

Tender + enlarged (hepatitis)

Small + hard (cirrhosis)

Spleen—enlarged (portal hypertension)

Anorectal exam:

I: Fistula (Crohn's)

Fissure (Crohn's)

Abscess (IBD)

Anal cancer

Rectal prolapse

Prolapsed hemorrhoids

Digital exam: Tumor/polyp felt

Blood on finger (tumor/IBD)

Pus/mucus (IBD)

Black motion (melena)

pale motion (obstructive jaundice/steatorrhea)

CASE SCENARIO

Answer 3.1:

Pain: When did it start?

Did it come on suddenly?

Have you had it before?

Where exactly is it?

How bad is it?

Is it constant or does it come and go?

Does it go anywhere else?

What makes it better or worse?

Any associated symptoms?

Vomiting: When did it start?

How often are you sick?

What color is it?

Any blood in it?

Bowels: When did your bowels last work?

What is your normal bowel habit?

Have you passed any wind (flatus)?

Have you passed any blood?

Answer 3.2:

General: Alert conscious and orientated in distress +/–

Pale/anemia +/–

Jaundice +/–

Dehydrated +/–

Cachexic +/–

Lips/mouth signs + dentition

Hands: Nails/palms/temperature of peripheries

Vital signs: P/BP/temp/RR/(tachycardia, low BP, pyrexia, tachypnea)

Abdominal:

Inspection: Abdomen moving with respiration

Distension +/–

Scars

Visible peristalsis

Mass

Umbilicus

Palpation: Tenderness/guarding/rebound

Organomegaly

Percussion for ascites

Auscultation: Auscultation for bowel sounds

Groins: (Hernia)

PR: (Tumor/empty rectum)

Answer 3.3: Intestinal obstruction.

Answer 3.4: In the Western world, most commonly caused by either intestinal adhesions or obstructed hernia (small bowel) or by large bowel tumor.

TUTORIAL 2: Symptoms and Signs of Urological Diseases

Answer 1.1:
- When did the bleeding start. How do you know it is blood?
- Is it every time you pass water or does it come and go?
- What color is it—bright red/dark red?
- Are there clots in it?
- Is it a small amount or large amount?
- Does the blood come when you start to pass urine, all through the stream or just at the end?
- Are you on any tablets or medications (beetroot)?
- Plus, routine questions: Frequency/nocturia/dysuria.

Answer 1.2:
- How long have you had the problem?
- Is it every time you pass urine or intermittent?
- Can you describe the difficulty to me? If cannot, then ask directly:
  - Are you passing more or less urine than usual?
  - Do you have difficulty in starting the stream, have to stand there a long time?
  - Do you have to strain hard to pass the urine?
  - Does the urine flow stop and start?
  - Do you dribble urine at the end?
  - Do you leak urine into your underwear?
  - Plus routine questions

Answer 1.3:
- How long have you had the problem?
- Is it all the time or comes and goes?
- Can you describe it to me? If not, help patient—is it burning or worse than this (strangury and its significance will be defined later)?
- Are there other symptoms, e.g. frequency/nocturia/dysuria?
- If indicated, enquire about sexually transmitted diseases (STD)?

Answer 1.4:
- How long have you had it?
- Did it come on suddenly or gradually?
- Do you have the dribbling all the time or intermittently?
- Is it just at the end of passing urine or do you leak in your underwear?
- Do you have difficulty in starting and keeping a good stream?
- Do you feel like your bladder is not empty after you have passed urine?
- Do you have any abdominal pain?
- Plus other routine questions.

Answer 1.5:
- When did you first notice it?
- How did you notice it (e.g. in the bath or while peeing)?
- Have you noticed any 'bits'/debris in your urine?
- Have you any abdominal pain/bowel symptoms?
- Any other urinary tract symptoms?

CASE SCENARIOS

Answer 2.1: Obstructive.

Answer 2.2: Irritative.

Answer 2.3: Strangury—suggests an inflammation of the urethra.

Answer 2.4: Irritative symptoms: Dysuria, frequency, nocturia, strangury plus penile discharge, possibly hematuria. A source of contact.

Answer 2.5:
Ask:
- Do you have a regular 'partner'?
- Have you had any casual relationships outside of your partner recently?
- Then ask the questions for the symptoms of STD.
- Then ask if the partner has any of these symptoms.

Note: If you do this with tact and sympathy you will be surprised at the ease with which the patient will discuss the problem, they will be very worried about the situation and will be glad to 'get it off their chest'.

Answer 3.1:
Pain: When did it start, has he had it before?
Where exactly is it?
Has it moved to anywhere else (better than radiate)?
How bad is it?
Is it constant or colicky, anything makes it better or worse?

Blood: When did he first notice the blood—in relationship to the pain?
Does he see it every time he passes urine?
How does he know it is blood?
Color and quantity?
Any clots?
Where is the blood in his stream—at the beginning, throughout or at the end?
Is he on any medications?

Routine urinary tract questions: Dysuria/frequency/nocturia.

Answer 3.2:
- Blood at the start of the stream is often from the urethra
- Blood at the end of the stream is often from the bladder or prostate

- Blood throughout the stream or in the middle of it can be from the kidneys, urethra or bladder.

Answer 3.3:

General:	Is he alert conscious and orientated?
	Is he in obvious distress (pain)?
	Is he pale (pain, anemia)?
	Is he flushed (pyrexia)?
Vital signs:	Tachycardia

Abdomen

Inspection:	Moving normally with respiration
	Distended
	Scars
	Visible mass
	Skin discoloration, e.g. erythema
Palpation/	
Percussion:	Tenderness/guarding/rebound, including loins and back
	Organomegaly, especially are kidneys ballotable
	Any groin mass (hernia) or lymph nodes in groin
Auscultation:	Normal bowel sounds

Genitalia:

Inspection:	Any swelling of scrotum
	Any skin discoloration
	Any penile abnormality, e.g. discharge
Palpation:	Testes normal/epididymis normal

Answer 3.4: Right-sided ureteric colic.

Answer 4: See Table 2.1

Table 2.1 Types, characteristics and frequency of renal calculi

Type	Appearance	Frequency (%)
Calcium oxalate	Brown with sharp projections 'Mulberry stone' (metabolic)	65
Mixed calcium, oxalate and phoshate	Smooth and white (metabolic)	15
Magnesium ammonium phosphate (struvite)	Most of staghorn calculi (infection)	10–20
Pure calcium phosphate	Whitish brown (renal tubular acidosis)	3–6
Uric acid	Smooth, hard and yellowish	5–10
Xanthine	Smooth, red	Rare
Cystine	Soft, yellow or green (cystinuria)	1–3

Remember the following, it will save you looking it up later:

Though renal calculi may be caused by metabolic disorders and infection, the majority are idiopathic with the patients having no major metabolic disorder found on investigation (stone analysis and biochemistry).

Oxalate stones are found in idiopathic hypercalciuria and are treated by low calcium diet and high fluid intake. Struvite, triple phosphate stones are associated with infection; treatment is by removal of the stones, correction of any underlying anatomical abnormality and by keeping the urine sterile. Cystine stones are treated by alkalinizing the urine and a high fluid intake. Uric acid stones are treated by alkalinizing the urine and allopurinol.

TUTORIAL 3: Symptoms and Signs of Vascular Diseases

Answer 1.1:

- How long have you had the problem?
- Describe what the pain is like.
- Have you had it before?
- Did it come on gradually or suddenly?
- What makes it worse, e.g. walking further?
- What makes it better, e.g. stopping and resting?
- Does the pain come on each time after walking the same distance?
- Is it becoming worse overtime, i.e. is it progressive (has the claudication distance decreased)?
- Have you injured or hurt your leg?
- Have you any back pain?
- Have you been bedbound recently or on a long distance flight?
- What about the other calf?
- If you think it is claudication then ask about other arteriosclerotic risks. For example, angina/MI/stroke/chest pain/fainting/weakness/numbness/pins and needles/loss of vision.
- If you think DVT ask for risk factors.
- Finally ask if they have any other problems or illnesses at present.

Answer 1.2:

- How long have you had the problem?
- Describe what it is like, where is it—toes/forefoot?
- Is this the first time you have had the problem?
- Have you injured the foot or noticed any skin changes, e.g. ulcer?
- Does it feel better when you hang your foot by the side of the bed, or walking on cold floor (a sign of rest pain)?
- Any history of claudication or other peripheral vascular disease risk factors: angina, muscle weakness, loss of vision.
- Relevant past medical history, e.g. heart attack/fainting/diabetes, etc.

Answer 1.3:
- How long have you had the ulcer?
- Show me where it is.
- How did it start: what do you think caused it?
- How does it bother you?
- Is there just one ulcer?
- Has it changed since you first noticed it?
- Then the risk factors which might cause an ulcer (arterial/venous/neuropathic).
- Any history of claudication/angina/MI/hypertension, etc.
- Relevant past medical history, e.g. diabetes, varicose veins, family history.

Answer 1.4:
- Is this the first time?
- What happened (note amaurosis fugax—transient monocular blindness).
- Any associated neurological symptoms and how long do they last—transient weakness/paresthesia/fainting/loss of sensation.
- Relevant past medical history, e.g. on warfarin, any previous heart valve surgery.

CASE SCENARIO

Answer 2.1:
- Show me where the pain is.
- Have you ever had it before, and if so, describe the features.
- If on walking—what distance/relieving/precipitating factors.
- Have you been on a long distance flight recently?
- Have you fallen and injured your leg?
- Do you have any back pain or pain moving down your leg?
- Have you had any serious illness recently?
- If you think the pain is claudication then you will ask about risk factors at this stage, i.e. hypertension/angina/MI, etc.
- If you think it may be a DVT, ask about risk factors if not done so already.

Answer 2.2:
General:

Face:	Alert and conscious and orientated?
	In pain or distressed?
	Pale or jaundiced?
	Well-nourished?
	Well-hydrated?
	Lips: Cyanosed/plethoric/intraoral pathology and dentition?
Hands:	Palmar pallor
	Clubbing

Vital signs:	Pulse/BP/RR/temp/peripheries
CVS:	Cardio: lips
	JVP
	Inspection of chest
	Apex beat
	Auscultation
	Leg edema

Remember, this is a 'vascular case', so you have to examine the upper limbs/neck/face for evidence of vascular disease:

Compare both upper limbs:

Inspection:	Color:	Normal
		Pale
		Congested
		Blotchy
	Ischemic changes:	Thinning of skin
		Hair loss
		Ulceration
Palpation:	Temperature
	Capillary refilling
	Pulses distal to proximal comparing both sides
	Radial
	Ulnar
	Brachial
	Axillary
	+/- Thrills

Auscultation for bruits

Palpate and auscultate carotid arteries in neck

Face:	Cyanosis/plethoric
	Arcus/xanthelasma
	Fundi

Appropriate neurological assessment if relevant Hx or local signs, e.g. weakness

RS:	Inspection
	Auscultation
	Percussion
Abdomen:	Pulsatile mass
	Bruit
Specfic:	Lower limbs (including full vascular assessment)
Look:	Compare both limbs – Any swelling/deformity/muscle wasting
	– Any bruising
	Change in color, e.g. pale/blue
	Varicose veins

Then look at right leg:

Any signs of ischemia – Thickened, dystrophic toe nails, ulcers, gangrene
– Look at pressure points

Feel: Temperature/tenderness (especially calf)
Pulses (dorsalis pedis, posterior tibial, popliteal, femoral)
Capillary refill
Sensation

Move: Limitation on movements
Muscle wasting
Fixed deformities
Buerger's angle/test

Then look, feel/move for other leg.

Neurological examination: Back and legs.

TUTORIAL 4: Symptoms and Signs of Endocrine Diseases

Answer 1.1:
- How long have you had the lump?
- How did you notice it?
- What was its size when you first noticed it? Has it increased in size? Does it change in size?
- Is it painful?
- Does it change with your menstrual cycle?
- Any associated nipple discharge?
- Do you have any family history of breast cancer?
- Then ask about the risk factors of breast cancer.

Answer 1.2:
- When did the pain start?
- Do you get it with every period?
- How long does it last for?
- Is the pain in one breast or both?
- Do your breasts feel lumpy when you have the pain?
- Does the lumpiness go away when the pain stops?
- What makes the pain better?
- What makes it worse?
- Do you get any nipple discharge at this time?
- Is the surrounding breast tissue tense/tender?

Answer 1.3:
- How long have you had the lump?
- How did you notice it?
- Show me where it is:
  The questions you ask then will depend on where the lump is and whether it appears to be in the region of the thyroid gland.
- If in region of thyroid, ask
- Is it getting bigger?
- Is it painful?
- Are you otherwise fit and well, if not, why not?
- How are your appetite and weight?
- Ask specific questions for hyper- and hypothyroid clinical status.

- If you think it is, say, a cervical chain lymph node or a parotid swelling, the questions will be similar with added specific relevant questions, e.g. throat/ear problems.

CASE SCENARIOS

Answer 2.1:
- When did you notice the lump?
- How did you notice it?
- Have you had lumps before? If so, when?
- Do you think it is getting bigger in size?
- Is it painful?
- Does it ever go away?
- Are you still having your periods? If so does the lump alter with your periods?
- Is there any discharge from your nipple?
- Is there any history in your family of breast problems?
- Then ask for risk factors of breast cancer:
  - Do you have any children?
  - Did you breastfeed your children?
  - Age at 1st pregnancy?
  - When did you get your 1st menstrual cycle (menarche)?
  - Have you already reached menopause? If so, at what age?
  - Are you/were you on any oral contraceptives or hormone replacement therapy?

Answer 2.2: When examining a breast use the 'Aide-Memoire': LOOK/FEEL/MOVE (always remember the 3 components)

> When examining the breasts: BREAST/AREOLA/NIPPLE and apply these to Look/Feel/Move. If you do this you are unlikely to miss an important finding.

The features suggesting the lump is malignant, using Look/Feel/Move are:

Inspection: Disparity in breast size
Visible lump
Skin tethering (may be more noticeable on lifting arms)
Nipple retraction
Reddening, irregularity or ulceration of skin adjacent to lump
Peau d'orange

Feel: Lump is
Hard in consistency
Irregular
Nontender
Blood expressed from nipple
Palpable hard/fixed axillary nodes

Move: Fixed to skin
Fixed deep to pectoralis muscle

Plus presence of supraclavicular nodes/enlarged liver/ascites.

Answer 2.3:

Look: No nipple or skin changes (lump usually not visible)

Feel: Well-defined edge
Smooth surface

Move: Not attached to skin
Not fixed deep
No axillary glands
Breast mouse (fibroadenoma): Moves about.

CASE SCENARIO

Answer 3.1:

- How long have you noticed the swelling?
- Did it come on suddenly or gradually?
- Is it tender or painful?
- Have you noticed any other symptoms or problems with your health since the swelling came on?

Then enquire after:

- Symptoms of hyperthyroidism:
  - Heat intolerance
  - Sweating
  - Palpitations
  - Anxiety
  - Weight loss (despite good appetite)
  - Diarrhea
  - Oligomenorrhea
- Symptoms specific for Graves' disease:
  - Diplopia (extraocular muscles affected by amino-glycan deposition).
  - Do you notice your eyes protruding out when you look at the mirror?
  - Do you have blurred vision (optic nerve atrophy)?

Answer 3.2:

General

- General inspection:
  - Slim
  - Restless
  - Irritable
  - Sweating
- Hands:
  - Warm and moist
  - Onycholysis
  - Thyroid acropachy (clubbing)
  - Palmar erythema
  - Fine tremor
  - Tachycardia
  - Irregularly irregular pulse (atrial fibrillation)

- Ocular:
  - Exophthalmos
  - Lid retraction
  - Lid lag
  - Chemosis (conjunctival edema)
  - Ophthalmoplegia
  - Optic nerve atrophy
- Legs:
  - Proximal myopathy
  - Pretibial myxedema
  - Hyperreflexia

Specific (Neck)

- Inspection:
  - Dilated neck veins (if there is retrosternal extension blocking venous drainage)
  - A swelling that moves on swallowing but does not move when patient sticks out their tongue
- Palpation:
  - A diffuse swelling of the neck that involves both lobes
  - Firm in consistency
  - Temperature may be increased
  - May be pulsatile
  - Not fixed to skin or underlying structures
  - No associated lymphadenopathy
- Percussion:
  - Retrosternal extension may be present
- Auscultation:
  - May have bruit (hyperactive thyroid).

Answer 4: Both lid lag and lid retraction are caused by over activity of the involuntary part of the levator palpebrae superioris muscle. If the upper eyelid is higher than normal and the lower lid is in its normal position, the patient has lid retraction. This gives a 'staring' gaze not to be confused with exophthalmos. Lid lag is when the upper eyelid 'lags' behind as it follows a finger moving from above downwards (dynamic test not just observation) (Fig. 4.1).

Answer 5:

 Normal

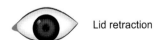 Lid retraction

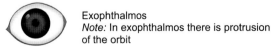 Exophthalmos
Note: In exophthalmos there is protrusion of the orbit

Fig. 4.1 Eye signs in thyroid disease

TUTORIAL 5: Difficulty in Swallowing and Heartburn

CASE SCENARIOS

Answer 1.1: Gastrointestinal system.

Answer 1.2:
- When did it start?
- How did he notice it?
- Has he ever had it before?
- Is it getting worse?
- Is the problem with solids or is it for liquids as well?
- Is it painful when he swallows and if so where?
- Does the food stick on the way down and if so where?

Answer 1.3:
- You should ask him all the questions which appear in your routine history taking protocol for the gastrointestinal tract, namely:
  - Have you been vomiting or feeling sick?
  - Have you vomited any blood? Have you had any acid regurgitation or heartburn? Have you any indigestion/abdominal pain/distension?
  - Are your bowels working regularly—any blood or slime? How is your appetite? Have you lost any weight?
- A suggested protocol is included in this tutorial as the answer to Question 1.8.

Answer 1.4:
- What does he vomit—liquid or food? Is there any food in it he has eaten days before?
- Is there any blood present?
- Is the vomiting becoming worse?
- Does it come out with a lot of force, i.e. projectile?

Answer 1.5:
- Establish his normal bowel habit and what it has now become.
- Did the constipation start after his difficulty in swallowing or has he had it for longer?
- Has he passed any blood or mucus with the bowels?

Answer 1.6: Whitish or yellow slime either in or on the bowel motion.

Answer 1.7: Ask him the rest of your history taking protocol or proforma, taking care not to miss out any of the questions.
So you will cover: Past medical history
Family history
Social history
Review of systems
Drugs and Allergies

Answer 1.8: Please refer to Table 5.1.

Answer 1.9: The patient is a 72-year-old retired laborer who is a heavy smoker. He presents with an 8-week history of gradually worsening difficulty in swallowing and vomiting. He can now only swallow liquids. He has also developed a cough and hoarseness of his voice.

Answer 1.10: Carcinoma of the esophagus.

Answer 1.11:
1. General exam: Face   Arms
              Hands   Legs
2. Vital signs
3. Specific system examination (in this case GI system)
4. The rest of the routine exam (i.e. neck/chest/CVS/RS, etc.)

Answer 1.12:
Face: Is the patient alert, conscious and orientated?
Is the patient in any distress, e.g. pain/respiratory distress?
Does the patient look pale or jaundiced?
Specifically examine his eye mucous membranes and sclera. Does the patient look cachexic (signs of weight loss are sunken cheeks, loss of temporalis and masseter muscle bulk).
Is he dehydrated?
Look at the lips for cyanosis, skin changes, e.g. angular stomatitis.
Look in his mouth—paleness of mucous membranes, cyanosis ulcers, tongue abnormalities, state of dentition.
Hands: Nail changes: Clubbing/koilonychia/leukonychia, etc.
Palms: Palmar pallor or erythema, sweating or dry, dupuytren's contracture, tremor, flap, muscle wasting.
Arms: Scratch marks, venous abnormalities, e.g. thrombophlebitis, proximal myopathy
Legs: Ankle/leg edema
Skin changes, e.g. pretibial myxedema.

Answer 1.13: Pulse/BP/temperature/respiration rate.

Answer 1.14:
Neck: Any masses/lymph nodes, in particular enlargement of the supraclavicular nodes
Chest: Any skin changes, e.g. spider nevi
Any dilated veins
Gynecomastia

Table 5.1 History taking protocol

Surgical history: Suggested protocol

Name: Age: Occupation:

Presenting complaint(s): Duration of each

History of presenting complaints:

Past medical history:
- Serious illnesses/operations/ever been in hospital/had anesthetic, if so, any problems
- Diabetes/jaundice/heart attack/high BP/stroke/Rh fever/TB

Family history: Mother died of, father died of? Brothers/sisters? Any family illness

Social history: Married?, children?, smoke, drink, home/financial circumstances diet, travel

Review of systems:

CVS:	Chest pain SOB Palpitations Ankle swelling	**RS:**	SOB/Asthma Cough Sputum +/– blood Fever/night cough
Abd:	Difficulty in swallowing Nausea/vomiting +/– blood Heartburn/acid reflux Indigestion/abdo pain/abd distention Change in bowel habit +/– blood Appetite Weight loss	**GUS:**	Frequency Dysuria Nocturia Hematuria Periods/Pregnancies Postmenopausal bleeding (+ if indicated: Hx of sexual contact)
CNS:	Headaches Fits/blackouts/dizziness Weakness/numbness/tingling Stroke/sleep well/depressed	***MS:**	Painful//stiff/swollen joints Neck/back pain Fingers white/blue in cold
Hemo:	Bruise easily Difficulty stopping bleeding Lumps under arms, in neck, groins Clots in legs/lungs: DVT/PE	**Endocrine:**	Swelling in neck Hands tremble Prefer hot/cold weather Increased sweating/fatigue Change in appearance/voice
DRUGS and MEDICATIONS		**ALLERGIES**	

*Musculoskeletal system

Answer 1.15:

Inspection: Movement with respiration (lack of movement may indicate peritonitis)

Distension (ascites, obstruction)

Evidence of weight loss (malignancy)

Scars? If present, ask to cough (may demonstrate an incisional hernia)

Evidence of skin color change, e.g. jaundice/bruising

Any skin lesions, e.g. pigmentation

Any obvious mass (malignancy, abcess, organomegaly)

Any visible pulsation (obstruction/very thin)

Any distended veins (portal hypertension)

Abnormal pulsations (aortic aneurysm)

Umbilicus? Normal and inverted (ascites/hernia)

(Remember you should list these parameters whether they are present or not—this acts as an 'aide de memoire', makes sure you do not miss any relevant findings and in the examination situation shows the examiner you are well taught and are thinking)

Palpation: Superficial—tenderness/guarding/rebound

Deep—mass

Specific organ palpation: Liver/spleen/kidneys

Percussion: Of mass/organ

Ascites—fluid thrill/shifting dullness

Auscultation: Bowel sounds/bruits

Examine groins: For hernia/enlarged lymph nodes

Examine genitalia

Anorectal examination: Inspection and rectal examination

Answer 1.16:
- Cardiovascular system
- Respiratory system
- Arterial/venous system: If indicated
- Neurological system: If indicated
- Musculoskeletal system: If indicated.

Answer 1.17: Some or all of the following may be present:

General: Pale

Jaundiced

Cachexic

Dehydrated

Hands: Pale palmar creases

Neck: Supraclavicular nodes

Abdomen: Obvious weight loss

Jaundice

Mass—liver

Distended—ascites—unusual

Palpation—upper abdominal mass

enlarged liver.

Answer 1.18a: Poor appetite

Catabolism of the malignant process.

Answer 1.18b: Anemia of malignancy/loss of blood/poor food intake.

Answer 1.18c: Metastatic spread to liver.

Answer 1.18d: Aspiration pneumonia

Lung secondary.

Answer 1.18e: Involvement of recurrent laryngeal nerve.

Answer 2.1: Ask her to tell you about her problems (i.e. let her talk first). If she has not covered the questions you specifically want answered, then you must ask her directly. Remember this is part of the skill of taking a history, let the patient tell you about her symptoms to start with without letting her divert to a lot of irrelevancies. This only comes with practice.

One way or the other, you need answers to the following:

- How long have you had this problem?
- Do you have it all the time or does it come and go?
- Is it getting worse?
- What makes it worse, e.g. bending over, in bed at night, hot drinks, alcohol, coffee, chocolate?
- What makes it better, e.g. sleeping sitting up, avoiding the things which make it worse, which ones?
- Do you get any acid or bile coming into your mouth?
- Do you get any water coming up into your mouth (water brash)?
- Have you any difficulty swallowing?
- Does food feel like it sticks?
- Have you any chest pain?
- Have you vomited or brought up any blood?
- Do you feel nauseated?
- All the other routine GI protocol questions, e.g. appetite/weight loss, etc.
- Are you on any drugs or medication?
- Are you taking any drugs or medication which help relieve the problem?

Answer 2.2: Gastroesophageal reflux disease (GERD).

Answer 2.3: GERD is caused by reflux of gastric acid through the cardioesophageal sphincter. This is normally prevented by a high pressure zone at the lower end of the esophagus, together with:

- The mucosa at the cardia acting as a plug.
- The acute angle between the stomach and the esophagus.
- The crura of the diaphragm acting as sling.

The acid reflux causes inflammation and then ulceration of the esophagus, which may eventually lead to a stricture of the esophagus.

The following factors may lead to GERD:

Anatomical: Obesity

Alteration in the angle of His

Alteration of the mucosal plug

Laxity of the crura

Physiological: Reduction in the lower esophageal sphincter pressure zone

Delayed gastric emptying

Gastric distension and increased abdominal pressure (e.g. pregnancy)

Gastric acid hypersecretion.

Also alcohol, stress, and smoking.

Answer 2.4: Figure 5.1: The picture shows the mucosal changes of reflux esophagitis with linear inflammation and ulceration, as seen through an upper gastrointestinal endoscope.

Answer 2.5: Figure 5.2: This is a barium swallow and shows a tapered narrowing at the lower end of the esophagus with dilation of the esophagus above it. These are the classical 'bird beak' or 'rat's tail' appearance of achalasia.

Answer 2.6: Achalasia is a condition caused by failure of relaxation of the lower end of the esophagus due to either partial or complete loss of the myenteric plexus (Auerbach's plexus).

Answer 2.7: Achalasia most commonly occurs in younger females (aged 20-40). They are very slow eaters and always finish behind the rest of the family. The dysphagia is slowly progressive often over a period of years. Usually the patient has difficulty with solids and liquids. After months or years they start to vomit, often 'old food'. They may eat standing up, have bad breath, and have bouts of coughing and aspiration.

Malignant change in the esophagus can occur after years.

With carcinoma of the esophagus, the disease is more common in elderly men, starts with dysphagia for liquids and then for solids and develops over a period of just a few weeks. Early weight loss and cachexia occur.

Answer 2.8: Very uncommon—a GP may never see a case in his working life, but it remains a favorite of both students and examiners!!

TUTORIAL 6: Dyspepsia

Answer 1: Indigestion is a term commonly used by patients—by it, they can mean a number of symptoms including epigastric discomfort or epigastric pain usually associated with food, belching, 'wind', a feeling of satiety, regurgitation and nausea. If the patient says he has indigestion you must ask what he or she means by that.

Most patients are familiar with the term indigestion, so it is a good starter question, define what they mean by it, but you may also have to clarify the situation by asking if they have any abdominal pain or discomfort associated with eating. A lot of patients do not know what you mean by dyspepsia so it is not a good starter question.

Now:
Dyspepsia is a common medical term which covers a number of upper abdominal symptoms including: Upper abdominal discomfort or pain, a feeling of abdominal fullness, early satiety, abdominal distension and bloating, belching and nausea (This is a medical term for a specific group of symptoms. It relates to a symptom complex rather than a diagnosis.)

Some gastroenterologists prefer to say 'uninvestigated dyspepsia'. If, when the patient has been fully investigated, no pathology is identified then it is labeled functional dyspepsia or nonorganic dyspepsia.

Next:
There are four subgroups of dyspeptic patients based on their predominant symptoms:
1. Ulcer-like dyspepsia
2. Reflux (or GERD-like dyspepsia)
3. Dysmotility like dyspepsia
4. Nonspecific dyspepsia.

The patient's symptoms do not always differentiate between organic and functional (nonorganic) disease, this can only be achieved reliably by investigation.

This may sound complicated to start with but it is important that you appreciate these fundamental differences before we go further.

CASE SCENARIO

Answer 2.1: Hello Mr F, I am Dr Smith and your GP has asked me to see if we can find out what is wrong with you:
- What exactly is the problem? (let him talk) and then ask appropriate lead questions, if necessary, i.e. if the patient does not volunteer the information.
- What do you mean by abdominal discomfort?
- Where exactly is the discomfort (show me)?
- How long have you had it?
- Is it there all the time or does it come and go?
- Is it associated with food?
- What makes it better?
- What makes it worse?
- Are you taking any medications, pills or drugs?
- If not volunteered ask about: Night pain and its relief, heartburn, nausea, vomiting and difficulty in swallowing.
- Ask specifically if he has vomited any blood or passed any very black bowel motions.
- Then ask the rest of GI protocol questions: Change in bowel habit, bleeding/appetite, weight loss.

Answer 2.2: Peptic ulcer disease.

Answer 2.3:
- Have you vomited any blood?
- Have you passed any black, tarry stools?
- Have you taken any aspirins or tablets that might contain aspirin, any steroids or tablets for arthritis?

Answer 2.4: Hematemesis is vomiting of blood, this may be fresh blood (bright red), older blood (dark red) or blood altered by the gastric acid—brownish, so called 'coffee grounds'.

To establish that it is actually blood that has been vomited the best way is to inspect the 'vomit'. If not possible, look on patient's clothes—ask if it contained 'clots' and why he thought it was blood.

To estimate the amount, ask the patient if he vomited say a 'cup full' or more than this—say a 'bowl full.'

Answer 2.5: Melena is blood that has passed through the gastrointestinal tract from a bleeding source in the upper gastrointestinal tract—usually proximal to the ligament of Treitz*. It is black and shiny (like tar on the road) and has an unmistakable smell (remember the triad: BLACK, TARRY and STINKS!).

(*look this up if you do not know what or where it is)

Answer 2.6:

General:	Alert, conscious and orientated (routine mental status)
Face:	Anemic (bleed, malignancy)
	Jaundiced (wrong diagnosis, secondaries)
	Nutritional status (malignant disease)
	Dehydration status (vomiting)
	Mouth, tongue, dentition (other signs e.g. angular stomatitis, aphthous ulcer, teeth poor—may need intubating for surgery)
Hands:	Pale palms (anemia)
	Clubbing/koilonychia (liver disease: Wrong diagnosis)
	Leukonychia (nutrition)
Vital Signs:	(Routine general status)

Neck:	Lymph nodes (CA stomach)
Chest:	Spider nevi (liver disease)
Axilla:	Acanthosis nigricans (CA stomach)

Specific:
Abdomen:

Inspection	(mass/distension/scars/veins/umbilicus)
Palpation	(tenderness, guarding/mass/liver)
Percussion	(mass/ascites)
Auscultation	(routine)
Groins:	(routine)
Rectal Ex:	(mass/melena).

Answer 2.7: Peptic ulcer disease.

Answer 2.8: A large duodenal ulcer is shown on the bottom left with a smaller ulcer on the top right, known as kissing ulcers.

Answer 2.9: Duodenal or gastric biopsy
HP status (*Helicobacter*).

Answer 2.10: Perforated duodenal ulcer
Peritonitis.

Answer 2.11: 'Shock'—presumably hypovolemic in nature.

Definition: Acute circulatory failure with inadequate or inappropriate perfusion causing cellular hypoxia.

Answer 2.12: Generalized peritonitis—inflammation of the whole of the peritoneal cavity (as opposed to localized peritonitis).

Answer 2.13:
Tenderness: Pain elicited by either superficial or deep palpation usually indicative of inflammation of the parietal peritoneum or stretching of the capsule of an organ.
Guarding: Tightening of the abdominal muscles, as a reflex to the pain induced by palpation.
Rebound tenderness: Sudden withdrawal of the manual pressure causes a sharp exacerbation of the pain of peritoneal inflammation.

Note: Do not elicit 'rebound' tenderness by palpation if you think the patient has got it!! This will cause the patient severe pain. He will not like it and you will lose his confidence (especially children). Asking the patient to cough or move about are 'gentler' ways of demonstrating rebound tenderness.

Answer 2.14: Air under the diaphragm or pneumoperitoneum.

Answer 2.15: Surgery.

Answer 2.16: Perforation of the anterior wall of the first part of the duodenum.

Answer 2.17: Oversew closure + omental patch + lavage.

Answer 3.1: Ask him to tell you about his symptoms. If he does not volunteer the information or you need more details, use the 'leading' questions below:
- What do you mean by indigestion?
- When did it start?
- Is it getting worse?
- Is it there the whole time or comes and goes?
- What makes it better/worse?
- Have you ever had it before?
- Do you have any other problems?
- How much weight have you lost?
- Why have you lost this weight?
- Rest of GI protocol questions.

Answer 3.2: An upper GI malignancy – stomach
– pancreas.

Answer 3.3:
- Epigastric pain: Dull, aching and sometimes radiating to the back.
- Loss of appetite, weight loss.
- Feeling of early fullness, nausea.
- Early vomiting if proximal or later if distal stenosis.
- The symptoms of anemia.

Answer 3.4:
- *H. pylori* gastritis.
- Atrophic gastritis (pernicious anemia).
- Partial gastrectomy.
- Gastric polyps.
- Familial adenomatous polyposis (FAP).
- Blood group A.

Answer 3.5: He looks cachexic and possibly jaundiced.

Answer 3.6: Concavity of the temporalis muscles.
'Hollow cheeks'—loss of bulk of masseter.

Answer 3.7a: Most probably metastatic spread of tumor called Troisier's sign (when associated with carcinoma stomach) or Virchow's node.

Answer 3.7b: May indicate transcelomic spread of tumor— occurs most commonly in ovarian and stomach cancer.

Answer 3.8:
Locally: Through the wall of stomach and into surrounding structures: Omentum, transverse colon, pancreas, left lobe of liver.

Linitis plastica is when the tumor spreads in the wall of the stomach, the so-called 'leather bottle' stomach.
Distally: Via the lymphatics to nodes along the greater and lesser curves (level 1) and then along the nodes along the celiac axis and its branches (level 2). Spread to para-aortic

nodes is level 3 involvement. Via the bloodstream to liver and omentum.

Transcelomically: To peritoneal cavity (Pouch of Douglas).

Answer 3.9: By the T, M and N staging system:
- Tumor
- Nodes
- Metastases.

TUTORIAL 7: Obstructive Jaundice

CASE SCENARIOS

Answer 1.1: You will probably start by saying something like "What is the problem?"

Let the patient talk but at an appropriate time make sure all the following points are covered, using leading questions where necessary:

Pain:
- Show me where the pain is.
- When did it start?
- Did it come on gradually or suddenly?
- Have you ever had it before?
- How bad is the pain—mild, moderate or severe?
- Have you had it all the time since it started or does it come and go?
- Since it started has the pain ever gone away completely – if so, for how long?
- How would you describe the pain—colicky, constant, sharp, and dull?
- Does the pain go anywhere else—say, to your back?
- Is there anything that makes the pain worse, e.g. movement?
- Is there anything which makes it better, e.g. lying still?
  (Do you feel anything else wrong with you at the moment or in recent months?)

Note: These questions are moving away from the simple mnemonic and are in a more sensible order.

If you ask here 'do you feel anything else wrong with you at the moment or recently' this is a good time to ask the rest of the GI protocol questions.

Nausea and vomiting:
- When did you start to feel sick?
- When did you start to vomit?
- Was this before or after the pain started?
- Have you had this before?
- How many times have you vomited?
- What is in the vomit, e.g. food, bile?
- Is there any blood in it?
- Is it very forceful?

Answer 1.2:
- Site?
- When did it start?
- Had it before?
- Sudden or gradual in onset?
- Type (sharp/dull)?
- Severity?
- Radiation?
- Aggravating factors?
- Relieving factors?
- Associated symptom?

Answer 1.3:
- Have you had any difficulty in swallowing?
- Have you had any acid regurgitation or heartburn?
- Have you had any indigestion over the last few months and what do you mean by this?
- Has your tummy blown up?
- Are your bowels working regularly and have they changed in the last few months?
- Have you passed any blood or slime with your bowel motions?
- How has your appetite been over the last few months?
- Have you lost any weight recently?
- Have you been able to eat since the pain started?
- Have you ever been yellow jaundiced?
- Have you noticed any change in the color of your urine or bowel motion?

Note: This is the basic protocol but with some additions considered appropriate for this case—you will learn the 'additions' with experience, they make your history more focused.

Answer 1.4:
- Dry mucous membranes.
- Sunken, lusterless eyes.
- Decreased skin turgidity.
  (Postural hypotension, low urine output, tachycardia, and hypotension are signs of severe dehydration)

Answer 1.5: Murphy's sign is the demonstration of tenderness on palpation over the gallbladder area and is indicative of inflammation of the gallbladder (acute cholecystitis).

Demonstrate by asking the patient to breath in while the examining hand exerts gentle upwards pressure under the right costal margin. If Murphy's sign is to be considered positive, the same maneuver must not elicit pain when carried out in the left costal margin.

Answer 1.6:
Acute cholecystitis—Acute onset of upper abdominal pain with nausea and vomiting, fever and positive Murphy's sign.
No PH of ulcer dyspepsia.
No signs of generalized peritonitis.

Answer 1.7: She has most likely developed infection in the common bile duct due to blockage by a gallstone(s), the clinical condition known as cholangitis.

Answer 1.8: See Figure 7.3.

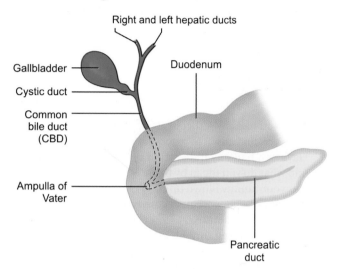

Fig. 7.3 Basic anatomy of biliary tree

Answer 1.9: Questions about the jaundice itself:
- When did you notice the yellow jaundice?
- How did you notice it?
- Has it become worse?
- Have you had it before?
- Have you noticed any change in the color of your urine?
- Have you noticed any change in the color of your bowel motion?
- Has your skin started to itch?
- Have you had any abdominal pain?
- Have you had any fever?

(These questions give pointers to the type of jaundice—obstructive/hepatocellular)

Then you should ask the risk factors for jaundice: This may help with the diagnosis:
1. Have you been in contact recently with anyone with jaundice? Has anyone in the family had jaundice? Have you ever been in hospital with jaundice? (infective hepatitis).
2. Do you drink alcohol and how much? (alcohol-induced cirrhosis).
3. Have you had any blood transfusions? (blood transfer of hepatitis B).
4. Do you take any medications? (side-effect of drugs).
5. Have you injected yourself with drugs? (IV drug abuse—hepatitis/HIV).
6. Have you had any casual sexual relations not with your normal partner? (Sexually transmitted disease).

7. Have you had or got any blood disease or abnormality and do they run in the family? (hemolytic blood disease).
8. Have you travelled abroad recently? (hepatitis A).

Answer 1.10:
- Scleral icterus
- Jaundice of skin or abdomen
- Scratch marks on arms/legs
- Dark urine
- Pale colored stools on rectal examination.

Answer 2.1:
- When did you first notice you had become yellow?
- Who noticed it?
- Has it become worse?
- Is it there the whole time or does it go up and down?
- Have you noticed any change in the color of your urine?
- Have you noticed any change in the color of your bowels?
- Has your skin been itching?
- When did the pain start?
- Where is it?
- Have you ever had it before?
- Is it getting worse?
- How severe is it?
- What sort of pain is it—dull/sharp?
- Is it there the whole time?
- What makes it better?

Then ask all the risk factors for jaundice:
- Hepatitis
- Alcohol
- Drugs and medications
- IV drug abuse
- STDs
- Blood transfusions travel
- Hemolytic or autoimmune disease.

Then ask all the other GI tract protocol led questions:
- Any difficulty in swallowing
- Any nausea or vomiting
- Any heartburn or acid reflux
- Any indigestion or abdominal distension
- Any change in bowel habit +/– blood
- Appetite and weight loss.

Answer 2.2:
1. Upper GI malignancy? Cancer head of pancreas.
2. Metastatic liver disease—jaundice.
3. ??? Gastric cancer.

This is the way you may list your differential diagnosis at the completion of the history and examination—it is conventional to put the most likely diagnosis first. The question marks are used to indicate gastric carcinoma is a possibility but much less likely.

Answer 2.3: 'When a patient has obstructive jaundice and the gallbladder is palpable—the cause of the jaundice is more likely due to a pancreatic neoplasm rather than stones in the CBD'. (If the patient has gallstones as the cause, the gallbladder is likely to be shrunken and fibrosed due to inflammation).

Answer 2.4: Said to be a history of painless, obstructive jaundice with anorexia and weight loss but remember about 90% of patients have some pain by the time they present—usually dull upper abdominal pain or pain in the back.

Answer 2.5:

Prognosis: Cancer of periampullary region/distal CBD = 20–40% 5-year survival.

Head of pancreas: <5% still alive at 5 years overall median survival from diagnosis <6 months.

For those undergoing resection median survival = 12–19 months (Ca head of pancreas: Only about 10% suitable for resection).

Answer 2.6:
- Endoscopic retrograde cholangiopancreatography (ERCP).
- Shows filling of a dilated CBD containing gallstones.

Answer 2.7:
- Contrast enhanced CT scan: Picture on right is a coronal reconstruction.
- Shows mass in head of the pancreas.

TUTORIAL 8: Abdominal Pain (The Pancreas)

CASE SCENARIOS

Answer 1.1: Place the examining hand on the patient's abdomen and press gently. Release the depressed fingers and if rebound tenderness is present, the patient feels a sudden increase in pain.

Rebound tenderness is a sign of peritoneal irritation or inflammation of the peritoneum or peritonitis. Remember peritonitis can be localized or generalized.

Rebound tenderness is an accurate sign, but very painful for the patient.

The guiding rule is not to perform the test for rebound if you think the patient will have a positive test!!

What is the alternative?
- Ask patient to cough—he/she will have pain in the area of inflammation and may move his/her hand to that area.
- Ask patient to roll over on the bed and he/she will again localize the pain to the area of inflammation.

Answer 1.2: Absence of bowel sounds means the normal peristalsis of the bowel has ceased. This is usually indicative of generalized peritonitis.

Remember that obstructive bowel sounds are high pitched and come in runs; high pitched, infrequent tinkling sounds indicate paralytic ileus.

The total absence of bowel sounds in an acute abdomen is a very useful sign to indicate generalized peritonitis, but remember with localized peritonitis, you will still hear bowel sounds.

Answer 1.3:

Differential diagnosis:
1. Acute pancreatitis:
   Hx: Acute onset epigastric pain soon becoming generalized, sometimes radiating to the back and sometimes relieved by sitting forward.
   Associated with anorexia, nausea and vomiting.
   Ex: Epigastric or more generalized tenderness, rebound and guarding.
   Absent or very scanty bowel signs.
   Systemic signs: Fever, jaundice, tachycardia, tachypnea, peripheral underperfusion—'shut down'.
   If severely hemorrhagic: Cullen's sign, Grey Turner's sign, Fox's sign (inguinal region bruising).
2. Peptic ulcer disease (either acute exacerbation or perforation).
   Hx: Dyspepsia for a long time, then presents acutely with a sudden onset of upper abdominal pain. If acute exacerbation, will remain localized; if perforation, will spread over whole abdomen.
   Ex: If acute exacerbation, local epigastric tenderness. If the ulcer is perforated, there are the clinical signs of peritonitis: Diffuse tenderness, 'board-like rigidity' and absent bowel sounds. Jaundice is not present unless the patient is grossly septic.
3. Acute cholecystitis:
   Hx: Long history of food-related upper abdominal discomfort, perhaps with previous episodes of acute inflammation (episodes of fever, associated with constant RUQ pain that may radiate to scapula) +/- jaundice. (In this scenario, the history does not sound like gallbladder disease and the signs of diffuse peritonitis do not occur unless the gallbladder is perforated).

Answer 1.4:
- Blood tests:
  - FBC (reduced Hb level in anemia, raised WCC in infection).
  - CRP ('C' reactive proteins) elevated in inflammation.
  - U&E (look for electrolyte imbalance/dehydration).
  - LFTs (look at liver enzymes and bilirubin levels).
  - Pancreatic amylase test (specific test for acute pancreatitis).

–   Blood cultures (identify cause of sepsis).
–   May need clotting screen and ABGs (if pancreatitis).
*   Urine dip stick
    –   Should be carried out routinely in all cases of acute abdomen, in this case may be negative but if the diagnosis was, say acute cholecystitis, may show bile in urine.
*   Imaging:
    –   Erect chest X-ray (look for air under diaphragm—perforated viscus).
    –   Abdominal X-ray: in pancreatitis may show an ileus (+ string of beads sign or the rarer sentinel loop sign).

*Answer 1.5: **Acute pancreatitis***
*   Amylase – 5 times above upper limit of normal is diagnostic of acute pancreatitis.
    3 times above normal is suggestive of acute pancreatitis.
*   Other abdominal conditions can cause a raised serum amylase.
    Common ones: • Perforated viscus
                  • Ischemic bowel. Amylase will be raised but will not be 5 times above normal.
    (There is evidence to suggest a s. lipase may be more specific and sensitive than the s. amylase but s. amylase is still the quickest and most commonly used).

Answer 1.6: Periumbilical bruising. If associated with pancreatitis, this usually indicates severe hemorrhagic pancreatitis and is called Cullen's sign.

Answer 1.7: Hemorrhagic 'bruising' of the flank.
    If associated with acute pancreatitis, this is called Grey Turner's sign. (TIP: How to remember Cullen's Vs Grey Turners: Cullen has a U in it [= umbilicus] and Grey has no 'U').

Answer 1.8:
*   By severity: Either mild/moderate or severe:
    –   Mild/moderate—Usually caused by gallstones.
    –   Severe—significant mortality (Imrie's criteria >3).

Answer 1.9: The history and clinical signs are unreliable in predicting whether the patient has mild/moderate or severe acute pancreatitis (and it is very important to know this to decide the optimum management).
*   Ranson's criteria and the Glasgow Prognostic Score are a set of parameters used to determine whether a patient is likely to have a mild or severe acute pancreatitis attack.
*   Remember the patient with severe pancreatitis can be clinically quite well, and then suddenly become very ill.

*   In every case of acute pancreatitis, the house officer (intern) should carry out a Ranson's or Glasgow score. The score will decide if the patient needs to be kept in a high dependency unit or the ICU under close invasive monitoring. If carried out, an APACHE II score of >8 indicates severe disease (see Module 3 Tutorial 5).

Answer 1.10:
*   Commonly alcohol and gallstones.
*   Rarer causes are: Mumps, steroids, biliary ascariasis, post-ERCP.

Answer 2.1:
*   Find out what type of alcohol he is drinking—beer, whiskey, and wine.
*   Quantify his alcohol intake.

Answer 2.2:
*   Quantitate in units of alcohol.
*   1 pint of beer = 2 units.
*   1 shot of whiskey = 2 units.
*   1 glass of wine (large) = 2 units.

Answer 2.3:
*   How long have you had diarrhea?
*   What does it look like?
*   What color is it?
*   Is it foul-smelling?
*   Any blood?
*   Any mucus?
*   Does it float? Do you have difficulty flushing the motions away?

Note: Check back with your answers in Tutorial 1.

Answer 2.4: Pale, bulky and offensive (smelly) stool indicate fat malabsorption.

Answer 2.5:
*   Means that patient may have developed diabetes mellitus (due to chronic damage to the pancreas, leading to loss of pancreatic islet tissue).

Answer 2.6: Erythema ab igne—caused by putting hot bottles on the abdomen to relieve chronic pain, e.g. in chronic pancreatitis, malignancy.

Answer 2.7: Pancreatic calcification.

Answer 2.8: Chronic pancreatitis.

Answer 2.9:
*   The secretion of unduly viscid pancreatic juice may allow protein plugs to form in the duct system, and these plugs calcify, subsequently to form duct stones.

- Impaired flow of pancreatic juice then leads to inflammation and stricture formation in the duct system with progressive replacement of the gland by fibrous tissue.
- Loss of acinar tissue is reflected eventually by steatorrhea, and, in time, loss of islet tissue may lead to diabetes mellitus.

Answer 2.10:
- Chronic pancreatitis—can never be reversed, but can be limited.
    - Stop them from drinking alcohol.
- Medical:
    - Treat the pain (specialist pain management).
    - Treat the malabsorption (pancreatic enzyme replacements).
    - Treat the diabetes mellitus (insulin).
- Surgical:
    - May be indicated if medical management has failed (will be discussed in Module 3).

TUTORIAL 9: Rectal Bleeding 1

CASE SCENARIO

Answer 1.1:
- What color is the bleeding?
- How much blood is there?
- When does he notice it—before or after defecation?
- Is it mixed in with the bowel motion?
- Has he had it before?
- Associated symptoms: Especially anal pain/discharge/mucus/pus/abdominal pain.

Answer 1.2:
- Any change in bowel habit?
- Any diarrhea/constipation?
- Any abdominal pain?
- Any change in appetite/weight loss?

Answer 1.3:
- Red blood usually comes from rectum/anal canal/sigmoid colon.
- Purple/dark blue blood is colonic in origin until proven otherwise.
- Black, shiny, tarry blood is melena—upper GI in origin.
- Slate grey bowel motion are caused by Iron (Fe) containing medications.

Answer 1.4:
- May indicate a cancer of the large bowel, for example—a change from a regular daily motion to alternating diarrhea, and constipation is classically said to indicate a malignant lesion of colon or rectum—actually a change to increased frequency is more significant.
- Colon and rectal cancers do not often present with constipation alone unless the patient is obstructed.

Answer 1.5:
- Because the patient's idea of a normal bowel habit is often very different!
- Ask if they have got diarrhea or constipation or both (and then define what they mean by diarrhea and constipation), then define their normal bowel habit and what it has changed to.

Answer 1.6: Because the differential diagnosis of the rectal bleeding will often be influenced by whether there is accompanying pain or not, e.g. classical hx of fissure in ano (streaks of bright red blood + severe cutting pain at anus).

Answer 1.7: Yes, family history of large bowel cancer/bowel polyps/FAP/HNPCC makes it more likely that the patient may have colon or rectal cancer.

Answer 1.8:
- Adenomatous polyp—refers to the histopathological type of the most common large bowel polyp. It is these types of polyps which can undergo the classical polyp-cancer sequence.
- Familial polyposis coli is a genetically inherited disease accompanied by the formation of multiple adenomatous polyps in the colon and rectum (and also sometimes in the small bowel and stomach) (FAP = defined as >100 polyps).
- Hereditary nonpolyposis colon cancer is polyp associated cancer occurring on an inherited basis but in a younger age group (40s) and on the right side of the colon. The number of polyps present is much smaller than in FAP.

Answer 1.9:
- A full general examination.
- A full abdominal examination.
- A full anorectal exam if possible; at least inspection and digital rectal examination.

Answer 1.10: The GP should refer to hospital a patient with rectal bleeding if:
1. He identifies a colorectal cancer.
2. He suspects from the history or examination that there is a malignancy.
3. He is unable to perform an anorectal examination which confirms that the cause is, within reasonable doubt, a benign cause which he feels happy to treat (e.g. hemorrhoids).
4. He suspects or identifies other pathology which requires hospital referral, e.g. inflammatory bowel disease.

Answer 1.11:
- To a general surgeon with a colorectal interest or,
- To a specialist colorectal surgeon if available or,
- To a gastroenterologist.
- An urgent referral should be made if the diagnosis is malignancy, or if this is suspected.
- Patient should be seen within 1–2 weeks.

Answer 1.12:
- Inspection.
- Digital exam.
- Proctoscopy.
- Rigid sigmoidoscopy or flexy sigy
(sometimes abbreviated to AR exam).

Answer 1.13:
- FBC.
- Bioprofile.
- Stool culture.
- CEA.
- Colonoscopy.

Answer 1.14:
- Macro: Everted, rolled edged ulcer.
        Polypoid, cauliflower lesion.
        Stenosing lesion.
        Flat polypoid lesion.
        Pedunculated polyp with malignant change.
- Micro: Adenocarcinoma (almost always).

Answer 1.15: See Figure 9.2
Just remember: Anus approximately 2%
                Rectum, rectosigmoid and sigmoid
                approximately 60%
                Left side approximately 70%
                Right side approximately 25%

Answer 1.16:
- Right side: More indolent—anemia/mass/late obstruction.
- Left side: Obstruct earlier, therefore pain and change in bowel habit earlier.

Answer 1.17:
- Locally through the bowel wall.
- Lymphatic to draining nodes
- Via blood to liver.
- Peritoneal cavity by transcelomic spread implantation.

Answer 1.18: Defines the degree of spread of the tumor, can be clinical staging (c) or pathological (p). Staging is used to plan management and provide a prognosis.

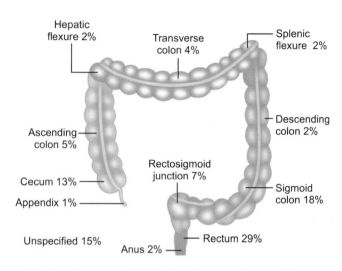

Fig. 9.2 Percentage distribution of colorectal cancer by site
(*Source:* Cancer, UK)

Answer 1.19: If you know the likely pathological spread of the tumor, you can define the imaging needed to stage the tumor.

Answer 1.20:
Local: By digital exam/CT/MRI/endoanal US + histo-pathology.
Lymphatic spread: May be CT/MRI/US but usually on histopathology.
Distal spread: CXR/CT/US/MRI.

Answer 1.21: See Figure 9.3

Answer 1.22: See Figure 9.4

Answer 1.23:
- Anterior resection of the rectum.
- Abdominoperineal resection (APER).

Answer 1.24: See Figures 9.5 and 9.6.

Answer 1.25: Height of the tumor in the rectum and whether you can obtain adequate distal clearance.

This probably needs a little explanation. When a large bowel cancer is removed, the operation should remove the tumor with clear proximal and distal margins together with the draining lymph nodes. In rectal cancers, it is established that there is little distal spread of the tumor margin and 2 cm of distal clearance is adequate. If the tumor lies at 7 cm from the anal verge this 2 cm of distal clearance can be achieved and the bowel ends joined back (anterior resection). If the tumor lies at 5 cm or below from the anal verge the distal clearance is inadequate and an APER is performed.

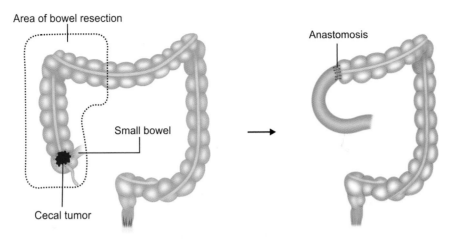

Fig. 9.3 Right hemicolectomy

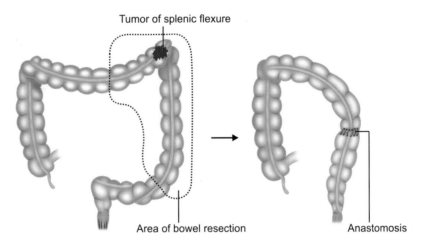

Fig. 9.4 Left hemicolectomy

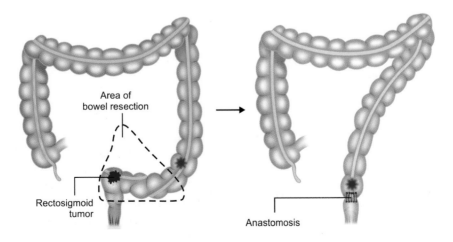

Fig. 9.5 Anterior resection of rectum (AR)

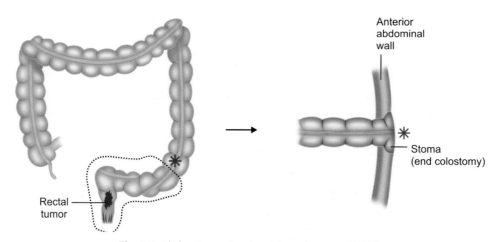

Fig. 9.6 Abdominoperineal excision of rectum (APER)

TUTORIAL 10: Rectal Bleeding/Anal Pain 2— Minor Anorectal Disorders

CASE SCENARIOS

Answer 1.1:
- Intermittent bright red bleeding on defecation.
- Classically said to 'drip' into toilet bowl.
- Itchiness around anus.
- Lumps on the anal area (either skin tags or prolapsed piles).
- Lumps coming down with defecation and going back.

Answer 1.2: Hemorrhoids are rarely painful unless prolapsed or thrombosed.

Answer 1.3: Bright red rectal bleeding is also a symptom of large bowel cancer or inflammatory bowel disease—if he describes an accompanying change in his bowel habit, this must be investigated further.

Answer 1.4: Hemorrhoidal symptoms are made worse by straining at stool. The fast, easy evacuation promoted by the bulky stools of a high roughage diet may be sufficient in itself to cure the symptoms.

Answer 1.5: Hemorrhoids are not varicose veins of the anal canal (otherwise the bleeding would be dark blue). Current views are that the suspensory fibers in the anal canal degenerate with straining and the cushions of the anal canal which contain arteriovenous connections slip out of place. This exposes them to the trauma of defecation and causes bleeding.

Hemorrhoids may be made worse by raised intra-abdominal pressure (e.g. in pregnancy).

Answer 1.6:
- **1st degree:** Only visible on proctoscopy (bleed or itch).
- **2nd degree:** Come down on defecation but go back spontaneously.
- **3rd degree:** Come down on defecation and can be reduced manually.
- **4th degree:** Remain down permanently.

Answer 1.7: Useful only in terms of deciding treatment:
- **1st degree:** Diet or injections.
- **2nd degree:** Diet/injections or if large enough: Banding.
- **3rd degree:** Banding or surgery.
- **4th degree:** Usually surgery.

(*Note:* The management will be discussed in more detail below.)

Answer 1.8:
- Inspection
- Digital examination
- Proctoscopy
- Rigid sigmoidoscopy (in that order).

Answer 1.9: Third degree.

Answer 1.10: The normal anal cushions hypertrophy, often with accompanying skin tag formation. The hypertrophied cushions indicate the presence of significant internal hemorrhoids. Often the patient will complain that their 'piles' are always prolapsed. When examined often they are referring to the skin tags and enlarged cushions rather than having 4th hemorrhoids. Similarly they may complain of lumps at the anal verge and again these are frequently the cushions or tags.

Answer 1.11: Refer Table 10.1.

Table 10.1 Treatment of hemorrhoids

1st degree (symptoms but seen only on proctoscopy)	High fiber diet +/– injection with 5% phenol in almond oil
2nd degree (come down on straining and retract spontaneously)	Small = Inject + fiber Large = Band + fiber
3rd degree (come down on straining—reducible manually)	No external component = Band Significant external component = Hemorrhoidectomy
4th degree (permanently prolapsed)	Hemorrhoidectomy

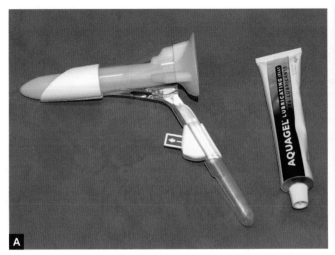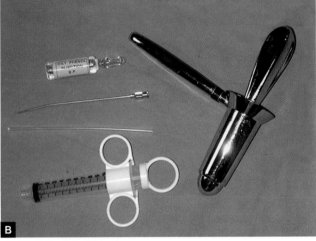

Figs 10.2A and B (A) Disposable proctoscope and lubricating jelly; (B) Nondisposable proctoscope and equipment for injecting hemorrhoids (Copyright RCSI with permission)

Answer 1.12: A short cylindrical instrument for examining the anal canal. It should be called an 'anoscope' (Figs 10.2A and B).

Answer 1.13: A 25 cm cylindrical instrument for examining the rectum. It would probably be better called a rectoscope (the rectum is 15 cm long). It is not always possible to pass the sigmoidoscope into the sigmoid colon (Fig. 10.3).

Answer 1.14: See Figure 10.4.

Answer 1.15: The anal canal is examined by a proctoscope. The rectum and sometimes the distal sigmoid by the sigmoidoscope.

Answer 2.1:

a. Anal pain:
   – When did it start?
   – When do you get it? (e.g. when your bowels work)
   – How bad is it?
   – How long does it last?
   – What makes it better?
   – Have you had it before?

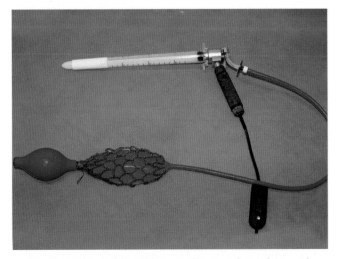

Fig. 10.3 Disposable rigid sigmoidoscope shown here with fiberoptic light source and bellows

b. Associated symptoms:
   – Is there any bleeding from the back passage—color and amount?
   – Has there been any change in your bowel habit?

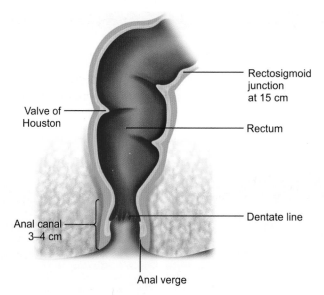

Fig. 10.4 Anatomy of the anal canal and rectum

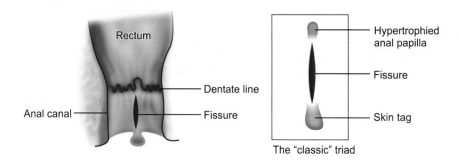

Fig. 10.5 Fissure in anoclassic triad

– Did the pain start after an episode of diarrhea or constipation?
– Do you feel anything coming down at the anus?
– Are you otherwise well, e.g. appetite/weight/fever?

Answer 2.2: A streak of bright red blood on the toilet paper.

Answer 2.3: Fissure in ano.

Answer 2.4: See Figure 10.5

Answer 2.5a: Idiopathic fissures are either posterior (most common) or anterior in the midline. If the fissure is 'off' the midline you should be suspicious of its etiology.

Answer 2.5b:
• Crohn's disease
• HIV

Answer 2.5c: The classical triad of:
• Fissure
• External skin tag
• Sentinel polyp.

Answer 2.5d:
• May be in midline but may be off the midline, e.g. 8 o' clock
• Often painless and multiple.
• Look bluish and are indurated.
• Often relatively painless.
• Associated with symptoms of Crohn's.
• Other anorectal manifestations of Crohn's, e.g. abscess, skin tags (but not always).

Answer 2.6:
1. Fecal bulking agent, e.g. bran or a mixture of a bulking agent and a mild laxative, e.g. normacol plus.
2. Local creams or suppositories containing local anesthetic and steroids, e.g. anusol or proctosedyl.
3. Topical nitrate neuromuscular blockers, e.g. 0.3% GTN paste.
4. Lateral subcutaneous sphincterotomy.
5. Endoanal advancement flap.

TUTORIAL 11: Lump in Breast

CASE SCENARIOS

Answer 1.1:
- When did you first notice the lump?
- How did you notice it?
- Has it become bigger or smaller?
- Does it change with your periods?
- Is it painful?
- Have you had lumps in your breast before?
- Is there any nipple discharge and, if so, what type?

Answer 1.2:
- Age.
- Family history.
- Early menarche/late menopause.
- Nulliparous.
- Breastfeeding.
- Age at first childbirth.
- Level of fat consumption.
- Obesity in postmenopausal women.
- Hormone replacement therapy.
- Radiotherapy.
- Oral contraceptive pill.

Answer 1.3:
Note: Your own medical school may have a different protocol for breast examination. The protocol shown below was agreed between the Penang Medical School and the Breast Surgeons at the hospital).

Examine with patient sitting on the edge of examination couch first.
Remember: LOOK, FEEL, MOVE BREAST, AREOLA, NIPPLE
Look: Right and left disparity/lumps/skin tethering.
  Abnormal skin changes, distended veins.
  Then AREOLA changes, then NIPPLE.
  Raise arms—look for tethering/mass.
Feel: By quadrants, systematically.
  Describe lump by set criteria: Site, size, shape, surface, etc.
  Do not forget:
Move: i.e. fixity to skin and pectoralis muscle.
  Then examine areolar and nipple.
  Examine normal breast first and then the other breast.
Feel axillae correct way: Anterior/posterior/medial walls and apex.
  Feel supraclavicular areas.
  Then lie patient down with head on 1 pillow, hand behind head and repeat whole sequence.

Finally check for ascites and liver enlargement by abdominal examination.

Answer 1.4:
There is disparity between the right and left breast with the nipple—areolar complex on the left side elevated by the tethered mass described below:
- Swelling in left upper inner quadrant.
- Marked skin tethering (Remember the sequence: Breast/areolar/nipple).

Answer 1.5:
Inspection: Breast distortion/disparity
  Skin tethering
  Peau d'orange
  Nipple retraction
  Blood-stained nipple discharge
Feel/Move: Hard
  Irregular
  Skin fixation
  Deep fixation
  Axillary lymph node enlargement
  + signs of distal spread—ascites/liver enlargement/bone tenderness.

Answer 1.6:
In situ - Ductal carcinoma *in situ* (DCIS) said to account for 20% of breast cancer diagnosed in USA, 90% of it on screening.
  Lobular (LCIS)—lobular carcinoma *in situ.*
Invasive ductal = 83%
Invasive lobular = 10%

Note: Graded from 1–3 well-differentiated to poorly differentiated.
Small % are special types—medullary/colloid/mucinous or tubular.

Answer 1.7:
Locally: To surrounding breast tissue.
  To skin.
  Deeply into muscle.
Distally: Via lymphatics to the axilla.
  Via lymphatics of internal mammary chain to the supraclavicular area.
  Via the bloodstream most commonly to the chest, liver and bones.

Answer 1.8: Triple assessment.

Answer 1.9:

1. **Full history and examination** (i.e. clinical assessment).
2. **Imaging:** Usually mammography +/– ultrasound.
   Ultrasound in patients aged 35 years or less may be better because of breast density.
3. **Tissue diagnosis:** FNAC
   or core biopsy (more recent trend)
   or open biopsy (rarely necessary).

Answer 1.10:

TNM staging: Being made more complicated every year. You should be familiar with a 'basic' version as listed below in Table 11.1.

Table 11.1 T, N and M staging of breast cancer	
Tis	CA *in situ*
T1	<2 cm
T2	2–5 cm
T3	>5 cm
T4a	Involvement of chest wall
T4b	Involvement of skin
T4c	= a + b
T4d	Inflammatory cancer
N0	No nodes
N1	Ipsilateral mobile axillary nodes
N2	Ipsilateral fixed nodes
N3	Internal mammary
M0	No distal metastasis
M1	Distal metastasis including supraclavicular nodes

Other terms sometimes used in classification of breast cancer are:

Operable breast cancer: Equivalent to: T1 T2 T3, N0-N1, M0
Locally advanced   Equivalent to: T4, N0-2, M0
Metastatic   Equivalent to: M1

In staging breast cancer, it would seem appropriate that all patients with a proven breast cancer should have at least a CXR and CT of the liver and possibly a bone scan. In 'operable breast cancer', the incidence of distal metastases is very small so in order to maximally utilize resources in many breast units abdominal CT and bone scan are only performed preoperatively, if symptoms suggest distal spread.

Answer 1.11:

- To determine to what extent the cancer has spread.
- To decide on appropriate management.
- To provide a prognosis.

Answer 2.1: A fibroadenoma.

Answer 2.2:

- Regarded as an aberration of normal breast tissue development, one-third becomes smaller in 2 years.

- Therefore, once diagnosis is confirmed can leave.
- Remove any >3 cm because of risk of phylloides tumor.

Answer 2.3:

- Explain to the young lady that you think the lump is nothing to worry about, i.e. benign and not a cancer.
- Explain that you need to confirm the diagnosis by putting a small needle into the lump to remove some cells to look at under the microscope [Fine needle aspiration cytology (FNAC)].
- Explain that if small (<3 cm) and the diagnosis is confirmed, it is safe to leave the swelling alone as it will probably disappear.
- If the patient wants it removed, this is acceptable but will leave a small scar.

Answer 3.1:

- When did the pain start?
- Is it in one or both breasts?
- What is its relation to the time of your period?
- Is it getting worse?
- Do you notice any lumpiness at the time you have the pain?
- Does the pain and lumpiness go away after your periods finish?
- Does the pain interfere with your life?
- Have you taken anything for the pain and if, so what? Does it help?
- Is there any nipple discharge?
- Is there any family history of breast problems and all the other RISK FACTORS for breast cancer discussed earlier?

Answer 3.2: Cyclical mastalgia.

Answer 3.3: Premenstrual nodularity and breast discomfort (cyclical mastalgia) are so common that they are regarded as part of the normal cyclical changes of the breast.

Lumpiness and nodularity can be diffuse or localized. Diffuse nodularity is normal particularly premenstrually. It is now accepted that the normal breast is lumpy. In the past, lumpy breasts were regarded as having fibroadenosis or fibrocystic disease, but the normal nodularity is not associated with any pathological abnormality. Focal nodularity is a common cause of breast lumps in women of all ages—the lump may vary with the menstrual cycle. The 'lumpiness' consists of diffused breast tissue thickening and often discrete cysts.

Answer 3.4: Exclude malignancy by triple assessment of the discrete lump. If symptoms are mild, reassurance alone may be sufficient. If more severe:

- Soft support bra day and night.
- Evening primrose oil.
- Danazol.
- Tamoxifen.

Answer 3.5: Explain the 'pathophysiology' we have discussed above, i.e. tell her it is regarded as 'normal' to have this problem and that the tests have shown she does not have cancer.

Assess how much trouble she is having and, if significant, ask if she would like to try some treatment (as delineated above).

TUTORIAL 12: Blood in the Urine (Urology 1)

CASE SCENARIO

Answer 1.1:
- Is this the first time you have seen red urine?
- Why do you think it is blood, what color is it—dark red, bright red, clots?
- How often does it happen?
- Where in the urine stream do you notice the blood, is it all through the stream, at the beginning or when you strain to finish?
- Have you any pain in your abdomen?
- Have you had any problems passing urine recently?
- Then ask directly the obstructive and irritative symptoms (*See* Module 1 Tutorial 2).
- Have you noticed a fever?
- How is your general health at present?
- How is your appetite and weight?
- Have you had any serious illness or operations?
- Are you taking any drugs or eating a lot of unusual foods—anticoagulants and analgesic abuse (aspirin) may cause bleeding, pyridium (in senna), rifampicin and beetroot discolor urine wine red.
- Have you injured yourself or been in an accident recently?
- Have you been involved in any vigorous exercise recently? (Jogger's hematuria).

Remember the past medical Hx, family history and social history may all provide important information as illustrated below:
- History of recent upper respiratory tract infection:
  - Glomerulonephritis, IgA nephropathy
  - Significant past medical or urological or surgical Hx of stone, UTIs, malignancy
  - Porphyria, TB, pelvic irradiation, bleeding disorders.
- History of tobacco use
  - Transitional cell carcinoma of bladder (TCC).
- Family history
  - Alport syndrome, GN, connective tissue diseases, stones, polycystic kidneys, coagulopathy, cancers.
- Occupational risk factors
  - Naphthylamine, benzidine or 4,4-aminobiphenyl in rubber, dye, petroleum—TCC

Answer 1.2:
Visualize the anatomy of the urinary tract—use the disease headings: Infective
Inflammatory
Neoplastic (benign and malignant)
and just work down from kidney to urethra.

Remember to add in the 'medical' and drug causes and trauma.

Hence

Kidney	infective	=	Pyelonephritis
			Glomerulonephritis
			Abscess
			TB
	inflammatory	=	Stone disease
	neoplasia	=	Carcinoma
	trauma	=	Direct blow from, e.g. accident
Ureter	inflammatory	=	Ureteric stone
	neoplasia	=	Ureteric tumor
Bladder	infective	=	Cystitis
			TB
	inflammatory	=	Bladder stones
	neoplasia	=	Tumor—benign and malignant
Prostate	neoplasia	=	benign: BPH, malignant: cancer
Urethra	infective	=	Sexually Transmitted Diseases
	neoplasia	=	Urethral tumor
	trauma	=	Direct inujry, e.g. fall

Answer 1.3: Pseudohematuria—causes:
- Drugs (pyridium, rifampicin)
- Vegetables (beetroots)
- Dyes in food
- Vaginal bleeding (menstrual bleeding) in female
- Medical diseases (obstructive jaundice, porphyria, hemoglobinemia, myoglobinemia).

Answer 1.4:
- Initial stream: Suggests urethra as source.
- Throughout the stream: Suggests bladder and above.
- End of stream: Suggests prostate/bladder neck and trigone.

Answer 1.5:
- Site
  - Renal angle, back
- Time and mode of onset
  - Sudden (stone) versus insidious (tumor)
- Severity
  - Very severe—renal/ureteric colic
  - Aching pain: Renal tumor, pyelonephritis
- Nature
  - Remember: Constant pain in renal colic
  - Colicky: Hollow organs
- Concurrent symptoms
  - Fever, chills rigors—pyelonephritis
  - Night sweats: TB, RCC

– Nausea and vomiting: Renal/ureteric colic
– Change of bowel habits: Bowel pathology
• Progression of pain
• Duration
• Relieving factors
• Exacerbating factors
• Radiation
– To groin or genitalia—ureteric colic
• Urinary symptoms
• Systemic reviews: GI symptoms, musculoskeletal system.

Answer 1.6: In this scenario, fever may be associated with:
• Infections—tuberculosis, endocarditis, osteomyelitis, abscesses, HIV infection.
• Cancers—Night sweats are an early symptom of some cancers: Lymphoma, renal cell carcinoma.

Answer 1.7:
Differential diagnosis: Renal carcinoma
Renal infection—acute
pyelonephritis, perinephric abscess
Renal stone

Answer 1.8: Just like the examination of the GI tract, you need to have a protocol
For urology, this will be very similar to the gastrointestinal tract protocol but with a few different emphases.
So:
General:
Face:	In pain?
	Cachexic/weight loss
	Flushed
	Dehydrated
	Jaundiced
	Anemic
	Lips and mouth
Hands:	Nail changes, no pale skin crease, palmar erythema
	Warm moist palms
	Abnormality of arms
Vital signs:	Pulse/BP/RR/Temp (Systemic disturbance—tachycardia, warm peripheries/temp/RR increased)
Neck:	Masses, nodes
Chest:	Full respiratory system examination because loin pain can originate in the chest
Back:	Most easily examined when examining back of chest
Abdomen:	Inspect/palpate/percuss/ausculate
	Groins + genitalia
	PR
	Legs

This is really just the same protocol as we have already learned except that the back, the groins and genitalia are emphasized.

In this case, we will be looking for specific signs which may point to one of the differential diagnoses.
Renal cell carcinoma
• Flank mass, left varicocele, signs of malignancy: Adenopathy, anemia, muscle wasting, liver mass.

Infection (acute pyelonephritis, perinephric abscess, TB)
• Fever, tachycardia, flank mass in abscess.

Renal stone
• May have signs of uremia
• Back: Signs of abscess (calor, dolor, rubor, tumor!).

Answer 1.9:
Symptoms
• Feeling weak and tired, lethargy.
• Having dizzy episodes and feeling faint.
• Intolerance to cold.
• Shortness of breath, palpitations, headaches, sore mouth and gums.
• Patients notice they are looking pale or others around them may say they are looking pale.

Signs
• Tachycardia
• Pallor
• Heart murmur
• Koilonychia.

Answer 1.10:
• Edema
• Hypertension
• Scratch marks
• Ecchymoses
• Pallor
• Tachypnea
• Lemon yellow.

Answer 1.11: Indicates underlying tenderness due to obstruction or inflammation.

Answer 1.12:
• Enlarged spleen
• Enlarged kidney
• Mass in tail of pancreas
• Mass in left colon
• Mass in stomach.

Answer 1.13:
• Site: Loin mass
• Ballotable on palpation
• Moves up and down on deep inspiration
• Examining hand can get above
• Not dull to percussion (overlying colon).

Table 12.1 Physical signs for differentiating between an enlarged kidney, spleen and gallbladder

	Shape	Get above	Direction on inspiration	Percussion	Ballotable	Others
An enlarged kidney	Round	Yes	Down	Resonance	Yes	
An enlarged spleen	Firm, smooth	No	Diagonally	Dull	No	Notch
Gallbladder	Smooth and hemi-ovoid	No	Down	Dull	No	
Hepatomegaly	Sharp or rounded edge, smooth or irregular surface	No	Down	Dull	No	

Answer 1.14a:

An enlarged spleen:

*   Moves down and medially on inspiration.
*   Cannot get above.
*   Dull to percussion.
*   May have palpable notch (30%).

Answer 1.14b:

*   Site—liver is in relation to the costal margin.
*   Cannot get above.
*   Moves down on early inspiration.
*   Dull to percussion.
*   Enlarged gallbladder is felt opposite tip of 9th rib.

Answer 1.15: See Table 12.1.

Answer 1.16: Causes of an enlarged kidney:

*   Distension of the pelvicalyceal system
    Hydronephrosis
*   Space occupying lesions
    Polycystic kidney
    Renal tumor
    Large simple cyst
    Abscess
*   Compensatory hypertrophy
*   Perinephric abscess.
    Most likely diagnosis in this case: Renal cell carcinoma.

Answer 1.17:

*   A varicocele.
*   The testicular vein on the left side drains into the left renal vein.
*   In this case, the left renal vein must be involved with the tumor with obstruction causing enlargement of the testicular veins.

TUTORIAL 13: Loin Pain (Urology 2)

CASE SCENARIOS

Answer 1.1:

*   When did the pain start?
*   Have you ever had it before?

*   Has it been there all the time since it started?
*   What sort of pain is it—severe, moderate, an ache?
*   Does it come and go—colicky?
*   What makes it better or worse?
*   Has it moved anywhere else?
*   Have you had any other symptoms with it, e.g. nausea, vomiting, fever?

Answer 1.2:

Skin: Herpes zoster (Shingles).
Respiratory system: Pneumonia/pleurisy.
Musculoskeletal/spine: Soft tissue trauma/lesion affecting thoracic nerve root.
Kidney: Renal/ureteric colic—stone/tumor/pyelonephritis.
Abdomen: Acute appendicitis/biliary colic/acute cholecystitis/dissecting AAA/perforated peptic ulcer/pancreatitis acute salphingitis/ruptured ectopic pregnancy.

This is thinking from 1st principles!

Answer 1.3:

1. Genitourinary system
2. Gastrointestinal system
3. Just possibly the musculoskeletal system (we know she has had back pain).

Answer 1.4: The protocol questions for GU/GI/MS systems:

GU: Pain on passing urine.
    Passing urine more frequently.
    Having to get up at night to pass urine.
    Blood in urine.
    Any change in color of urine—cloudy/smelly?
    Periods/pregnancies.
GI: Difficulty swallowing.
    Acid regurgitation/heartburn.
    Indigestion/distension.
    Change in bowel habit/blood/mucus.
    Appetite/weight loss.
MS: Tell me about your back pain—where/how long/ diagnosis?
    Any other joint pains?

Answer 1.5:

General: Alert, conscious and orientated.

    In distress/pain.

    Pale or jaundiced.

    Well-nourished.

    Dehydrated.

    Flushed.

    Lips and mouth abnormalities.

Hands: Warm and moist.

    Palmar pallor.

    Finger nail changes.

Vital Signs: Pulse/BP/temperature/RR.

Specific: **Abdomen:**

  Inspection: Moving with respiration

      Distension

      Skin changes/scars

      Visible mass/veins/pulsations

      Umbilical abnormalities

  Palpation: Tenderness/guarding/rebound

      Organomegaly

  Percussion: Dullness/ascites

  Auscultation: Bowel sounds

  Groins and hernia orifices

  External genitalia

  Rectal examination

  Vaginal examination?

Back **Look:** Skin changes/deformity.

   Feel: Tenderness/temperature/sensory changes.

   Move: Back/legs.

Answer 1.6a:

Lumbar region: A vertical line is dropped from the mid-clavicular point and crossed by a horizontal line drawn between the tips of the 12th ribs and by a line joining the anterior superior iliac spines. The lumbar region lies between these two lines (Fig. 13.1).

  Renal angle is the area posteriorly bordered by the 12th rib and the lateral border of the erector spinae muscle (Fig. 13.2).

  The loin or flank are not really medical terms but are often used by patients and doctors.

  'Medical' definition of loin—the part of the body on either side of the spinal column between the ribs and the pelvis (posteriorly). 'Medical definition' of flank—the side of the body between the ribs and the pelvis.

Note: You should be very specfic in using these terms as they are often wrongly used interchangeably.

Answer 1.6b: Sit the patient forward and put the palm of your left hand over the renal angle. Use the clenched fist of your right hand to knock against (punch) the dorsal surface of the left hand. If the patient experiences pain with this

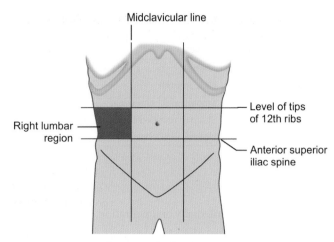

Fig. 13.1 The lumbar region

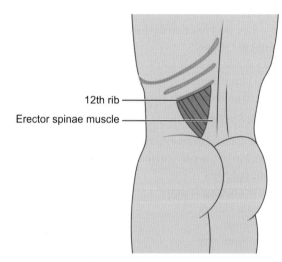

Fig. 13.2 The renal angle

test, it indicates the kidney is tender, usually indicating pyelonephritis or hydronephrosis.

Note: Many physcians do not like the decription as a 'punch test'—it sounds like you are deliberately going out to hurt the patient, and sometimes it is overdone and does hurt the patient.

Answer 1.6c: Extend from T12 to L3. Right kidney is 2 cm lower than left (displaced by liver). Posteriorly the kidneys lie in the renal angle (formed by the 12th rib and lateral margin of the vertebra).

Answer 1.6d: The kidneys are not normally palpable unless the patient is very thin. The right kidney is easier to feel than the left because it lies lower. Position the patient supine and close to the edge of the bed. Examine for both kidneys from the patient's right side. Remember where the kidneys lie anatomically so make sure you palpate over this area and not out in the 'flank or loin'—common mistake of beginners.

When examining the left kidney put the palmar surface of your left hand into the left flank with the fingertips in the renal angle and put the fingertips of your right hand under the costal margin just outside the lateral border of the rectus sheath.

Examining for the right kidney put your left hand into the loin posteriorly and the fingers of the right hand under the costal margin.

Ask the patient to take a deep breath in. What you are feeling for is the lower pole of the kidney as it comes down with respiration. If you move your posterior hand towards the anterior hand you will feel the lower pole of the kidney between your fingers. This is 'balloting'.

If the kidney is enlarged, this is much easier to do (After description given in Epsteins Clinical Examination, 3rd ed., Eds: Epstein, Perkin, Cookson and de Bono, Mosby, Edin. 2003).

Answer 1.7: The guiding rule as to whether you should perform a rectal examination is to ask yourself is the rectal examination likely to produce findings which will change your diagnosis or intended management. If not, do not do it—the examination is unpleasant and embarrassing for the patient, e.g. if you have already decided the patient has appendicitis, then a rectal examination is not necessary. In this case, rectal examination is unlikely to make a difference to either your diagnosis or management.

Answer 1.8: The history and particularly the physical signs would point to a renal cause for the pain, and therefore, a vaginal examination is not necessary. Only if you were still worried the cause may be gynecological in origin, is it necessary to do so.

Answer 1.9:
- Acute pyelonephritis
- Hydronephosis.

Answer 1.10a: Inflammation of the pelvicalyceal system and renal parenchyma caused by bacterial infection.

Answer 1.10b: Accumulation of pus in the renal pelvis and calyces.

Answer 1.10c: Dilatation of the pelvicalyceal system usually due to distal obstruction of the urinary system.

Answer 2.1:
- When did the swelling start?
- How did you notice it:
  – Is it one side or both?
  – Is it getting bigger?
  – Is it painful?

Answer 2.2:
- Hydrocele
- Hernia
- Tumor (much less likely).

Answer 2.3:
- Does the swelling ever go away, e.g. when you lie down?
- Can you reduce it?
- Are there any urinary tract symptoms?
- Is there any history of trauma?
- General health—appetite/weight loss?

Answer 2.4:
- General
- Abdominal
- Inguinoscrotal area.

Answer 2.5: Remember if you can get above the swelling in the scrotum you will go into your 'scrotal exam protocol'.

If you cannot get above the swelling, it is inguinoscrotal and you will go into your 'inguinal hernia exam protocol'.

Examination of male genitalia:
- Patient supine to start with.
- Examiner preferably wearing gloves (nonsterile).

Inspection:
1. INSPECT the penis, including the glans and meatus-dorsal and ventral surface. Look for size, shape, skin color, discharge, any discrete abnormality, e.g. ulcer/lump—use appropriate protocol to describe (e.g. SSS, etc. or BEDD, see Appendix 1). Retract prepuce if indicated.
2. INSPECT the scrotum from front and then lift up and look underneath; looking for any difference in size or shape (LvR), any skin abnormality, any mass, ulcer.
3. PALPATE—palpate the contents of the scrotum starting with the normal side first. Compare right to left side.
   Identify and Palpate:
   Testis
   Epididymis
   Spermatic cord (feel vas deferens and vessels).
4. If swelling is felt: Determine four facts:
   a. Is the swelling confined to the scrotum (i.e. can you get above it?).
   b. Can the testis and epididymis be defined?
   c. Is the swelling transilluminable?
   d. Is the swelling tender?
5. Define the characteristics of any swelling using the standard protocol (Size/Shape/Surface, etc).
6. Finally: Stand the patient up:
   Is the swelling still palpable or is a new one present? (e.g. varicocele) Can you get above it (i.e. is it inguinoscrotal or scrotal)?

Answer 2.6: Inspection shows that there is swelling of the left scrotum which appears to extend up to the inguinal area. The right scrotum appears normal. There are no obvious skin changes.

Answer 2.7: A hydrocele.

TUTORIAL 14: Vascular Disease (Arterial): Calf Pain of Chronic Onset and Leg Pain of Sudden Onset

CASE SCENARIOS

Answer 1.1:
- When did the pain start?
- Do you have the pain everyday or does it come and go?
- Where is it?
- Is the pain only there when you walk?
- How far do you walk before it comes on?
- What makes it better?
- What makes it worse?
- Is it just in one leg?
- Have you injured your leg?
- Do you have any pain in your back or abdomen?
- How is your general health?

Answer 1.2: Intermittent claudication.

Answer 1.3: You ask him directly about the other disease symptoms with which generalized atherosclerosis is likely to cause or be associated with:
- Do you have any chest pain or angina?
- Have you had a heart attack?
- Do you have high blood pressure?
- Have you had any problems with your eyes, e.g. blurred vision?
- Have you had a stroke, blackouts or weakness or numbness of your arms or legs?
- What is your diet like?
- Have you put on weight?
- Have you had your cholesterol checked?
- Are you diabetic and is there a family history of diabetes?
- Is there a family history of heart problems—define this.
  Then complete the whole of the rest of the history taking protocol (PMH/SH/ROS/medications and allergies).

Answer 1.4:
- Whether he smokes (how many cigarettes per day and time in years) and drinks alcohol (quantitate in units).
- What was his job and is he financially secure?
- Does he live in a house with stairs?
- Who looks after him?

Answer 1.5:
- Risk factors for atherosclerosis.
- How will he cope if he needs surgery?

Answer 1.6: Chest pain/breathlessness/palpitations/ankle swelling—if not asked before (+ appropriate follow-up questions to define the symptom or sign if positive answer is given).

Answer 1.7: If not already asked in presenting history, ask about headaches, fits, blackouts, dizziness, numbness, tingling, weakness of arms or legs, stroke.
Sleep problems and depression.
Problems with eyes—blurring of vision/transient blindness.

All are important because they are related to manifestations of peripheral vascular disease (PVD).

Answer 1.8:
- His β blockers are for his known hypertension.
- Daily aspirin (a platelet inhibitor) is taken to cut down the incidence of stroke and heart disease.

Answer 1.9: Mr P is a 68-year-old retired accountant with known hypertension. He gives a 3-month history of pain in his right calf coming on when he walks 100 meters and relieved by rest.

He has smoked 40 cigarettes per day for 30 years and drinks around 30 units of alcohol per week. He has had no other serious illnesses. He takes beta blockers and aspirin.

Answer 1.10: Atherosclerosis is the process of fatty degeneration and thickening which affects medium and large arteries and which is characterized by plaque formation. There are four stages in the pathogeneses:
1. Damage to the endothelial cells of the tunica intima of the artery occurs (because of hypertension/diabetes/smoking). The damaged cells attract platelets and an inflammatory reaction is setup with deposition of macrophages and lipoproteins.
2. A 'fatty streak' develops in the vessel wall consisting of foam cells which are macrophages filled with lipoproteins.
3. Fibrin deposits on the inflamed area and develops into the fibrous plaque.
4. If the plaque is stable it may simply grow and either narrow or occlude the vessel or it may become unstable and rupture resulting in either emboli or formation of thrombosis on the surface of the ruptured plaque (look at Pathophysiology of Atherosclerosis by Andrew Wolf: www.youtube.com/watch?v_rktoF7BHRiQ).

Answer 1.11: See Figure 14.1

Answer 1.12: See Figure 14.2

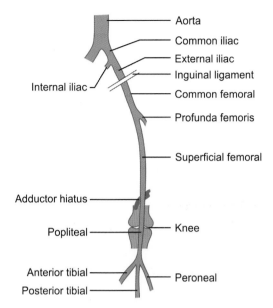

Fig. 14.1 Anatomy of the main arteries of the lower limb

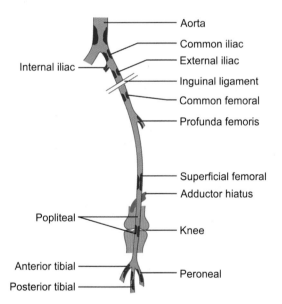

Fig. 14.2 Main sites of atheroma deposition in lower limb

Answer 1.13:
General:

Face:	Alert, conscious and orientated?
	In pain or distressed?
	Pale or jaundiced
	Well-nourished
	Well-hydrated
	Cyanosed/plethoric
	Lips, mouth, dentition—any abnormality.

Hands:	Finger nail changes, palmar crease pallor, palmar erythema, moist palms arms.	
Vital signs:	Pulse, BP, RR, temp, peripheries.	
CVS:	cardio: Lips	
		JVP
		Inspection of chest
		Apex beat
		Auscultation
		Leg edema.

Remember this is a 'vascular case' so you have to examine the upper limbs/neck and face for the physical signs of vascular disease:

Compare both upper limbs:

Inspection:	Color:	Normal
		Pale
		Congested
		Blotchy
	Ischemic changes	- Thinning of skin
		- Hair loss
		- Ulceration

Palpation:	Temperature	
	Capillary refilling	
	Pulses: Distal to proximal comparing both sides	
		Radial
		Ulnar
		Brachial
		Axillary
		+/– Thrills

Auscultation for bruits.

Palpate and auscultate carotid arteries in neck.

Face:	Cyanosis/plethoric
	Arcus/xanthelasma
	Fundi

Appropriate neurological assessment if relevant Hx or local signs, e.g. weakness

RS:	Inspection
	Auscultation
	Percussion
Abdomen:	Pulsatile mass
	Bruit
Specfic:	Lower limbs (including full vascular assessment)
Look:	Compare both limbs – Any swelling/deformity/ muscle wasting
	– Any bruising
	Change in color, e.g. pale/blue
	Varicose veins

Then look at right leg:

Any signs of ischemia	– Thickened, dystrophic toe nails, ulcers, gangrene
	– Look at pressure points.

Feel: Temperature/tenderness (especially calf)

Pulses (dorsalis pedis, posterior tibial, popliteal, femoral)

Capillary refill

Sensation.

Move: Limitation on movements

Muscle wasting

Fixed deformities

Buerger's angle/test

Then look, feel/move for other leg.

Answer 1.14: Atherosclerotic peripheral vascular disease (PVD) of a chronic nature.

Answer 1.15: See Figure 14.4.

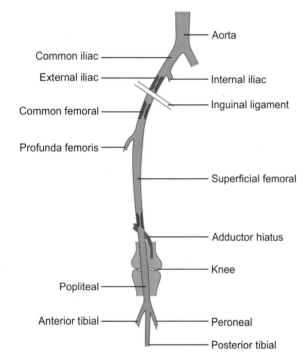

Fig. 14.4 Sites of atheroma in patient Mr P

Answer 1.16: Dystrophy is any condition related to abnormal development, often used in relation to degeneration. In the foot affected by PVD, the dystrophic changes refer to the absence of hair, shiny skin and thickened nails—all abnormal developments caused by reduced blood supply.

Answer 1.17:

a. Femoral pulse is located in the groin 1–2 cm below the midinguinal point (half way between the anterior superior iliac spine and the symphysis pubis). Its relationship to the femoral vein and nerve is vein/artery/nerve (VAN)—medial to lateral.

b. Popliteal pulse is located in the popliteal fossa just lateral to midline. Often difficult to feel especially in men. Examine with knee flexed—fingertips of both hands in popliteal fossa—move gently medially to laterally.

c. Posterior tibial lies just posterior to the medial malleolus (about 1 cm).

d. Dorsalis pedis: Lies on the dorsum of the foot between the 1st and 2nd metatarsals immediately lateral to the extensor hallucis longus tendon.

Please note these locations are made deliberately simple but are just as accurate as the more long winded descriptions found in some textbooks.

Answer 1.18: Refer Table 14.1.

Table 14.1 Risk factors for atherosclerosis and their medical management	
Risk factor	*Management*
Dyslipoproteinemia	Diet/statins
Smoking	Immediate and absolute cessation
Hypertension	Beta blockers or other antihypertensives
Obesity	Diet
Sedentary lifestyle/stress	Appropriate exercise regime/reduce stress
Diabetes	Appropriate, supervised management
Hypercoagulablity	Antiplatelet Rx; aspirin/clopidogrel
Age	
Family history	Screening

Always think of the risk factors and their management in this way (very easy to remember), known as best medical therapy (BMT).

Answer 2.1:

- Where is the pain—show me please.
- When did the pain start? What were you doing?
- Did it come on gradually or suddenly?
- Have you had it ever since or does it come and go?
- How bad is the pain? Has it become worse since it started?
- Has the pain moved?
- Have you ever had it before?
- Ask if he has had any trouble with his heart or blood pressure or a history of strokes.
- Has he any serious illness, ask specifically for diabetes.
- Has he been in hospital before?
- Was he fit and well before this started or did he have other problems?
- Is he on any drugs or medications?

Answer 2.2: Acute limb ischemia—probably embolic in origin.

Answer 2.3:
General:

Face:	Alert and conscious and orientated?
	In pain or distressed?
	Pale or jaundiced?
	Well-nourished?
	Well-hydrated?
	Cyanosed/plethoric?
Hands:	Palmar pallor
	Clubbing.
Vital signs:	Pulse, BP, RR, temp, peripheries.
CVS:	Cardio: Lips
	JVP
	Inspection of chest
	Apex beat
	Auscultation
	Leg edema.

Compare both upper limbs:

Inspection:	Color—Normal
	Pale
	Congested
	Blotchy
	Ischemic changes – Thinning of skin
	– Hair loss
	– Ulceration.
Palpation:	Temperature
	Capillary refilling
	Pulses: Distal to proximal comparing both sides
	Radial
	Ulnar
	Brachial
	Axillary
	+/– Thrills

Auscultation for bruits
Palpate and auscultate carotid arteries in neck.

Face:	Cyanosis/plethoric
	Arcus/xanthelasma
	Fundi.

Appropriate neurological assessment if relevant Hx or local signs, e.g. weakness.

RS:	Inspection
	Auscultation
	Percussion.
Abdomen:	Pulsatile mass
	Bruit.
Specfic:	Lower limbs
	(including full vascular assessment).
Look:	Compare both limbs – Any swelling/deformity/ muscle wasting
	– Any bruising

Change in color, e.g. pale/blue
Varicose veins
Then look at right leg
Any signs of ischemia – Thickened, dystrophic toe nails, ulcers, gangrene
  – Look at pressure points.

Feel:	Temperature/tenderness (especially calf)
	Pulses (dorsalis pedis, posterior tibial, popliteal, femoral)
	Capillary refill
	Sensation.
Move:	Limitation on movements
	Muscle wasting
	Fixed deformities
	Buerger's angle/test.

Then look, feel/move for other leg.

Remember this is a 'vascular case,' so at some stage you have to examine the upper limbs/neck, face for evidence of vascular disease. In this case, it will be better to assess the lower limbs first and then carry out a quick assessment of the rest of the cardiovascular system.

The protocol has been reproduced in full so you become used to its content.

Answer 2.4: Acutely ischemic right leg (pale/cold/swollen/ absent pulses) probably of embolic cause (atrial fibrillation/ sudden onset) but against background of chronic peripheral vascular disease (dystrophic changes).

Answer 2.5: Refer Table 14.2.

Table 14.2 Symptoms and signs of acute limb ischemia

Symptom/sign	Reliability
Pain	May be absent in complete block and is also present in chronic ischemia
Pallor	Varies with degree of block
Pulseless	Depends on level and degree of block
Perishing cold	Unreliable—leg takes up ambient temperature
Paresthesia	Sign of impending irreversible ischemia
Paralysis	Indicates irreversible change—reliable

Source: Garden, Churchill Livingston-Elsevier, 2007

Remember that the six P's are nonspecific except for parethesia and paralysis but are a good way of remembering what to look for.

Answer 2.6: At first the completely ischemic limb is marble white because of intense arterial spasm.

Over the next few hours, the spasm relaxes and the limb becomes mottled with bluish red areas which blanch on pressure (called nonfixed mottling). At this stage, the limb is salvageable.

Over the next few hours, the mottling becomes darker and does not blanch (fixed mottling). By this stage, the limb is not salvageable.

The calf muscle tenderness on squeezing indicates muscle ischemia and is an indication of the leg becoming nonsalvageable.

TUTORIAL 15: Vascular Disease 2: Leg Ulcers and Diabetic Foot

CASE SCENARIOS

Answer 1.1:
- Can you show me the ulcer?
- When did you first notice it?
- What do you think has caused it?
- Had you injured the leg?
- Has the ulcer become bigger?
- Is it painful?
- Is there just one ulcer?
- Is there any discharge?
- Has it healed over since you first noticed it?
- How long have you had the varicose veins?
- Have you ever had a thrombosis or clot in your leg?
- How is your general health?

Answer 1.2:

The ulcer on Mrs N's leg is immediately above the medial malleolus of the left leg (the gaiter area). (Site)
It is about 2 cm in diameter (Size)
It is ovoid in shape (Shape)
Its base contains red granulation tissue (Base)
Its edge appears sloping (Edge)
Depth—shallow: 1–2 mm (Depth)
Discharge—not seen (Discharge)
Surroundings—dark pigmentation,
reddening and thickening of skin (Surroundings)

> **Remember:** Look: site + size + shape + BEDDS
> Feel
> Move

Answer 1.3: A venous ulcer.

Answer 1.4:

Other causes are: Arterial
Mixed arterio/venous
Trauma
Neuropathic
Infective
Collagen vascular disease associated
Hematological
Malignant.

Answer 1.5: Refer Figure 15.2.

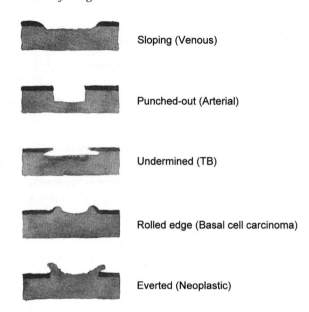

Sloping (Venous)

Punched-out (Arterial)

Undermined (TB)

Rolled edge (Basal cell carcinoma)

Everted (Neoplastic)

Fig. 15.2 Configurations of skin ulcers

Answer 2.1: Gangrenous toes.

Answer 2.2:
- When did you first notice anything wrong with your foot?
- How did it start off and what happened afterwards?
- Is it painful?
- Did you injure yourself?
- Did you go to the doctors?
- How long have you been a diabetic?
- What medications do you use for your diabetes?
- How do you decide how much insulin to use?
- How are you feeling in yourself at the moment?
- Do you have a fever?
- Do you have any problems with the other leg?

Answer 2.3: The right 4th and 5th toes are black and dry with a line of demarcation distal to the metatarsophalangeal joint. The skin of the other toes and dorsum of the foot is reddish blue, shiny and hairless. The nails are thickened and deformed.

Answer 2.4:
- The diabetic foot is liable to infection, ulceration and gangrene.
- The underlying pathology is a combination of ischemia, neuropathy and immune suppression caused by the diabetes.
- Poor blood supply to the foot is caused by the involvement of the small arteries of the foot in the microangiopathy of the diabetic process. This is often made worse by the

presence of atherosclerosis in the larger vessels of the foot and leg.

- Diabetic neuropathy affects the sensory, motor and autonomic nerves.

Sensory neuropathy: Because of the neuropathy the patient does not feel pain in his foot. He becomes susceptible to minor acute and chronic trauma because he does not notice them, e.g. shoes rubbing against pressure points. The lack of pain sensation is also why patients often present late.

Motor neuropathy: This affects the long and short flexor and extensor muscles of the calf and foot, leading to weakness and wasting. The toes become dorsiflexed making the heads of the metatarsals prominent and susceptible to pressure injury.

Autonomic: Because the foot does not sweat properly it becomes dry, scaly and fissured and liable to infection. A combination of abnormal proprioception from the sensory neuropathy and abnormal blood flow in the ankle and foot (caused by loss of autonomic control) results in the development of Charcot joints.

Answer 2.5: A Charcot joint or Charcot arthropathy is the progressive destruction of bone and soft tissues of weight-bearing joints caused by a mix of neurovascular and neurosensitive abnormalities.

Most affected are the foot and ankle joints and present as a swollen 'hot' joint. Joint deformities with pathological fractures and dislocations occur. The etiology nowadays is usually diabetes but also can be due to syphilis, alcoholism, leprosy, spinal cord damage, syringomyelia and renal dialysis. (*emed.medscape.com/article/1234293-overview*)

Answer 2.6: Simple to remember if you just think of the 'prominent' parts of the foot which come into contact with a harder surface, e.g. the ground/footwear/mattress in bed so the pressure points are:

- Tips of toes
- Heads of metatarsals
- Heel
- Lateral malleolus in bed
- Lateral border of plantar surface of foot.

Answer 2.7: Look back to the protocol you have developed in Module 1, Tutorial 14: Look, Feel, Move

Look (Inspect)
Look at both legs first: Compare size/shape/swelling
Color, skin changes
The look at each leg in turn: Dystrophic changes
Ulcers/gangrene/pressure point/webs of toes.

Feel (Palpate)
Both legs for temperature
then capillary filling/pulses/sensation for each leg.
Move
Test movements of joints/power and tone of main muscle groups.
Noting muscle wasting/deformity.

Answer 2.8a: Ulcer on heel—almost certainly caused by pressure on heel in elderly person lying in bed.

Answer 2.8b: Ulcers on tips of toes at pressure points, probably poorly fitting shoes.

Answer 2.8c: Infected gangrene of R first and second toes with edema and redness of dorsum of foot.

Answer 2.9:
Atherosclerosis: Eyes: arcus, hypertensive retinopathy
carotid/radial/brachial pulses for presence/absence/thrill/bruits
blood pressure
Examination of CVS
Abdomen: Pulsatile mass/bruits.
Diabetes: Weight/hydration/endocrine facies
Eyes: diabetic retinopathy
Skin: necrobiosis lipoidica
Cutaneous candida
Injection sites.

TUTORIAL 16: Head Injuries

CASE SCENARIOS

Answer 1.1:
- Primary survey: Remember by mnemonic 'ABCDE'
  - **A**irway with cervical spine control.
  - **B**reathing with institution of ventilation if necessary.
  - **C**irculation with hemorrhage control.
  - **D**isability—neurological and pupil assessment.
  - **E**xposure and environment.

Answer 1.2: The assessment of conscious level will come in 'D' after you have dealt with any lifesaving problems in ABC.
In the initial survey, this will consist of:
- Are eyes open
- Talk to patient
- Response to painful stimuli.

You will then perform a Glasgow Coma Scale (score) when you assess his head injury (HI) in your secondary survey.

Answer 1.3: Refer Table 16.1

Table 16.1 Glasgow coma scale (score)

Eye opening		Verbal response		Motor response	
Spontaneous	4	Orientated	5	Obeys command	6
To speech	3	Confused	4	Localizes pain	5
To pain	2	Inappropriate words	3	Flexion to pain	4
None	1	Incomprehensible words	2	Extension to pain	2
		None	1	None	1

Total Score = 15

Minor HI score = 14–15   Moderate HI = 9–13   Severe < 8

What you actually do:

1. *Eyes:* Look at patients' eyes, are they spontaneously open: if not, ask him to open and close his eyes (shout), if does not, rub his sternum (pain), see if opens his eyes.
2. *Verbal response:* Shout at him and ask him if he knows where he is and his name. Note his response—answers correctly/answers but in confused manner/answers in a confused manner wrongly/answers in 'gobbledygook'.
3. *Motor response:* Shout at him and ask him to move arms or legs. See if responds appropriately. If not, pinch his arm or leg, ask if this hurts him and see if he responds to this by either flexing it (withdraws leg) or extending it.

Answer 1.4:
- Eyes = 4
- Verbal = 4
- Motor = 6
- Total = 14

Can write down E4 V4 M6 (must be itemized for progression)

Answer 1.5:
- Severe GCS <8
- Moderate 9–13
- Minor >14/15

Answer 1.6:
a. Reliable objective way of recording the conscious state of a person.
b. Provides a continuous assessment of conscious state.
c. Provides a guide to management (<8 needs intubation).
d. Value in predicting outcome.

Answer 1.7:
- Pupillary examination.
- Neurological exam.

- Pulse, temperature, blood pressure, respiration rate (Vital signs).
- Search for CSF leak/blood from nose and mouth and ears.
- Survey of scalp for penetrating injury.

These form part of the secondary survey.

Answer 1.8: Pupil size and reaction to light: The nurses are more familiar with this than the doctors but you must know how to carry out this examination and the relevance of the abnormalities found to the head injury.

When performing a pupillary examination, the examiner should make the conscious patient focus on a distant object straight ahead. In the unconscious patient, assess in the position they are 'found in'.

A pupillary assessment includes:

1. Examination of size and equality of pupils:
   Pupil size: Width or diameter of each pupil in mm
   Use standardized gauge
   Normal diameter is approx. 3.5 mm (2–5 mm)
   Both pupils should be equal (+/– 1 mm).

2. Pupil shape:
   Pupil shape is reported as round, irregular or oval. Round is normal.
   Irregular may be the result of ophthalmic procedures, e.g. cataract or lens implant. Oval may be an early indication of raised ICP from pressure on cranial nerve 3.

3. Pupillary response to direct light:
   Assessed by shining a low beam flashlight (pen torch) inwards from the outer canthus of each eye (do not shine directly into pupil—causes glare).
   Record speed of response of each pupil as brisk/sluggish/nonreactive.
   Normal = Brisk
   Sluggish may indicate early raised ICP.
   Nonreactive usually indicates severe rise in ICP or severe brain damage.
   A complete pupillary reactivity examination also includes an assessment of the consensual pupillary response and accommodation.
   The consensual response is the normal constriction of the other pupil which occurs when a light is shone in one eye. When you are assessing pupillary reactivity, you should wait a minute or two between eyes for the consensual effect to wear off. If you ask a conscious person to focus on an object some 6 inches away from the eyes then both pupils will constrict—this is the normal accommodation response.
   The neurological examination should include:
   Movement of all four limbs.

Assessment of power and tone of all four limbs. Assessment of all reflexes—biceps/triceps/wrist/knees/ankles + plantar responses.

In particular, you are looking for asymmetry of these parameters.

Assessment of cranial nerves.

Answer 2.1: Extradural hematoma

Answer 2.2: Extra or epidural hematoma is a collection of blood outside the dura but within the skull, most often in the temporal region (due to middle meningeal artery laceration) (Figs 16.1 and 16.2). It is uncommon occurring in only 0.5% of all head injuries and 9% of severe HI. It has a better prognosis than other intracranial hematomas and appears as biconvex or lens shaped on CT.

Mechanisms of injury: Usually due to fractured temporal or parietal bone. Usually by trauma to temple beside the eye in motor vehicle accident (MVA), a fall or a sporting injury.

Answer 2.3: Usually following HI with or without loss of consciousness or drowsiness. Only about 30% have the classical lucid interval (hours to days) followed by deterioration in conscious level associated with the symptoms of rising ICP (progressive headache, vomiting, confusion, fits).

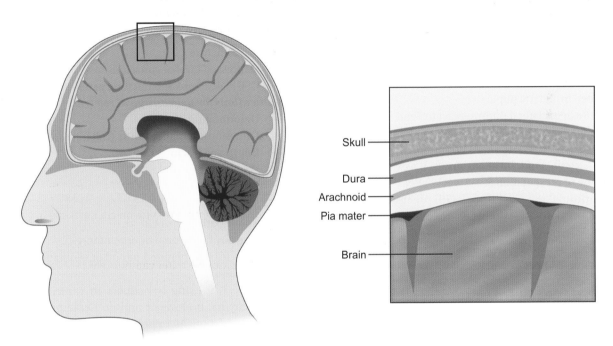

Fig. 16.1 The meninges of the skull and associated spaces

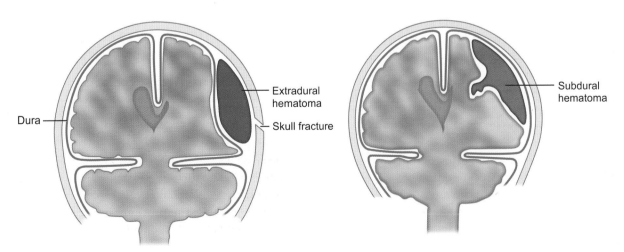

Fig. 16.2 Extradural and subdural hematoma

Signs: Hemiparesis

Brisk reflexes with up-going plantars

As becomes more severe: Deepening coma, bilateral spastic paresis, deep and irregular breathing, bradycardia, hypertension, ipsilateral pupil dilation (late).

Answer 3.1: Chronic subdural hematoma.

Answer 3.2: Collection of blood between the brain surface and the dura. Usually by tearing of bridging veins. Much more common than extradural hematoma and prognosis is worse because of coexisting brain injury.

An acute subdural (SDH), usually caused by a high speed impact to skull—from fall/MVA/assault. Clinical presentation depends on size of the hematoma and the degree of any associated parenchymal brain injury.

Findings are:

1. Altered level of consciousness.
2. Dilated ipsilateral pupil.
3. Failure of ipsilateral pupil to react to light.
4. Hemiparesis on opposite side to hematoma.

Chronic SDH: 25–50% have no history of head trauma; if present, usually mild. Insidious onset: If associated with HI, usual time of presentation is 4–5 weeks after.

Symptoms are insidious with decreased level of consciousness, balance problems, cognitive dysfunction and memory loss, motor deficit and aphasia. May fit.

Signs: Hemiparesis, Hemianopia, Papilledema, 3rd nerve dysfunction—unreactive dilated pupil/laterally deviated eye.

Answer 3.3a: GCS = 6   E1 V1 M4

Answer 3.3b: GCS = 13   E4 V3 M6

Answer 4:

Assessment:

1. Airway/breathing and circulation concerns addressed first. Remember this will include avoidance of hypoxia and hypotension which will exacerbate the HI.
2. Then assess the GCS, the papillary size and response, and a neurological assessment of the limbs.
3. Then make sure the patient is on a head injury chart so these parameters are continuously assessed— demonstration of a change is more important than a single reading.

Management: Remember the primary injury occurs as a direct result of the trauma, it may be diffuse or focal, of varying severity and is essentially irreversible.

Secondary brain injury occurs after the primary trauma and is a result of hypotension, hypoxia, pyrexia, infection and raised ICP.

The basis of management of HI should be:

Minor injury: To identify those who are at risk of developing secondary complications by your history and examination and then deciding if they need:

a. Skull X-ray
b. Should be admitted or not
c. Should be referred to a neurosurgeon.

a. ***Indications for skull X-ray:***

- Loss of consciousness or amnesia
- Focal neurological signs
- Suspected CSF leak or blood in nose or ears
- A penetrating wound
- Difficulty in assessing the patient, e.g. drunk or child.

b. ***Indication for admission:***

- Focal neurological signs
- Skull fracture
- Depressed level of consciousness
- CSF leak, depressed fracture, penetrating wound.

c. ***Indications for neurosurgical referral:***

- Deterioration
- Drowsiness in patient with skull fracture
- Depressed fracture/CSF leak
- Penetrating wound
- Failure to improve after 12–24 hours.

Severe injury:

1. In a stable patient do a CT.
2. Remove any hematoma by craniotomy.
3. Admit to ICU for planned period of ventilation to ensure oxygenation.
4. Measure ICP using transducer in ventricles or brain parenchyma, if elevated and no hematoma reduce by hyperventilation, mannitol and sedation.
5. Undertake intensive nursing care and physiotherapy.
6. Communicate with relatives.
7. Rehabilitate.

TUTORIAL 17: Preoperative Assessment and Postoperative Complications

PART 1: PREOPERATIVE ASSESSMENT

Answer 1.1: Because these illnesses may have a direct bearing on how the patient is managed, e.g. is operative surgery the correct option, or is he too high a risk and will allow an ASA or POSSUM risk assessment to be calculated (If you do not know what these are, look them up on the web). The illness may also affect his preoperative preparation, e.g. COPD, diabetes.

Answer 1.2: Because the previous surgery may be related to this presentation, e.g. adhesive obstruction or perhaps recurrent disease.

Old operation notes may need to be sought to identify what he has had done previously and any complications which may have occurred.

Answer 1.3: Because the patient may have had previous anesthetic problems and you and the anesthetist need to know about this, e.g. difficult intubation, scoline apnea. This information may be lifesaving but is all too often omitted from the routine history. Go and look at 5 surgical histories on the ward and see if the house officer has asked this question!

Answer 2:
- Were you admitted to hospital with the jaundice, and if so for how long?
- Were you told what the jaundice was due to?
- How did you get the jaundice? Were any other family members jaundiced at the same time?
- Have you had any vaccinations or blood tests for jaundice?
- Ask about all the risk factors for jaundice.

Answer 3: He may have significant liver failure which would compromise his surgery, and the use of certain drugs. If he is a hepatitis carrier and is operated on, you will then be putting your fellow staff at risk if appropriate precautions are not carried out.

Answer 4:
- Full viral hepatitis screen.
- Liver function tests.

Answer 5: Ensure that the ward staff are aware of his hepatitis status so that appropriate care can be taken during blood taking and specimen handling.

Ensure that the theater staff is aware he is a hepatitis carrier so that double gloving can be used, care with instruments and appropriate bagging and marking of specimens.

Answer 6:
- When did you have the chest pain and describe it.
- Did you see a doctor?
- What did he say was wrong with you?
- Were you in hospital?
- What treatment did you have?
- Are you still having problems with chest pain—if so please describe.
- What medications/tablets are you on?
- Plus other protocol questions for CVS.

Answer 7:
- CXR
- ECG
- Echocardiogram.

Answer 8: Inform your senior of the cardiac history and the results of the investigations. The consultant will probably seek the advice of the cardiologist before operating.

Make sure that the anesthetist is aware of the problem at an early stage.

Answer 9:
Diabetes:
- Poor control increases risk of wound infections and other complications.
  What should be done?:
  - Assess type of diabetes and fasting blood sugar level.
  - Obtain list of medications that patient currently takes. If poorly controlled, speak to your senior and arrange for the medical diabetologist to see the patient. If well-controlled speak to the anesthetist about perioperative management

(Diabetic management of the surgical patient will be discussed in Module 3)

Hypertension:
- May have impaired renal function.
- Likely to have other cardiovascular problems. If uncontrolled is likely to have operative and postoperative problems, e.g. MI, stroke.
- What should be done?:
  - Assess BP status with 4-hourly chart.
  - Assess for other cardiac diseases.
  - Control of BP prior to surgery with, if necessary, medical advice.

Stroke:
- Probably has underlying cardiovascular disease.
- Could also have a current source of embolus that may dislodge during surgery and cause, e.g. another stroke, acute limb ischemia.
- What should be done?:
  - Determine current neurological status.
  - Full assessment of cardiovascular system.
  - If necessary, provide thromboprophylaxis prior to surgery.

Rh fever:
- The rheumatic fever may have resulted in rheumatic heart disease and also means the patient is at risk for bacterial endocarditis.
- What should be done?:
  - Full cardiovascular physical examination (listen for murmurs).
  - ECG.
  - Echocardiogram (look at heart function, presence of any bacterial vegetations).
  - Prophylactic antibiotics should be given prior to starting surgery to prevent bacterial endocarditis.

Tuberculosis (TB):

- Patient might have active TB that can disseminate (e.g. via the respirator in the OT).
- Trauma of surgery can induce reactivation of TB.
- Poor lung function may already exist and will impair postoperative recovery.
- What should be done?:
  - If any suggestion of active TB delay the surgery and seek urgent assessment by respiratory physician.
  - If 'old' TB: Assess respiratory status and inform the anesthetist.

PART 2: POSTOPERATIVE COMPLICATIONS

Answer 10:
- Pulmonary atelectasis or bronchopneumonia
- Wound infection
- Intra-abdominal abscess
- Urinary tract infection
- Inflamed IV site superficial thrombophlebitis
- Thromboembolism
- Blood transfusion reaction
- Septicemia.

Answer 11:
- Due to blockage of the bronchi from retained secretions and if it persists, bronchopneumonia develops.
- Poor coughing because of pain/oversedation may be involved.

Answer 12:
- Early postoperative pyrexia usually in first 24 hours (may be high—39°C)
- Shortness of breath.
- Dry cough.
- Raised respiratory rate/tachycardia.
- Chest X-ray may be negative early on.
- Green sputum may occur later.

Answer 13:
- Physical signs on full chest examination.
- CXR.
- Sputum for culture.
- Blood gases.

Answer 14:
- Prevent by good analgesia and physiotherapy including incentive spirometer.
- Nebulized saline for 'hydration'.
- If severe may need bronchoscopy.
- If unresponsive may need antibiotics.

Answer 15: Incidence dependent on type of operation—clean (thyroid/breast surgery) or 'dirty' (colorectal). Varies from 0–40% depending on procedure.

Surgical technique and sterility, the patients susceptibility to infection (nutrition, immune status) and length of surgery are other factors.

Answer 16: Usually occurs after day 5 postoperatively. History of increasing pain and tenderness in the wound. Pyrexia, local tenderness, edema, wound—hot and red. Serous wound discharge, pus or just induration (anaerobic).

Answer 17:
- Clinical examination.
- Raised white cell count; bacteriology swab.

Answer 18:
- If there is a collection, drain it—may involve:
  - Removal of sutures/clips
  - Opening up the wound, or even
  - Formal exploration of wound
- Daily dressings
- Healing by secondary intention or secondary suture
- Antibiotics only if cellulitis/septicemia or anaerobic induration.

Answer 19:
- Pelvic
- 'Abdominal'
- Subphrenic
- Liver.

Answer 20: Collection of pus in the pouch of Douglas associated with a perforated viscus, infected hematoma or an anastomotic leak.

Answer 21:
- Pyrexia and malaise at day 4–10 postoperatively.
- Mucus passed rectally/pus through rectum or vagina.
- Tender, boggy mass on rectal exam.
- Confirm diagnosis with CT.

Answer 22: Percutaneous drainage.

Answer 23:
- Following severe generalized peritonitis either adequately or inadequately treated by surgery.
- Anastomotic leaks (often associated with inflammatory bowel disease).

Answer 24:
- Pyrexia, malaise, tachycardia, abdominal tenderness, abdominal ileus usually after day 4 or 5.
- Symptoms and signs of septicemia.
- Occasionally presents with cellulitis, wound drainage.

Answer 25:
- Clinical examination
- Raised WCC
- Abdominal CT.

Answer 26:
- Percutaneous drainage.
- Enteral/parenteral nutritional support.
- Antibiotics.
- Sometimes relaparotomy and drainage plus or minus intestinal diversion (stoma).

Answer 27:
- May follow generalized peritonitis, e.g. after perforated appendix, duodenal ulcer or perforated diverticular disease.
- May be an infected hematoma following surgery/trauma.

Answer 28:
- Swinging pyrexia 7–21 days after surgery (Fig. 17.2) pain in the upper abdomen/shoulder tip, breathlessness.
- Examination may be negative or there may be pain/tenderness in RUQ, liver may be enlarged. Perhaps chest signs of pleural effusion/atelectasis.

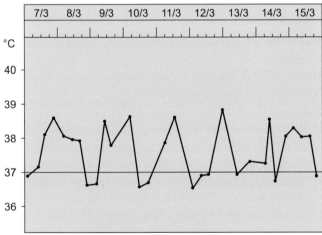

Fig. 17.2 Swinging pyrexia associated with subphrenic abscess

Answer 29: In the pre-ultrasound/CT days, the diagnosis was on clinical grounds +CXR: 'pus somewhere, pus nowhere else, pus under the diaphragm'.
Now: CT or ultrasound.
Raised WCC.

Answer 30:
- US-guided percutaneous drainage
- Sometimes need antibiotics
- Operative drainage, rarely nowadays.

Answer 31:
- Spread through the portal vein from abdominal sepsis (e.g. in appendicitis, diverticulitis)
- Spread from a septic focus in the abdomen via the hepatic artery
- Local extension from adjacent organ, e.g. gallbladder.

Answer 32: Malaise postoperative, swinging pyrexia, RUQ pain, jaundice, and tender enlarged liver.

Answer 33:
- Elevated diaphragm, pleural effusion, lower lobe collapse on CXR.
- Raised WCC, abnormal LFTs—Blood cultures.
- US scan or CT.

Answer 34:
- Percutaneous drainage.
- Appropriate antibiotics.

Answer 35:
- Most often associated with urethral catherization
- Any episode of hypotension with decreased renal perfusion, low urine output and stasis can be a cause.
- Also the presence of 'risk factors': Anatomical renal tract abnormalities, bladder outlet obstruction, stones, bladder diverticula, pregnancy, and diabetes.

Answer 36:
- More often in females: postoperative day 1 onwards
- Symptoms of frequency, urgency, dysuria, hematuria
- Suprapubic pain, renal angle pain, rigors, septicemia
- Urine may be cloudy, smelly and may contain blood
- MSU/CSU: Micro, culture and sensitivity.

Answer 37:
- High fluid intake and urine flow.
- Antibiotics.
- Remove catheter if possible.
- If no response, investigate urinary tract for risk factors.

Answer 38:
- Poor technique.
- IV line becomes 'tissued' or left in too long (many units will have a protocol for routine resiting, say every 48 hours).
- Failure to inspect the site regularly.
- May be sterile phlebitis but may become infected usually with *Staphylococcus* species.

Answer 39: Patient complains of pain at the IV site, IV infusion runs slowly or stops, redness, tenderness and cellulitis at drip site.

Answer 40:
- Resite IV line.
- Local pain relief—warmth of 'poultice'.
- Antibiotics if sepsis.
- Send off catheter tip for bacteriology.

Answer 41:

Virchow's triad   Increased blood coagulability
Decreased flow in veins—stasis
Intimal damage to blood vessels by
pressure, trauma.

Risk factors   Long operations, hip/pelvic operations
Obesity, smoking, cancer, IBD, OCP,
Previous DVT, commonly in calf/pelvis.

Answer 42:
- Flicker of pyrexia.
- Complains of calf tenderness.
- Limb may be tender swollen and warm.

Answer 43:
- Clinical examination.
- Duplex scan.
- Rarely venogram.
- Remember 'D Dimers' but only really to rule out.

Answer 44:

Prophylaxis: Subcutaneous heparin
Early mobilization
Anti-embolic stockings
Calf pumps
Good hydration.

Treatment: Stockings
Anticoagulants
Analgesia
Mobilization.

Use of twice daily ward round observation and DVT risk protocols.

Answer 45:
- The source is usually a calf DVT that has extended into femoral/pelvic veins or from the pelvic veins themselves.
- Embolus passes through the right heart into the pulmonary arterial circulation.
- Clinical effect depends on the size of the embolus and where it lodges small embolus at lung periphery gives localized infarct and pleuritic pain.
- Large embolus in maim pulmonary arteries gives circulatory collapse.

Answer 46:
- Chest pain
- Shortness of breath
- Pleuritic pain on deep breathing
- Hemoptysis

- Tachycardia, pyrexia, signs of DVT
- Circulatory collapse with gallop rhythm, hypotension and raised JVP.

Answer 47:
- Clinical examination
- CXR—may be negative/decreased lung markings/wedge opacity
- ECG: Q3/T3 S in 1
- ABG's: low pO_2, low pCO_2
- CT angiography scan
- Now rarely V/Q scan.

Answer 48:

'Minor' peripheral PE: Analgesia, anticoagulants, oxygen

Major central PE: Resuscitation
Therapeutic angiograms
Thrombolytic therapy
If all fails urgent surgery: Inflow
embolectomy or bypass.

Answer 49:

If minor: Reaction to pyrogens or recipient antibodies to donor white cells.

If major: Incompatible blood.

Answer 50:

Minor: Flicker of pyrexia 1–2 hours after start of transfusion plus rash.

Major: Pain at transfusion site/chest/abdomen flushing, rigors, bronchospasm, hypotension.

Answer 51:
- Mild pyrexia with no other signs or mild pyrexia with rash, it is safer to stop the transfusion and contact the hematology laboratory rather than continue with close observation (+antihistamine) as some would suggest.
- *Major reaction:* Take blood and giving set down send to lab with new patient blood sample plus urine. Give hydrocortisone/adrenaline (1:1000–0.5 mL IM), oxygen.
- Pulse, BP, urine output, clotting times.
- Immediate senior help.

Answer 52: Overwhelming infection spreading from a primary source into the bloodstream.

Usually due to Gram negative organisms or *Staphylococcus* or *Streptococcus* Gram negative septicemia common after biliary, urological or bowel surgery.

Answer 53: Looks ill with tachycardia, hypotension, rigors. May be very warm peripherally and then become cold and under perfused.

Answer 54:
- Examine abdomen, chest, wound, urine, CVP line for cause.

- Send blood cultures.
- Send other indicated samples: for example, urine, catheter tip, sputum, pus FBC, electrolytes, and perhaps ABGs.

Answer 55:
- IV antibiotics.
- IV circulatory support; fluids, inotropes.

- Urinary catheter and hourly urine output.
- Further imaging as indicated, e.g. CT for abdominal sepsis.
- Treat identified cause urgently with surgery if indicated.

Answer 56: Refer Table 17.5.

Patient complaint	Cause	Etiopathology	Presentation	Diagnosis investigation	Management
Pyrexia	Pulmonary collapse Bronchopneumonia	Retained secretions, sputum plugs, poor coughing, pain/oversedation	1st 24 hrs postoperative high temperature; SOB/dry cough, RR up, tachycardia	Clinical Ex of chest CXR–may be –ve early on. Sputum for culture. ABG's	Prevent with good analgesia/physio. Nebulized saline for hydration. May need bronchoscopy or antiboitics
	Wound infection	Type of surgery: Clean versus dirty, surgical technique and sterility, immune status, nutrition, length of surgery	Usually after day 5 postoperative. Pain in wound tenderness, redness, edema, hot. Discharge: serous, pus. Indurated in aerobic infection	Clinical Ex. WCC up Bacteriology from wound swab	Drain collection by dropping sutures, opening Wd or exploration of Wd. Daily dressings. Healing by 2nd intention or 2nd suture Antibiotics if cellulitis or septicemia
	Intra-abdominal abscess/sepsis: subphrenic	Collection after peritonitis or infected hematoma	Swinging pyrexia 7–21 days postoperative Pain in RUQ Pleural effusion	CXR/US/CT WCC up	Percutaneous drainage Antibiotics open surgery
	Pelvic abscess	POD collection after peritonitis/hematoma/leak	4–10 days postoperative: malaise, pus or mucus PR/PV, boggy mass on PR	CT WCC	Percutaneous drainage
	Abdominal sepsis	Interloop/subviscus after peritonitis/anastomosis leak	Malaise, abdo tenderness, ileus, septic after day 4–5 cellulitis/discharge	Clinical exam. Raised WCC CT	Percutaneous drainage, nutritional support. Surgery/stomal diversion
	Liver abscess	Spread from abdo sepsis via portal vein or hepatic artery	Swinging pyrexia, malaise, RUQ pain, jaundice, big liver	CXR: Effusion. WCC up, LFT's abnormal US/CT	Percutaneous drainage antibiotics
	Urinary tract infection	Associated with catheterization, low urine output, low renal perfusion, diabetes, anatomical factors, e.g. stones	Day 1 onwards dysuria/hematuria, suprapubic pain, rigors, cloudy smelly urine	MSU CSU Micro, C+S	High fluid intake, antibiotics, remove catheter, may need Ix urinary tract
	Inflamed IV site	Poor technique, drip 'tissued', may become infected (*Staph.*)	Pain at IV site, infusion runs slow/stops, redness, tenderness, cellulitis	Bacteriology swab Catheter tip for culture	Resite IV line, local heat Antibiotics, if cellultis
	Thromboembolism: DVT	Virchow's triad Risk factors: Cancer/IBD/prev DVT/long surgery hip/pelvic ops Obesity/smoking	Flicker of pyrexia, calf tenderness, swelling, warm Present as PE	Routine clinical Ex on ward rounds Duplex scan	Prophylaxis: Stockings, subcutaneous heparin, mobilization Rx: Stockings anticoagulation
	Pulmonary embolism	Source is DVT or pelvic veins	Depends on size of embolus and where lodges Chest pain, SOB, pleuritic pain, hemoptysis Signs of DVT Collapse	Clinical Ex CXR/ECG/ABGs/CT scan, angiography	Minor: Oxygen, anticoagulants, analgesia Major: Rescusitation, therapeutic angios, thrombolysis, surgery

Table 17.5 Pyrexia

Contd...

Contd...

Patient complaint	Cause	Etiopathology	Presentation	Diagnosis investigation	Management
	Blood transfusion reactions	Minor: Reaction to white cell pyrogens or recipient a/b's Major: Incompatable blood	Minor: pyrexia/rash 1–2 hours after start of transfusion Major: Pain at IV site/in chest/abdomen, flushing, rigors, bronchospasm, hypotension	New blood and urine samples, clotting screen, FBC, bioprofiles	Minor: If any doubt stop transfusion Major: Stop transfusion, replace IV line, give hydrocortisone or adrenaline Contact lab and seniors Close monitoring
	Septicemia	Infection spreading Into bloodstream from primary source: often biliary, bowel, urological surgery gram –ve, *Staphylococcus Streptococcus*	Tachycardia, hypotension rigors, warm then cold peripheries	Clinical exam of chest/ wound, urine, CVP, blood cultures culture of urine, pus. catheter tip, sputum as indicated	IV antibiotics IV fluids, inotropes Monitoring after imaging for source. Surgery, if indicated

Abbreviations: SOB, shortness of breath; temp, temperature; RR, respiratory rate; CXR, chest X-ray; ABGs, arterial blood gases; Ex, examination; WCC, white cell count; Wd, wound; PR, per rectum; PV, per vagina; US, ultrasound; CT, computed tomography; RUQ, right upper quadrant; LFTs, liver function tests; MSU, midstream urine; CCU, clean catch urine; CVP, central venous pressure

TUTORIAL 18: Postoperative Complications (2)

Answer 1: See Table 18.1

Table 18.1 Complication: Wound pain					
Patient complaint	Cause	Etiopathology	Presenting features	Diagnosis investigation	Management
Wound pain	Pain due to incision	Inadequate analgesia Type of incision	Early postoperative distressed/restless tachycardia/raised BP	Exclude other causes	Prophylaxis with local anesthetic in wound, adequate, appropriate analgesia, epidural/PCA
	Hematoma	Poor technique Clotting problems	Swelling, bruising, leakage early or late	Clinical, occasionally ultrasound	Early and expanding: reoperate Late: leave alone/drain/open wound
	Wound infection	Type of surgery dirty/ clean. Technique	Usually after day 5 pain/ redness/fever/induration fluctuance/discharge: serous or pus	Wound swab	Open wound by removing stitches/ clips Irrigation + daily dressing antibiotics if cellulitis/anaerobic septic
	Fistula	Type of operation Technique Comorbidity	Pain, redness, induration Discharge depends on origin of fistula	Bacteriology Fistulogram, CT	See under complication: Fistula

Abbreviations: BP, blood pressure, PCA, patient-controlled analgesia

Answer 2: See Table 18.2

Table 18.2 Complication: Chest pain					
Patient complaint	Cause	Etiopathology	Presentation	Diagnosis investigation	Management
Chest pain	Cardiac	MI	Central, severe, constant (>15 minutes) radiation, numbness, tingling, cold, shut down, hypoxic	Hx+Ex, vital signs, ECG, CXR, enzymes	High flow O_2, IV access, IV morphine (5 mg) + antiemetic, aspirin 300 mg orally, cardiologist
		Arrhythmia	Palpitations, dull chest pain, dizziness	Ex, ECG	Cardiologist
		Angina	Dull, central ache with exertion. Ppt by stress response, fluid overload, hypotension, not giving previous angina medication	Exclude MI	Sit up, high flow O_2, sublingual GTN, cardiologist

Contd...

Contd...

Patient complaint	Cause	Etiopathology	Presentation	Diagnosis investigation	Management
	Pulmonary	Pulmonary embolus	Central chest pain/pleuritic, breathless, sweating, cyanotic, tachycardia, hypotension, JVP up Risk factors—DVT	Hx and Ex, vital signs, PO_2 down, ECG—S wave in V1, Q3, T3, CXR—may be nothing, ABG's, CT	O_2, BP support Anticoagulation thrombolysis Pulmonary embolectomy
		Atelectasis pneumonia aspiration	Pyrexia/coughing + sputum pleuritic pain	Chest exam (reduced air entry, bronchial breathing), CXR sputum	Prophylaxis (physio/antibiotics) O_2, physio, nebulization Antibiotics, bronchoscopy
	Gastric/ esophageal	Acid reflux	Bloating, flatulence, heartburn	Hx	PPI, Gaviscon
		Acute gastric dilation	Vomiting coffee grounds, abdominal distension, ulcer type pain	Hx, abdo X-ray	NG intubation
		Peptic ulcer			PPI
	Musculo-skeletal	Chest incision, cough, trauma	Pain worse with movement	Local tenderness	Analgesia

Abbreviations: DVT, deep vein thrombosis; NG, nasogastric; MI, myocardial infection; ECG, electrocardiography; GTN, glyceryl trinitrate; JVP, jugular venous pressure; CXR, chest X-ray; ABGs; arterial blood gases; PPI, proton-pump inhibitors

Answer 3: See Table 18.3

Table 18.3 Complication: Abdominal pain					
Patient complaint	Cause	Etiopathology	Presentation	Diagnosis investigation	Management
Abdominal pain	Anastomotic leak	Incidence higher in low rectal anastomosis, Crohn's resections	Pain, pyrexia, tachycardia, hypotension, > from day 5, Signs of localized/general peritonitis	Clinical, CT + contrast (in rectum)	Localized: NBM, IV fluids, antibiotics watch + wait; Generalized: Immediate fast resuscitation: IV fluids, antibiotics inotropes, CVP, catheter: Back to theater
	Intestinal obstruction	Early adhesions	Colicky abdo pain, nausea, vomiting, distension, obstructive bowel sounds	CXR, erect + supine abdo X-ray, CT	NBM, IV fluids, ? NG tube, check U+E, occasionally needs further surgery
	Postoperative hemorrhage	Primary, secondary	Tachycardia, BP down, pale, shut down, blood from drain	Hb, PCV	NBM, IV fluids, X match, back to theater
	Perforated viscus	Stress, perf du, intestinal trauma, diathermy	Sudden onset, Shocked, signs of peritonitis	Plain X-rays, CT	Laparotomy
	Pancreatitis Acute cholecystitis	Stress of surgery	Localized/general peritonitis, pyrexia, tachy, BP down	Amylase, plain X-rays chest and abdo, CT	Treat cause
	Intestinal ischemia	Embolus, thrombosis	Risk factors: PVD, AF, post CABG, abdo pain, peritonitis	Clinical, CT, at laparotomy	Laparotomy
	Intra-abdo abscess/ sepsis	Dirty op, poor technique, stomal problems	Pyrexia/rigors, tachycardia, hypotension, localized tenderness, cellulitis, pus in wound/drain	FBC/U +E, blood cultures, appropriate swabs/ bacteriology, plain films, CT	Drainage: CT-guided, laparotomy, antibiotics

Abbreviations: CT, computed tomography; NBM, nil by mouth; CVP, central venous pressure; NG, nasogatric; FBC, full blood count; U + E, urea and electrolytes ; PVD, peripheral vascular disease; AF, atrial fibrillation; CABG, coronary artery bypass grafting; abdo, abdominal; perf du, perforated duodenum; BP, blood pressure; Hb, hemoglobin; NBM, nil-by-mouth; PCV, packed cell volume

Answer 4: See Table 18.4

Table 18.4 Complication: Leg pain

Patient complaint	Cause	Etiopathology	Presentation	Diagnosis investigation	Management
Leg pain	Deep venous thrombosis (DVT)	Virchow's triad trauma/stasis/ hypercoagulable Risk groups: Age/ malignancy/ Previous DVT/bed rest/OCP	Usually after day 3 postoperative, pain in calf, spike of temperature, swollen leg, tender calf, leg warm, rarely reddening, ankle edema, signs of PE	Clinical examination: Compare to other side Measure calves, duplex scan (in A+E: D-dimers), rarely need venography	Prophylaxis: TED stockings, subcutaneous heparin, mobilization, calf pumps Rx: below knee: LMW heparin Extension into femoral vein: Full anticoagulation
	Trauma	Soft tissue injury or bony fracture	Fall in bathroom or out of bed, local tenderness, bruising, pain on movement	History + local signs: e.g. fractured hip, radiology	Anti-inflammatory drugs, support, mobilization, bony injury: Rx as appropriate
	Lumbar disc prolapse	Immobilization coughing/sneezing/ straining	Pain radiating down leg from back to buttocks to leg	Previous history numbness/ paresthesia in affected dermatome, loss of ankle jerk	Bed rest/analgesia, early mobilization, physio, rarely surgery

Abbreviations: OCP, oral contraceptine pill; PE, pulmonary embolism; LMW, low molecular weight

Answer 5: See Table 18.5

Table 18.5 Complication: Wound discharge

Patient complaint	Cause	Etiopathology	Presentation	Diagnosis investigation	Management
Wound discharge	Bleeding	Usually primary hemorrhage, early postoperative ?poor hemostasis	Slow superficial ooze, visible vessel on wound edge, rarer: significant arterial bleeding e.g. arteriotomy	Remove dressing, inspect wound, look for clot, signs of hemorrhage elsewhere (i.e. clotting problem— rare) check clotting screen if worried	Ooze: Apply pressure dressing and recheck, visible vessel under run, major arterial bleeding—seek urgent senior help, may need further surgery
	Wound infection	Type of surgery: Clean/dirty Poor technique	Discharge may be pus/ serous/serosanguinous other signs of wound infection: pain/redness/fever/ induration/fluctuance	Bacteriology swab, blood culture if bacteremic	Open wound by removing suture, irrigation, daily dressings, antibiotics if cellulitis/anaerobic/septic
	Dehiscence = wound breakdown, can be partial = skin/ subcutaneous or complete –thro all layers - "burst abdomen"	Wound infection, poor technique, contributing factors: Poor nutrition, immune suppression, steroids	Often painless, occurs "suddenly", complete dehiscence occurs at about day 10 postoperative	May look superficial with skin/ subcutaneous separated, sometimes viscera are visible	If superficial wound, toilet and gauze packing; if complete: cover with sterile pack, reassure patient, put up IV line, take back to theater and resuture
	Fistula	Breakdown of intestinal anastomosis/ischemic/ traumatized viscera—often gives abscess which then fistulates to surface, may be fecal (small bowel/ large bowel or gastric or pancreatic or urine)	Wound or drain site appears infected—may leak, serous fluid/pus to start then fistula fluid	Establish nature of discharge (e.g. urea will show if urine) Define anatomy Fistulogram/CT	Protect skin, apply stoma bag/device, measure output, replace fluid and electrolytes, enteral feeding or TPN May need further surgery

Abbreviation: TPN, total parenteral nutrition; CT, computed tomography

Answer 6: See Table 18.6

Table 18.6 Complication: Nausea and vomiting					
Patient complaint	Cause	Etiopathology	Presentation	Diagnosis investigation	Management
Nausea and vomiting	Anesthesia	Drug induced, e.g. opiates, PCA	Usually in first 24 hours postoperative	Exclude other causes	Try antiemetic, e.g. stemetil: 12.5–25 mg IV/IM q4–6 hourly or metoclopramide 10 mg
	Related to surgery	Ileus Prolonged surgery, drugs, electrolyte disturbance	Nausea, vomiting, abdo distension, abdo discomfort, hiccoughs	Distended abdo, infrequent high pitched tinkling bowel sounds, air fluid levels on abdo X-rays	NBM, NG tube, antiemetics, IV fluids correct electrolytes, observe
		Intestinal obstruction abdo surgery fibrinous adhesions Acute gastric dilatation	Colicky pain, nausea, vomiting, abdo distension, no flatus	Abdo distension, obstructive bowel sounds, air fluid levels on plain X-rays, CT.	NBM, NG aspiration, IV fluids, correct electrolytes, observe for signs of ischemia or fail to settle, may need surgery
		Following abdominal surgery, trauma, immobilization, CPAP	Nausea, vomiting, hiccups, abdo distension, 'shock'	Abdo X-ray, electrolytes	Nasogastric intubation, correct fluid and electrolyte balance
	Medications	Opiates, especially pethidine, NSAIDs, antibiotics		Look at medication chart—have antiemetics been used	Antiemetic, consider changing drug
	Electrolyte disturbance	Hyponatremia		Overload with 'water' postoperative, volume depletion, electrolytes, urine osmolality, urine Na	Reverse cause
	Pseudo-obstruction Colonic obstruction without mechanical cause	Metabolic-low K/ uremia, prolonged immobilization- orthopedic patients Drugs/trauma/sepsis	Nausea, abdo distension	Plain abdo X-rays Water soluble gastrografin enema	Colonoscopy with suction, rarely operative

Abbreviations: PCA, patient-controlled analgesia; NG, nasogastric; NBM, nil by mouth; NSAIDs, nonsteroidal anti-inflammatory drugs; CPAP, continuous positive airway pressure; abdo, abdominal; CT, computed tomography

Answer 7: See Table 18.7

Table 18.7 Complication: Constipation					
Patient complaint	Cause	Etiopathology	Presentation	Diagnosis investigation	Managenent
Constipation		Immobility, drugs— opiates, dehydration, diet—no fiber	No bowel action	Exclude mechanical obstruction	Diet, mobilization Bulking agents—fybogel, irritant laxative-senna or osmotic laxative— lactulose

Answer 8: See Table 18.8

Table 18.8 Complication: Postoperative breathlessness

Patient complaint	Cause	Etiopatholgy	Presentation	Diagnosis investigation	Management
Breathlessness or 'SOB'	Respiratory	Atelectasis Small airways plug with secretions Aspiration Pneumonia	SOB, tachycardia, pyrexia	Chest Ex CXR	Physio, nebulized bronchodilator
		Pneumothorax CVP insertion, nephrectomy, incision/cervical spine operation	Reduced air entry, hyper-resonance, pain, tracheal deviation	Clinical Ex, if time CXR	Needle decompression, chest drain
		Pleural effusion cardiac, infection, infarction, subphrenic can be blood/chyle/pus	SOB	Chest exam, CXR/CT, diagnostic aspiration	Small: leave, large: aspirate + Rx of specific cause
		Pulmonary embolus	SOB/chest pain hemoptysis/collapse	Symptoms Clinical Ex/CXR/CT	Oxygen, anticoags, thrombolysis, embolectomy
		ARDS: Sepsis, massive blood transfusion, aspiration gastric contents	SOB, tachypnea, cyanosis, restlessness, confusion	Likely cause from clinical exam, O_2 saturation, ABGs, CXR	Rx cause, fluids/inotropes, antibiotics, ventilation + PEEP
	Cardiac	Pulm edema associated with cardiac failure: MI/arrythmias/valvular disease	SOB Cyanosis, chest pain	Cardiac exam ECG, CXR enzymes	Stop fluid overload, CVP monitoring, diuretics, inotropes
	Wound pain	Thoracic/Upper abdo Incisions with inadequate analgesia	SOB, tachypnea, pain in wound	Type of incision, amount of analgesia given, exclude other causes of SOB	Analgesia: oral/parenteral, epidural PCA—patient controlled analgesia
	Blood loss	Severe overt as in haematemesis, melena, severe concealed as in operation associated arterial or venous	Tachycardia, hypotension, pale, cold, clammy	Vomiting blood Blood/melena per rectum, blood in drains	IV fluids Blood Rx cause
	Sepsis	SOB, tachypnea associated with septic 'shock' from primary source in abdomen, e.g. anastomotic leak or chest, e.g. CVP line or urinary tract (UTI)	SOB, tachypnea, tachycardia, hypotension, hot peripheries, cold peripheries, source for sepsis,	Clinical exam, blood cultures, Other indicated specimens, pus, urine, catheter tip	IV fluids, IV antibiotics, inotropes, interventional drainage of septic source, e.g. operation or image-guided

Abbreviations: SOB, shortness of breath; Ex, examination; CXR, chest X-ray; CVP, central venous pressure; ABG, arterial blood gases; ECG, electrocardiography; MI, myocardial infarction; Pulm, pulmonary; abdo, abdominal; ARDS, acute respiratory distress syndrome; PCA, patient-controlled analgesia; PEEP, positive end-expiratory pressure

General management for all patients with postoperative breathlessness:
Sit up
Reassure/
High flow oxygen/

Hx and examination,
O_2 saturation monitoring
P/BP continuous monitor
ECG,
Portable CXR.

Answer 9: Risk factors are:

Aging

Underling disease – Neuropsychiatric disorders
– Parkinson's disease
– Drug addiction
– Alcoholism.

Medications

Types of surgery – Gynecology
– Eye surgery
– Urology
– Cardiac surgery (emboli).

Environment Intensive care unit
Unfamiliar surroundings of hospital ward.

Pain

Sleep disorders

Anxiety and distress

Answer 10: Etiopathology of postoperative confusion:

1. **'Organic'** Hypoxia
Hypotension
Sepsis
Dehydration and electrolyte disturbance, e.g. hyponatremia
Metabolic: Hypoglycemia, hypercalcemia
Drugs—residual anesthetic drugs, e.g. ketamine, opiates antibiotics and steroids
Cerebral embolism
Delirium tremens (DTs) acute alcohol withdrawal, drug withdrawal

2. Unexplained neuropsychiatric delirium.

Answer 11:

1. Obtain quick history (from the nurses), carry out a physical exam and survey of the postoperative charts (pulse/BP/O_2 saturation) fluid intake and output/drug charts, this is aimed at identifying any of the above 'organic pathology' and its cause. You will be particularly looking to see if the patient has evidence of sepsis, chest infection, dehydration, a cerebrovascular accident or a myocardial infarct.

2. If you find evidence of any of the above, the management will be directed at the specific cause.

3. Send off blood for urgent FBC/urea and electrolytes/blood glucose/CXR and ECG.

4. If there is no obvious specific organic cause, institute early treatment with IV psychotropic drugs: Haloperidol or diazepam.

5. Contact your senior. Tell him what has happened and what you have done and ask him to come and see the patient.

6. Do not forget to look at the results of your investigations as soon as possible.

(*After Jean Mantz: institute-anesthesia-reanimation.org/IMG/pdf/agitation.pdf*)

Answer 12:

Prerenal	Hypotension
	Hypovolemia
Renal	Nephrotoxic drugs
	(e.g. gentamicin, steroids)
	sepsis, myoglobinuria
Post-renal	Blocked urethral catheter
	Ureteric injury.

Answer 13:

1. Careful monitoring of urine output—hourly in immediate postoperative period and then four-hourly.

2. Careful and correct management of fluid balance charts—input and output. With at least twice daily review of these.

3. Routine use of parameters for assessing 'volume status'-clinical exam, CVP, daily weight.

4. Daily urea and electrolytes and review of these.

5. Avoid episodes of hypo and hypertension by routine monitoring and early action.

6. Anticipate the patient who may have problems. Optimize cardiac function by monitoring it regularly using pulse/BP/oxygen saturation/ECG/CVP and if necessary intra-arterial or Swan Ganz lines (or now newer flow based method such as esophageal US). Giving early inotropic support where necessary. Early involvement of ICU and intensivists.

7. Avoid nephrotoxic drugs where possible or monitor levels carefully if being used, e.g. aminoglycosides.

8. Use careful sterile techniques to avoid sepsis (e.g. with CVP lines). Identify sepsis early and treat adequately—intervention/antibiotics.

Answer 14:

1. Look at the routine charts—P/BP/CVP and at other dinamap parameters, if available, e.g. O_2 saturation/ECG. Identify any abnormalities.

2. Look at the fluid balance charts and assess the recent trend in his urine output and fluid input.

3. Examine the patient for signs of hypotension and hypovolemia and any indication for the cause of these, e.g. bleeding/sepsis.

4. Send off urgent FBC, chemical bioprofile and if indicated ABGs.

5. Institute appropriate management of the causes you have identified, be these any of the pre-renal and post-renal causes you have listed above (you are not expected to be familiar with details of management at this stage—this will be further discussed in Module 3).

(*After Davidson and Rai, Student. BMJ. April, 1999*)

TUTORIAL 19: Blood Transfusion

CASE SCENARIOS

Answer 1.1: No. Remember that blood transfusions can cause complications, e.g. reactions, antibodies, cardiac failure. There is no evidence that cardiovascular function is improved by hemoglobin levels above 10 g/dL.

Answer 1.2:

- Transfusion trigger is defined as the Hb or hematocrit level at which most patients require red blood cell transfusion. The lower limit of transfusion trigger for general medical and surgical patients is 7.0 g/dL or hematocrit 21%.
- Current data suggests that restraining transfusions favors positive outcomes except when significant underlying cardiac disease is present.

Answer 1.3a: Yes, he needs transfusion because his hemoglobin level is below the 'trigger level' and the benefits of the transfusion (for example, in oxygen carrying capacity) are likely to outweigh the chances of a transfusion complication.

Answer 1.3b: Packed red cells. He may also require platelets and fresh frozen plasma (FFP) if active bleeding continues.

Note: Whole blood is an inefficient way of giving red cells and hemostatic factors. Whole blood is usually only used when there is a need for rapid large volume transfusion (e.g. road traffic accident).

Answer 1.3c:

- Red blood cells
- Platelets
- Fresh frozen plasma (FFP)
- Cryoprecipitate
- Plasma fractions: Human albumin
  Prothrombin complex concentrates
  Immunoglobulins.

Answer 1.3d: Type and screen involves determining the patient's ABO and Rh(D) status and screening a sample of the patient's serum for clinically significant antibodies.

The sample is held for up to 7 days and if blood is needed it can be provided in 15 minutes (need to exclude major ABO incompatibility).

Group and hold is same as type and screen.

Cross matching takes 1 hour and involves type and screen and direct testing of the patient's serum for compatibility with RBCs taken from the blood to be transfused.

The antibody screening may take hours.

Note that most hospitals have a protocol for whether the patient needs to be cross matched for an operation or whether 'group and hold' is sufficient. By avoiding unnecessary full cross matching, a huge amount of blood products and money is saved.

Answer 1.4: When the blood sample is taken, adopt the following regime:

1. Identify the patient (preferably with ID band).
2. The sample must be fully labeled before leaving the bedside and should never be prelabeled. (Include: name and hospital ID no.).
3. The X-match form must be fully completed: Name/DOB/ Hospital number.

Before commencing a transfusion, the following regime must be followed. The checks must be performed by two individuals, at least one of whom should be an SRN (State Registered Nurse) or a medical officer. Check:

1. Full patient identity on the wrist band with the compatibility label on the unit of blood and the report form.
2. The ABO and RhD type on pack, label and report form.
3. The donation number on pack, label and report form.
4. The expiry date of pack.
5. Examine the pack to make sure there is no hemolysis or leak.
6. If all is correct, the compatibility form is signed by both nurses/and or doctor, put in notes and the copy is returned to lab.

Answer 1.5: Explain the reason for the transfusion. Explain the common side effects of blood transfusion, i.e. minor transfusion reactions, anaphylaxis, major transfusion reactions and infective complications.

Tell the patient the symptoms of these and that he/she must report such symptoms immediately to the nurses if they occur while the blood is being given.

Make sure that the patient has no religious beliefs or advanced directives which express the wish that they do not wish to receive allogeneic blood. Tell the patient they will be on pulse, BP and temperature chart.

Answer 1.6:

- The use of the patient's own blood for transfusion.
- Only indicated if the patient expresses wish.
- Only indicated if the patient is likely to need blood.
- Sepsis and myocardial disease are absolute contraindications.
- Must be done well in advance and the blood can only be stored for 5–6 weeks.

Answer 2.1: Group O Rh –ve. Can be used in all recipients because there are no red cell antigens, no Rh antibodies and the anti-A and B plasma antibodies are removed in processing.

Answer 2.2: Massive transfusion refers to the transfusion of the equivalent of the circulating blood volume in 24 hours (in adult = 10–12 units). May be associated with transfusions in trauma, gastrointestinal bleeding and obstetrical problems.

Answer 2.3:
- Thrombocytopenia
- Coagulation factor deficiency
- Hypocalcemia
- Hyper and hypokalemia
- Hypothermia
- ARDS.

Answer 3.1:

Full name: Admission date:

DOB:

Gender:

ID no:

Ward/room and consultant I/C:

Type and amount of transfusion required:

Date of request:

Date transfusion required:

Blood group if known:

Patient's diagnosis

Reason for transfusion

Any previous transfusions

Answer 3.2: See Table 19.2

Answer 3.3: The following details must be checked by you (the HO) and the nurse who must be an SRN or supervised by one:
1. Check the patient identity band on his/her wrist (name and number) with the compatibility label, the unit of blood and the request form.
2. Check the ABO and RhD type on the pack, label and the request form.
3. Check the donation number on the pack, label and request form.
4. Check the expiry date of the pack.
5. Examine the pack for signs of hemolysis or leakage.
6. If ALL the above are correct, the compatibility form is signed by both the nurse and yourself, entered into the patient's notes and the copy returned to the lab.

Answer 3.4: Take baseline pulse/BP/RR and temperature before starting blood transfusion.

Record pulse/BP/RR/temperature 15 minutes after start of each packet and hourly while transfusion continues (maximum 4 hours).

Answer 3.5: A febrile nonhemolytic reaction—usually due to white cell antibodies in the recipient plasma reacting with donor leukocytes.

Answer 3.6:
- Stop the transfusion, put up new giving set with 0.9 N saline running.
- Recheck the identity against unit of blood.
- Inform the lab.
- Record in notes.
- For pyrexia, give paracetamol
- If rash/itch is troubling patient, give IV hydrocortisone 100 mg or piriton 10 mg IV.

Answer 3.7: Either an acute hemolytic reaction (major incompatibility) or an acute anaphylactic reaction.

Answer 3.8:
1. Stop the infusion and start a slow IV infusion with 0.9 N saline through a new giving set.
2. Put patient on oxygen (100%).
3. Double check labeling of blood.
4. Send blood for FBC, platelets, clotting screen, repeat compatibility and electrolyte bioprofile.
5. Telephone the hematologist and tell him what has happened.
6. Send suspect packet back with blood investigations.
7. Repeat coagulation profile and electrolytes 2 hourly.
8. Monitor ECG, especially if potassium is raised.
9. Catheterize the bladder and monitor urine output.

Further management:
- Maintain urine OP 1.5 mL/kg/hr; if necessary with fluid challenge or furosemide.
- If urine output drops below this, assume renal failure and seek specialist help.
- If hyperkalemic, use insulin glucose drip or calcium resonium, seek help.
- If disseminated intravascular coagulation (DIC) occurs seek urgent advice from intensivist or hematologist.

Answer 3.9: Continuous monitoring with dinamap in HDU or ICU (pulse/BP/O_2 sat/ECG). Check following:
- Electrolytes 2 hourly
- Coagulation screen 2 hourly
- Urine output 1 hourly.

Table 19.2 Cross match, blood and blood products request form (completed)

UNIVERSITY HOSPITAL

Name : Arthur W

RN : Ward 9

Unit no. : PG 192345

D.O.B. : 12/6/43   Sex: (M) / F

Admission date : 31/05/07   Room no. :

Doctor : Mr. L

Request date : 6/6/07   Time :

Time received :

CROSS MATCH, BLOOD AND BLOOD PRODUCTS REQUEST FORM   7591

TEST REQUESTED   PLEASE MARK [✓] APPROPRIATE BOX(ES)

Diagnosis	Reason for transfustion	Blood Group A, Rh +ve	
Neoplasm Stomach Post Surgery	Postoperative Hb = 7.2	Hb	Platelet
		7.2	

Any previous transfusion? (Yes) / No	If yes, state date of last transfusion 2/6/07	Complication? Nil known

Transfusion required

☐ (a) Urgent

[✓] (b) Date 7/6/07 .... Time 9 pm ...... am/pm

☐ (c) Reserve for 46 hours   Packed cells
                              from 3 pints

☐ Blood given immediately without crossmatch (to save life)

☐ Whole blood .... ☐ Platelet concentrate ....

[✓] Packed cells .... ☐ Cryoprecipitate ....

                              ☐ Fresh frozen plasma ....

☐ Group screen and hold

Signature ....

Chop and name of
Consultant .... Dr L.

TUTORIAL 20: Acute Abdomen: Abdominal Pain and Vomiting (Intestinal Obstruction)

Answer 1.1:
1. When did it start?
2. Where is it? Show me.
3. Does it go anywhere else? Show me.
4. Have you ever had it before?
5. What is it like—dull/sharp/ache?
6. How bad is it—worst you have ever had/mild/severe?
7. Did it come on suddenly or gradually? What were you doing?
8. Does it come and go or is it there the whole time? Does it come in waves?
9. What makes it worse, e.g. moving, breathing?
10. What makes it better, e.g. lying still/any medications, vomiting?
11. Do you have any other symptoms come on with it, e.g. diarrhea, vomiting?

Answer 1.2:
- Visceral pain comes from stretching or inflammation of hollow organs.
- It is dull in character and nonlocalizing.
- Foregut visceral pain is localized to the epigastrium, mid gut to the umbilicus and hind gut to the suprapubic or lower abdominal area.
- So this lady's pain is likely from the mid gut.

Answer 1.3:
- Tell me about the vomiting, when did it start/how many times have you vomited/what color is it/does the vomit smell?
- Have your bowels worked since the pain started, if so, was it diarrhea? If not have you passed any flatus? Any blood or mucus?
- Has your tummy blown up—become distended?
- The rest of the routine questions from GI protocol: Any difficulty swallowing/reflux or heartburn/any indigestion, has your bowel habit changed over the last few month? How is your appetite, have you lost weight recently? Then ask PMH/FH/SH/ROS.

Answer 1.4: The watery green vomit is green because it contains bile, therefore, the pylorus must be open, i.e. the obstruction is distal to the pylorus. Brown vomit which is feculent in nature (smells of feces) is from the small bowel and usually indicates complete obstruction.

Answer 1.5: Intestinal obstruction:
- Probably caused by adhesion, due to previous surgery.
- Likely small bowel because of the relative acute onset of symptoms.

Answer 1.6:
General: Signs of distress—pain
Pale
Signs of dehydration
Abnormal vital signs:
Evidence of peripheral circulatory collapse.

Abdomen:
Inspection:
- Scars: Ask to cough (? Incisional hernia)
- Visible peristalsis
- Abdominal distension
- Abdomen moves equally on respiration - if not probably has peritonitis.

Palpation:
- Tenderness/guarding/rebound
- Mass
- Hernial orifices (obstructed femoral hernia often missed in women).

Percussion: Ascites.
Auscultation: Hyperactive runs of high pitched bowel sounds typical of intestinal obstruction.

Rectal examination: Empty rectum: or characteristics of the feces.

Answer 1.7:
- Intestinal obstruction—most likely small bowel and secondary to adhesions. Justification for this diagnosis is because she has the classic symptoms and signs, i.e. abdominal pain/vomiting/abdominal distension and constipation. She has a midline scar, and may therefore, have adhesions.
- She does not have a history or physical signs to suggest the obstruction may be due to a large bowel tumor.

Answer 1.8:
- Blood: FBC—look for anemia, raised WCC (indicates sepsis)
Urea and electrolytes - dehydration (raised urea)
- electrolyte imbalance
- both due to loss of fluid into bowel
Serum amylase - do in all adult acute abdomen unless diagnosis is obvious.
- Imaging: Erect chest X-ray—air under diaphragm (perforation)
Erect and supine film of abdomen—classical signs of obstruction (many radiologists will now say to use supine abdo X-ray followed by CT, if available).

Answer 1.9:
- Sodium : 135–145 mmol/L
- Potassium: 3.5–5.0 mmol/L
- Urea: 2.5–6.7 mmol/L
- Chloride: 97–100 mmol/L
- HCO_3: 21–28 mmol/L
- Creatinine: 70–150 μmol/L.

Answer 1.10:
- Urea raised because patient is dehydrated, losing fluids into the bowel
- Potassium low because patient is losing potassium by vomiting.

Answer 1.11:
Face: Sunken orbits, lack luster eyes, dry tongue.
Hands and arms: Loss of skin turgor.
Tachycardia and hypotension (if severe).
Cold peripheries (if severe)—Hands cold and clammy.
Urine output low.
Weigh the patient (5% loss in weight indicates 5% body water loss)—clearly this is not of use when you first see the patient.

Low urine output is now regarded as less reliable because there may be other causes for this.

Answer 1.12: Crystalloids—use Ringer's Lactate/Hartmann's solution + added potassium.

Use to rehydrate and to correct the hypokalemia (i.e. replace fluid deficit).

Answer 1.13:
- 1st image—plain film of the abdomen—erect.
- 2nd image—plain film of the abdomen—supine.

Answer 1.14:
- Small bowel obstruction.
- 1st image – Presence of multiple air-fluid levels, centrally placed and step laddered in fashion.
- 2nd image – No air-fluid levels.
    – Presence of dilated bowel at the center of the abdomen with visible valvulae conniventes (small bowel mucosal folds).

Answer 1.15:
- Adhesions
- Strangulated hernia.

Answer 1.16:
- Conservatively – NG tube—aspirate the small bowel contents hourly.
    – Fluid and electrolyte replacement.
- Surgically – Adhesiolysis—remove adhesion and untwist bowel.

Answer 1.17:
- Increasing abdominal tenderness—as evidence of bowel ischemia.
- Failed conservative management after 48 hours.

Answer 1.18: A fibrinous band adhesion with visible viable proximal small bowel and distal gangrenous small bowel.

Answer 1.19: See below and next page for specimen table (Table 20.2).

Answer 1.20: See appropriate sections of Table 20.2

Table 20.2 Acute abdominal pain: Core knowledge—after Epstein in Clinical Examination 2nd Ed, 1997, Mosby, Edin.							
Condition	*Location of pain*	*Character of pain*	*Aggravating factors*	*Relieving factors*	*Associated symptoms*	*Physical signs*	*Diagnostic test*
Acute appendicitis	Periumbilical Moves to RIF	Initially colicky becomes continuous	Movement, coughing	Lies still	Anorexia, vomiting 1–2X's, occasionally diarrhea	Flushed, RIF tenderness, rebound, guarding	?CT scan
Acute cholecystitis/ biliary colic	Epigastrium, RUQ, may go to back	Sudden or gradual onset, usually constant	Movement		Fever, previous indigestion, fat intolerance	Tender in RUQ +ve Murphy's sign	Plain X-rays ultrasound
Intestinal obstruction	Small bowel = periumbilical Large bowel = lower abdomen	Colicky			SB : Vomiting LB : Vomiting late, absolute constipation	Abdominal distension, visible peristalsis	Erect and supine abdo films: Distention + air fluid levels CT scan
Ureteric colic	Loin to groin	Severe colicky/ constant/ intermittent		Rolls around	Vomiting, sweating	Usually no abdo signs, sometimes hematuria	KUB, CT urogram

Contd...

Contd...

Condition	Location of pain	Character of pain	Aggravating factors	Relieving factors	Associated symptoms	Physical signs	Diagnostic test
Acute pancreatitis	Upper abdo then moves all over	May start dull and become severe		Usually, lie still, sometimes may be sitting forward	Nausea, vomiting systemic—fever tachy, BP down	Sometimes local tenderness to start then diffuse tenderness guarding, rebound, no bowel sounds	S. amylase, after 4 days urinary amylase
Perforated peptic ulcer	Sudden onset epigastric then radiates over whole abdo	Severe	Movement	Lies still	Vomiting	Fever, tachy, hypotension, board like rigidity no bowel sounds	Erect CXR, erect abdo film may show free gas, CT more accurate
Acute diverticulitis	Lower abdo or LIF	Gradual onset becomes localized in LIF	Coughing, moving	Lies still	PH of diverticulosis with abdo pain constipation, diarrhea	Local tenderness, guarding rebound if perforates, generalized peritonitis signs	Contrast enhanced CT
Ruptured abdominal aortic aneurism	Previous back/loin/lower abdo then sudden onset lower abdo pain	Sudden onset severe				Pulsatile mass Tachycardia Hypotension Shut down	Only if doubt rediagnosis: CT
Ruptured ectopic pregnancy	Lower abdo/Shoulder tip/diffuse abdo	Severe	Movement	Lies still	Sexually active missed period	Tachycardia, hypotension, signs of peritonitis	Positive pregnancy test, TV ultrasound

Abbreviations: RIF, right iliac fossa; CT, computed tomography; RUQ, right upper quadrant; KUB, kidney ureter bladder; SB, small bowel; LB, large bowel; LIF, left iliac fossa; TV, transvaginal

TUTORIAL 21: Swellings in the Neck

CASE SCENARIO

Answer 1.1:
- When did you notice the swelling?
- Has it changed since you first noticed it?
- How did you notice it?
- Is it painful? Have you developed any swellings anywhere else?

Answer 1.2:
- Are you otherwise fit and well?
- How is your appetite?
- Have you lost any weight?
- Have you any difficulty swallowing?
- Have you developed a cough?
- Do you prefer hot or cold weather?
- Has there been any change in your voice or skin?
- Has your bowel habit changed?
- Are your periods regular?
- Has anyone else in the family a similar lump?

Answer 1.3a:
- Prefers cold weather but sweats a lot.
- Appetite very good but loses weight.
- Becomes nervous and anxious.

- May develop diarrhea.
- Periods become infrequent.

Answer 1.3b:
- Becomes very slow, lethargic and tired.
- Gains weight.
- Feels cold and prefers hot weather.
- Becomes constipated.

Answer 1.4: Euthyroid.

Answer 1.5: Goiter is an enlargement of the thyroid gland.

Answer 1.6:
- Ask the patient to swallow or take a sip of water: The gland moves up on swallowing.

Answer 1.7:
- On inspection, look for swelling of both lobes.
- Define the isthmus on palpation, then palpate each lobe from behind and delineate each 'solitary swelling'.

Answer 1.8a:
- Any neck swellings and their anatomical position (e.g. anterior triangle) and approximate size.
- Any scars.
- Any skin discoloration.
- Any distended veins or arterial pulsation.
- If swelling present: Ask patient to swallow.
- If midline or close to midline, ask to protrude tongue.

Answer 1.8b:
- Palpate from behind.
- Confirm the anatomical position of the swelling and if it is in thyroid gland by swallowing. Check if you can get below the swelling (often forgotten).
- In this case, the lump is in the thyroid: Hence, define its characteristics, size/shape/consistency, etc.
- See if it is attached to the skin.
- See if attached to deeper structures.
- Feel the carotid pulses.
- Systematically feel each group of lymph nodes in the neck and supraclavicular area.
- Move back to the front and re-examine with palpation if necessary (sometimes easier to define solitary swelling from front). Feel for the trachea.

Answer 1.8c: If you cannot get below the swelling, check for retrosternal extension by percussion over the upper chest across the manubrium.

Answer 1.8d: Listen over the gland for a bruit (increased blood supply—in thyrotoxicosis) or stridor.

Answer 1.8e:
- Every student knows this but not often seen and when present is likely to upset the patient, so be cautious.
- Ask patient to elevate their arms and see if their face becomes congested (red) or cyanosed and whether they become breathless or if a stridor is heard with a deep breath.

Note: It is a sign of thoracic inlet obstruction.

Answer 1.9a: Likely to be a multinodular goiter.

Answer 1.9b: This is termed a "solitary thyroid nodule"—differential diagnosis is dominant nodule of multinodular goiter, adenoma, malignant nodule or a thyroid cyst—favorite exam question!

Answer 1.9c: Diffuse goiter likely to be Grave's disease.

Answer 1.9d: Rare: Likely to be a thyroiditis.

Answer 1.9e: Likely to be an anaplastic malignancy.

Answer 1.9f: Hyperthyroidism

Answer 1.9g: Retrosternal extension of multinodular goiter (MNG).

Answer 1.9h: Thoracic inlet obstruction.

Answer 1.10:
1. Dominant nodule of multinodular goiter.
2. Solitary thyroid cyst.
3. Adenoma.
4. Malignant nodule.

Answer 1.11: You look for the following clinical signs:

a. **Hyperthyroidism:**
   Face: Anxious/nervous/sweaty Exophthalmos/lid retraction/lid lag/divergent gaze/diplopia/chemosis

   Note: Exophthalmos: Sclera visible below the eye, lid retraction: sclera visible above the eye.
   Hands: Sweating/tremor/clubbing/onycholysis (Plummer's nails).
   Arms: Proximal muscle weakness.
   Pulse: Tachycardia/atrial fibrillation.
   Legs: Pretibial myxedema/generalized hyperreflexia: assess ankle jerks.

b. **For myxedema:**
   Face: Coarse, dry skin, peaches and cream complexion, periorbital puffiness. Loss of eyebrows at lateral end, thin coarse hair.
   Hands: Cold, dry palms.
   Arms: Puffiness of wrists. Legs: Delayed ankle jerk.

Answer 1.12: Euthyroid.

Answer 1.13:
- FBC
- TSH, T3/T4, thyroid antibodies
- Biochemical profile including serum calcium
- Ultrasound scan of the neck
- Fine needle aspiration of the nodule (FNAC).

Answer 1.14a: See Figure 21.1

Anterior triangle:	Base = Inferior border of mandible
	Anterior = Midline of neck from Mandible to sternal notch
	Posterior = Anterior border of sternocleidomastoid
Posterior triangle:	Base = Middle third clavicle
	Anterior = Posterior border of sternocleidomastoid
	Posterior = Anterior border of trapezius

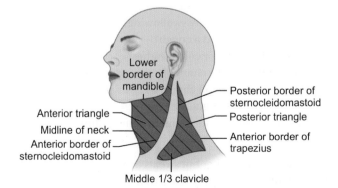

Fig. 21.1 The anterior and posterior triangles of the neck

Answer 1.14b: Because the pretracheal fascia, which envelopes the thyroid is attached to the cricoid cartilage.

Answer 1.14c:
- Often used interchangeably.
- Some say exophthalmos is eye protrusion with an endocrine cause, proptosis is eye protrusion with non-endocrine cause.
- Some say it is the amount of protrusion measured by ophthalmometry: <18 mm = proptosis, >18 mm = exophthalmos.

Answer 1.14d: Cause is uncertain. Occurs only in Graves' disease. There is an inflammatory infiltrate of the orbital contents.

Answer 1.14e: Raised areas on the anterior surface of lower limbs. Can be reddish, brown or skin colored. Uncommon!

TUTORIAL 22 : Swelling in Groin

CASE SCENARIO

Answer 1.1:
1. When did you first notice the swelling? What were you doing when you first noticed it? Has it been there ever since? Has the swelling changed since you first noticed it?
2. Does the swelling disappear on lying down or can you reduce it manually? (Suggests that it is an uncomplicated hernia).
3. Does the swelling go down into the scrotum? (If it does, it is more likely to be an indirect hernia. However, a swelling that remains in the inguinal region could either be an indirect or direct hernia).
4. Have you ever had an episode when the hernia becomes irreducible ('stuck out'), associated with abdominal symptoms like pain, vomiting, abdominal distension or not passing wind or feces? (Suggests an episode of possible obstruction and may indicate the need for early surgery.)

Answer 1.2a:
- Firstly find out how much of a problem the hernia is for the patient in terms of interfering with his normal daily life. Then identify any underlying cause(s) which may have been influential in precipitating the onset of the hernia. For example: Causes of repeated raised intra-abdominal pressure from straining to pass urine or constipation (both these symptoms, if present, will require evaluation).
- History of chronic smoking—chronic bronchitis, history of COPD, chronic cough, bronchial asthma.
- Occupation (heavy lifting).

- Clearly these factors will need addressing either before or after the patient has his hernia repaired.
- Then enquire about significant comorbid factors that may contraindicate surgery or make the surgical intervention high risk, for example, cardiorespiratory problems. Such cases may require a conservative approach unless complications like obstruction or strangulation develop.

Answer 1.2b: Enquiry should then be made to ascertain if there have been any symptoms or signs which suggest the hernia has become obstructed, i.e. episodes of irreducibility associated with symptoms of abdominal distension, vomiting, colicky abdominal pain and absolute constipation. If yes, will warrant early surgery.

Answer 1.3: Please note that the examination protocol for 'hernia' will differ from doctor to doctor, book to book and medical school to medical school. The protocol suggested below may be criticized by some physicians. The main points of difference in protocols are listed below with a brief explanation as to why the particular recommendation is made:
1. The patient is initially examined lying supine on the bed with the head supported by one pillow. Many will recommend that the patient be examined initially 'standing up'. In practice, it is much more difficult to carry out the steps of the hernia examination with the patient standing. If the hernia examination with the patient supine is conclusive, it may not be necessary to re-examine the patient in the standing position. However for the purposes of the protocol, it is suggested that the student examines the patient supine, notes the findings and then re-examines the patient standing up.

   Note: The main indication for examining the patient standing up is in the patient who gives a history suggestive of a hernia but in whom the examination in the supine position is inconclusive. In these cases, when the patient is 'erect' and is asked to cough, the swelling may become visible.
2. *Exposure:* Medical students are traditionally taught that during examination for a hernia the patient should be exposed from the 'nipples to the knees'. This is not acceptable—such exposure will likely embarrass the patient and is just not necessary. Fully expose the groin areas, covering the genitalia with the bed sheet until it is necessary to examine these areas. The patient will recognize that you are protecting his/her modesty and will gain confidence in you (a very important and often forgotten aspect of medicine).
3. The 'deep ring occlusion test' is traditionally taught to medical students to differentiate between an indirect

and direct hernia. In practice, many surgeons do not use this test because it is so inaccurate [a wide deep ring is often not occluded by the finger(s) and a false negative is obtained]. Many surgeons prefer the scrotal invagination test which is not usually taught in medical schools because it is said to hurt the patient. In this protocol, we have retained the use of 'deep ring occlusion test' because of its value in understanding the 'anatomy' of an inguinal hernia. The student should be familiar with the 'scrotal invagination test' but may not include it in the protocol as a routine, however, the individual doctor may choose to adapt it in later practice.

Suggested protocol:

Patient supine and adequately exposed (see above):

Look:

1. Any visible swelling? Note position and size.
2. Any other relevant signs, e.g. scars, change in color of skin.
3. If swelling is present, ask patient if they can reduce it for you and then proceed as follows. If they are unable to reduce, see instructions in Note 2.
4. Ask patient to cough: Look to see if a swelling appears, if so, look very carefully and see if the swelling comes down lateral to medial (indirect) or posteroanterior (direct). This is probably the most 'accurate' test of all, so do it carefully.

Palpate:

1. If swelling present, ask the patient to reduce again.
2. Place hand flat on the line of the inguinal canal and ask patient to cough, note if there is a cough impulse or a swelling appears and in which direction the impulse or swelling travels.
3. Identify the anatomical landmarks of the inguinal ligament: Anterior superior iliac spine (ASIS) and the pubic tubercle. Note the latter lies in the crease at the bottom of the abdomen and not in the groin crease. Ascertain if the swelling is above and medial to pubic tubercle—inguinal hernia or below and lateral—femoral hernia.
4. Identify the midpoint of the inguinal ligament (half-way between the ASIS and the pubic tubercle)—one cm. above this is the position of the deep inguinal ring.
   With the swelling reduced place one or two fingers of your right hand over the deep ring and press firmly. Ask the patient to cough. If the swelling is controlled the hernia is indirect; if the swelling appears medial to the fingers it is direct (but see point 3 above). This is called the 'deep ring occlusion test').
5. Scrotal invagination test (see point 3 above): 'Free the scrotum.' Invaginate the little finger (gently) into the neck of the scrotum and pass it upwards to the position of the external ring to enter the inguinal canal. Ask the patient to cough. Can you feel a swelling coming into the canal? If so does the swelling hit the tip of your finger (indirect) or back of your finger (direct)?
6. Complete the examination by examining the scrotum and testis.
7. Examine the other groin and scrotum in exactly same way.

Ask the patient to stand:

- If no swelling visible, ask the patient to cough.
- Look for cough impulse or swelling.
- Note the size and position of swelling in relation to pubic tubercle.
- If a swelling is seen, ask the patient to reduce it and hold it reduced for you.
- Identify your landmarks, occlude the deep ring and ask the patient to cough again, does it remain controlled (indirect).

Note 1: If on standing, a swelling is seen that is painful or difficult to reduce by the patient, do not progress with the standing examination any further, just do the examination with the patient lying down.

Hint: When the patient is standing, probably the best way of feeling a swelling or cough impulse is to stand at the side of the patient or behind him and put your left hand on his inguinal canal for the patient's left side and right hand on the inguinal canal for right side.

Note 2:

- If you are examining a patient with a large scrotal swelling visible on standing or lying down, you are best to examine him lying down first.
- Ask him to reduce the swelling—if he can, proceed with the 'hernia protocol.'
- If he cannot, you have to decide one thing—can you get above the swelling, if so, it is a 'scrotal problem' and you examine accordingly.
- If you cannot get above the swelling then it is an inguino-scrotal swelling and is an indirect inguinal hernia until proven otherwise.

Answer 1.4:

- A hernia is the protrusion of a viscera or tissue through a normal or abnormal opening in the body.
- The hernia has a mouth, a neck and a sac. The sac consists of a body and fundus.

Answer 1.5: See Figures 22.1 and 22.2

- The inguinal canal runs from the deep ring downwards and medially to the external ring.
- The anterior wall is the external oblique aponeurosis.

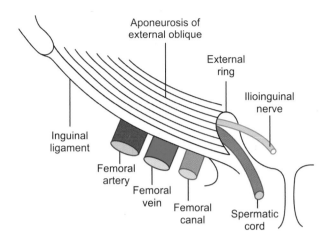

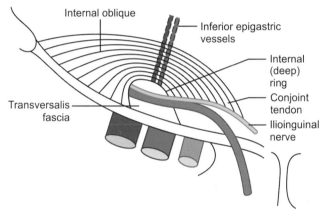

Fig. 22.1 Anatomy of the inguinal canal

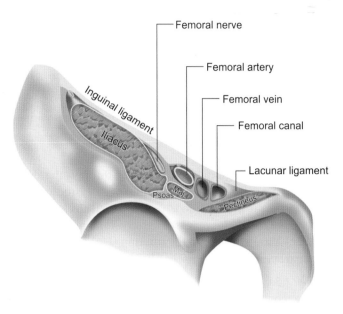

Right hemipelvis showing femoral canal anatomy

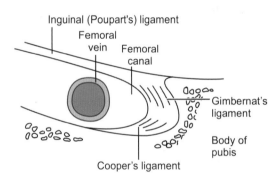

Fig. 22.2 Anatomy of the femoral canal

- The posterior wall is the transversalis fascia laterally and the conjoint tendon medially.
- The superior wall or roof is the arching fibers of the internal oblique and transversus muscle.
- The inferior wall is the inguinal ligament.

Answer 1.6a:
- Anterior superior iliac spine (ASIS).
- Pubic tubercle.

*Answer 1.6b: **ASIS**:* Follow the iliac crest anteriorly from its highest point. The first prominent bony landmark felt is the ASIS.

Pubic tubercle:
1. Probably the most efficient method is to identify the lower abdominal skin crease (which is present in every abdomen—no matter how fat or thin). Feel in the midline of this crease for the bony prominence of the symphysis pubis and then move laterally 1.5 cm to identify the pubic tubercle.
   Note: The pubic tubercle does not lie in the neck of the scrotum (where 'beginners' commonly palpate but well above this on the lower abdominal wall).

Other methods which you can try are:
2. Palpate downwards from the umbilicus in the midline until you come to the bony prominence of the pelvic inlet—the symphysis pubis is in the midline. The pubic tubercle is the bony prominence about 1.5 cm lateral to it.
3. Follow the inguinal ligament medially from its attachment to the ASIS. It is attached medially to the first bony prominence you encounter—the pubic tubercle.

Some would recommend the following:
Ask the patient to adduct his or her thigh under resistance. Follow the adductor longus tendon superiorly to where it is attached to the Riders tubercle, a roughened bony area on the pubic bone. The pubic tubercle is the bony prominence just superior to this attachment of the adductor longus.

This method is quite complicated to do but is very useful in one situation: Sometimes the visible swelling of what you think is an indirect inguinal hernia appears to lie below and lateral to the pubic tubercle (i.e. in the position of a femoral hernia).

If you carry out the above maneuver using the adductor longus to identify the pubic tubercle the 'swelling' lifts up and is then clearly identifiable as above and medial to the pubic tubercle. You may not understand this until you come across the situation clinically!!

Answer 1.6c: It is 1 cm above the mid-point of the inguinal ligament.

Answer 1.7: See Figure 22.3

An indirect inguinal hernia comes through the deep inguinal ring and lies lateral to the inferior epigastric artery.

A direct sac pushes into a weak transversalis fascia and lies medial to inferior epigastric artery. If large an indirect inguinal hernia may lie in the scrotum (Fig. 22.4). A direct inguinal hernia never enters the scrotum.

Answer 1.8a: An uncomplicated hernia that does not reduce spontaneously or manually.

Answer 1.8b: A hernia that is irreducible because of the size of the hernia or because of adhesions of the contents of the hernia to the sac. However, the contents are not strangulated or obstructed.

Answer 1.8c: An irreducible hernia complicated by the contents becoming obstructed.

Answer 1.8d: An irreducible hernia when the blood supply of the contents of the sac are compromised, i.e. reduced or cut off.

Answer 1.8e: Congenital hernia due to the presence of a patent processus vaginalis presenting in a baby or young child.

Answer 1.8f: An inguinal hernia that extends into the scrotum. This is always an indirect inguinal hernia as direct hernias do NOT extend into the scrotum.

Answer 1.9:
a. Symptomatic patient with no significant comorbidity to make him an unacceptable operative risk.
b. Patient with a hernia that is irreducible and giving symptoms or signs suggestive of either obstruction or strangulation.

Answer 1.10:
1. Herniotomy: Removal of the sac.
2. Herniorraphy or hernioplasty: Procedure carried out to correct the underlying cause, i.e. Strengthening of posterior wall of inguinal canal.

Answer 1.11:
• The 'Lichtenstein' mesh repair.
• Less often: Nylon darn.
• The classical 'Bassini' repair in which the conjoint tendon is stitched to the undersurface of the inguinal ligament has now been superseded.

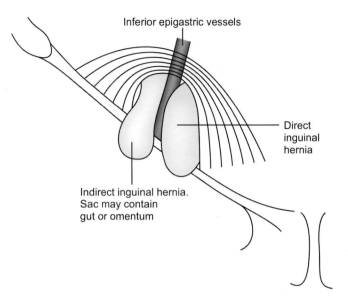

Fig. 22.3 Relationship of direct and indirect inguinal hernia to the inferior epigastric artery

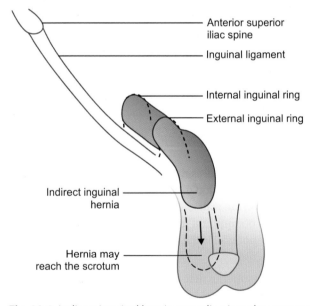

Fig. 22.4 Indirect inguinal hernia extending into the scrotum

Answer 1.12:
• Open hernia repair is the classical conventional repair. An external groin incision is used to open the inguinal canal and to perform the herniotomy and herniorraphy.
• Laparoscpic repair is the newer so called 'key hole surgery'. It is carried out via either transperitoneal or pre-peritoneal approach and involves the use of small incisions, a camera and operating ports to perform the repair.

Answer 1.13:
• My name is Dr Smith and I am the house surgeon who will be looking after you when you have your hernia operation.

Your surgeon, Mr Cox, has asked me if I will explain the operation to you and get you to sign the consent form.

- Could I ask you first if you know what a hernia is and how the operation will be done? (Whatever, the condition, always find out first what the patient knows about his diagnosis and intended treatment, may be nothing, may be a great deal—at least then you know where you are).

Patient says he just knows he has a hernia and that he needs an operation:

- You have a swelling in your groin which is caused by some of the contents of your abdomen coming out through an opening in the abdominal wall. This condition is called an inguinal hernia and the cause is a weakness of the abdominal wall.

- Your surgeon has advised you to undergo an operation to repair the hernia as it can cause complications in the future.

- The operation in your case will be carried out under general anesthesia, so you will be asleep during the operation. You will not be allowed to have anything to eat or drink for 6 hours before your operation. I will be marking the site of your operation with a cross (please do not rub it off). The anesthetist will visit you before the operation and you can ask her any questions you wish.

- An incision (cut) about 3 inches long will be made in your groin. During the surgery, the contents of the hernia are put back in the abdomen, the sac of the hernia is cut off and closed. The weakness of the abdominal wall is then strengthened using a nylon mesh.

- If the surgery is done in the morning, you will probably be discharged home in the evening of the same day provided that everything is satisfactory. You will be provided with painkillers and a list of what you can and cannot do. If your cut is closed with clips or nonabsorbable sutures arrangements will be made for your GP's nurse to remove them. You will be given an appointment for a check follow-up at the hospital in six weeks.

- This is a very safe operation but it is possible for the following complications to occur in a small number of cases. Inability to pass water after the operation and needing a tube in the bladder: bleeding with local swelling in the groin region and scrotum; redness or infection of the skin wound; very rarely infection which could lead to the mesh needing to be removed; there is a small incidence of recurrence of the hernia .

- Do you understand what I have explained to you?

- Have you any questions you would like to ask about the operation and what happens afterwards?

- Would you like me to speak to your relatives?

- Please read the consent form and if you are happy and have no further questions, please sign it.

Differential Diagnosis/Investigations/Basic Management

TUTORIAL 1: Upper Gastrointestinal

Patient 1: Difficulty in swallowing.
Patient 2: Heartburn.
Patient 3: Weight loss and abdominal pain.

Instructions: In this module, we will be moving on from history and examination to differential diagnosis, investigation and in some cases management.

Many of the clinical scenarios will be the ones, we have already used in Module 1.

To get the most out of the directed self-learning, it is very important that you carry out the preparation work diligently. Please do this yourself and not in groups. This is what you should do for each tutorial:

a. Reread the chapter on the tutorial topic in your standard surgical textbook.
b. Read any lecture notes you may have, if relevant.
c. Try and then answer the tutorial questions without recourse to the book or your notes—much as you do in a Modified Essay Question (MEQ) examination.
d. Then check with the book, your notes, or seek help from your tutors to make sure you have the correct answers and understand them. Complete or alter the tutorial answer sheet accordingly.
e. Keep a file of your questions and answers.

Please remember the aim is for you to learn as you go along.

The tutorials are better carried out one by one over an extended period of time so that deeper learning is maximized.

Question 1: Case scenario
Difficulty in swallowing. You will recall this patient from Module 1.

Mr T is a 72-year-old labourer who presents to you with an 8-week history of difficulty in swallowing. He can only eat liquid food. He also notices his voice has become hoarse. Lately he has had a productive cough at night. He has a long history of heartburn. He has been a heavy smoker for 50 years and drinks 3 bottles of beer everyday.

Question 1.1: From the history described earlier, what do you think is the differential diagnosis in this patient?

Question 1.2: List the features in the history which will allow you to decide which is the likely cause of the dysphagia.

Question 1.3: List the findings on physical examination, you may find in a patient with esophageal cancer.

The following are the findings when Mr T is examined:
Mr T is thin and cachexic. He has obviously lost weight. He looks slightly anemic. His supraclavicular nodes are enlarged. There is a decrease in air entry to his right lung base. His liver is palpable and firm on abdominal examination.

Question 1.4: List the investigations you will order to confirm your diagnosis and write alongside why you would do each one.

This is Mr T's chest X-ray (Fig. 1.1).

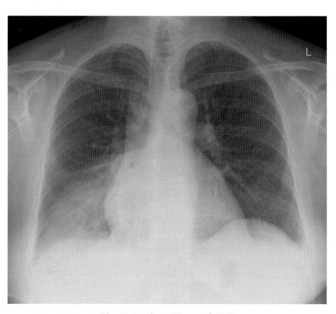

Fig. 1.1 Chest X-ray of Mr T

Question 1.5: What do you see? What has caused this change?

Question 1.6: What is this instrument (Fig. 1.2)?

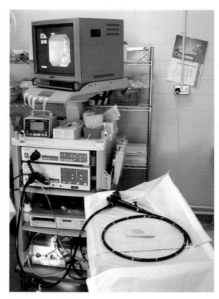

Fig. 1.2 Copyright RCSI with permission

Question 1.7: Write down exactly how an upper gastrointestinal endoscopy is performed, including the methods of sedation/anesthesia. Use bullet points or numbers.

Note: Go and see a few done in endoscopy theater.

Question 1.8: Write down in bullet points how you, the House Officer, will consent this patient for an upper gastrointestinal endoscopy. Do this in non-medical terms exactly as you would explain it to a patient.

Question 1.9: What is shown in this picture which was taken at Mr T's endoscopy (Fig. 1.3)?

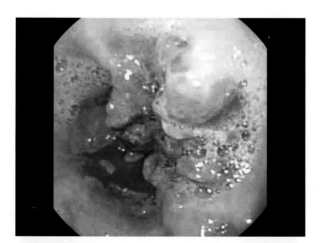

Fig. 1.3 Reprinted from Surgery (Oxford) 29,11, Griffin MS and Wahed S, Oesophageal Cancer. pp. 557-62, 2011, with permission from Elsevier

Question 1.10: How long is the esophagus?

Question 1.11: How do you measure where the lesion is in the esophagus?

Question 1.12: Briefly discuss the histopathology of the lining of the esophagus and what changes it may undergo.

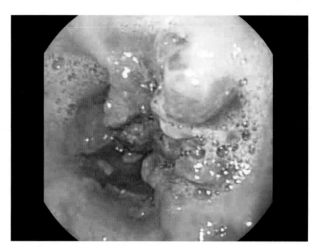

Fig. 1.4 With permission Elsevier as in Fig. 1.3

The Figure 1.4 above shows a Ca esophagus at 30 cm from the incisors.

Question 1.13: List (in outline only) the staging protocol for esophageal cancer.

Question 1.14: What investigations will allow you to stage Mr T's cancer?

Mr T is found to have a T3 N2 MI cancer of his esophagus. This means the tumor has spread to the adventitia of the esophageal wall (T3), involves 3–6 regional lymph nodes (N2), and there are distal metastases (M1) (it is not really necessary to know the full staging details as an undergraduate, but if you wish to look further at this go to: *www.cancerresearchuk.org/cancer-help/type/ oesophageal-cancer*.

Question 1.15: What are your comments on this staging in terms of management and outcome?

Question 1.16: What are the two main parameters which decide if the patient with esophageal cancer is suitable for operation?

Mr T is deemed inoperable because of the extent of his disease. However, he still has considerable dysphagia.

Question 1.17: List the modalities which are available for palliating Mr T.

Question 1.18: The management of cancer of the esophagus will be covered in Module 3. However, to lay some 'foundations' make an outline drawing of the operations used for:

a. Cancer at the esophagogastric junction
b. Lower third esophagus
c. Middle third esophagus
d. Upper third esophagus.

together with the name of the operation.

You may have to look after patients who have been operated on for this disease, when you are a house officer. It is necessary for you to know what the operation are (Not the operative details)—otherwise you will not be able to talk to the patient about his treatment and look out for the complications.

Question 2: Case scenario

Heartburn: You will recognize this history from Module 1 Tutorial 5.

> Miss Q is a 40-year-old obese lady with a 3-month history of burning sensation in her chest especially when she lies down at night. When it started, it was intermittent but now she gets it every night. She also has episodes in the day time after she has eaten. She has a lot of belching which is sometimes accompanied by acid in her mouth. She has noticed, it is worse when she eats chocolate and drinks coffee. She gets a burning in her chest when she drinks hot drinks and has a whisky.

Question 2.1: What is your diagnosis?

Question 2.2: There are two main causes of the clinical syndrome of GERD. What are they?

Question 2.3: What abnormality is shown on the barium swallow/meal X-rays shown in Figures 1.8 and 1.9?

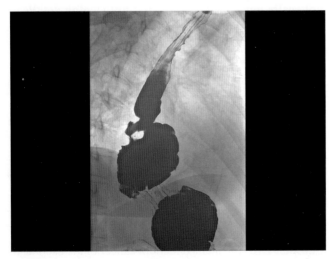

Fig. 1.8

Question 2.3a: Figure 1.8

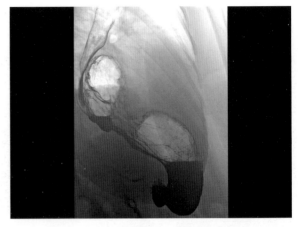

Fig. 1.9

Question 2.3b: Figure 1.9

Question 2.4: What do you see on this Chest X-ray (Fig. 1.10)?

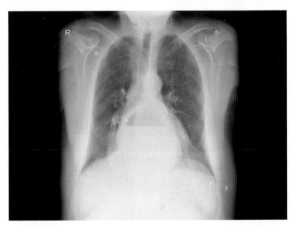

Fig. 1.10

Question 2.5: What investigation is this? What do you see (Fig. 1.11)?

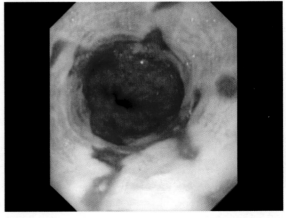

Fig. 1.11

Question 2.6: What investigations will you order for Miss Q?

Question 2.7: Figure 1.12 is an image from the endoscopy. What does it show?

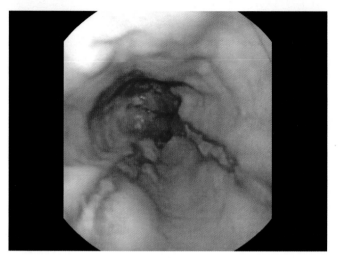

Fig. 1.12

Question 2.8: Discuss briefly how you would treat this patient medically—use bullet points only.

Question 2.9: What is pH manometry? How do you perform it?

Question 2.10: Is it helpful in GERD?

Question 2.11: What are the indications for surgery in GERD?

Question 2.12: Make a drawing of the most commonly used operation for GERD.
    What is it called?
    What surgical approach is used? (Not details.)

Question 3: Case scenario
Weight Loss and Abdominal Pain

Mrs V is a 37-year-old teacher. She has had difficulty in swallowing for years and also of retrosternal discomfort. Her symptoms have become worse recently. For years, she has been a slow eater, always the last to finish in her family. Now she finds both fluids and solids get stuck. She occasionally vomits old food and has lost some weight.

Question 3.1: What investigation will you do first?

Upper gastrointestinal endoscopy shows a slightly dilated esophagus with lack of peristaltic waves. The endoscope seems to stick at the cardia, but then passes into a normal stomach. There is no evidence of a cancer. A barium swallow and meal is ordered:

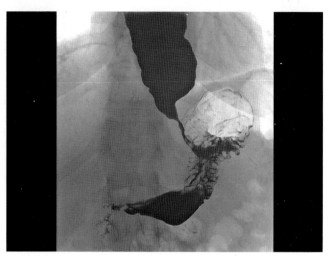

Fig. 1.14

One of the pictures taken is shown in Figure 1.14.

Question 3.2: Describe what you see.

Question 3.3: The video taken as the swallow takes place show shows the barium enters the stomach very slowly. These investigations suggest the patient has achalasia. How could we confirm the diagnosis?

Question 3.4: What is esophageal manometry? Describe how it is done.

Question 3.5: How do you treat achalasia? Make a bulleted list.

Question 4: Case scenario

A 70-year-old man presents with weight loss, lethargy and a dull upper abdominal ache. On examination, he is anemic, but has no glands in his neck or supraclavicular area. There seems to be a fullness in his epigastrium; his liver is not palpable and rectal examination is normal.

Question 4.1: What is your differential diagnosis?

Question 4.2: What investigations will you order?
    Look at Figures 1.15 and 1.16. Figure 1.15 is an endoscopic view of the gastric antrum.

Question 4.3: Describe what you see in Figure 1.15.

Question 4.4: What sort of X-ray is Figure 1.16 and what do you see?

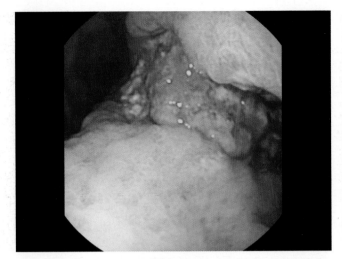

Fig. 1.15

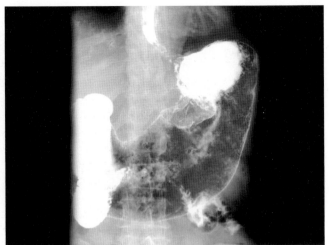

Fig. 1.16

Question 4.5: What other procedures would be performed at the endoscopy?

Question 4.6: How do you stage gastric cancer? What is the prognosis? Make a table.

Question 4.7: Draw the operations which may be performed for cancer of the stomach together with their names.

TUTORIAL 2: Hepatobiliary and Pancreas

Patient 1: Jaundice and abdominal pain.
Patient 2: Jaundice and weight loss.

Please read your lecture notes, the appropriate chapter in your surgical textbook and Tutorial 7 on *Obstructive Jaundice* from Module 1. Then try and answer the case questions below. Look up what you do not know or are not sure about.

Then REDO the tutorial and enter the questions and corrected answers into your records.

Question 1: Case scenario 1

Jaundice and Abdominal Pain

A 35-year-old lady is admitted to the surgical ward with a 12 month history of fatty food intolerance and intermittent upper abdominal pain. One week prior to her admission to hospital, she had an episode of severe upper abdominal pain which lasted for 8 hours and then went away. Twenty-four hours later her husband noticed she had become 'yellow'.

Question 1.1: What do you think the jaundice could be due to, i.e. what is your differential diagnosis at this stage?

The patient says that she has noticed some upper abdominal discomfort especially after she has eaten-fried food. She has also had a lot of belching and some heartburn. The pain she had last week came on suddenly and is the worst pain, she has ever had. She was very sick—green colored fluid. She took some paracetamol and went to bed and the pain went away. A day later her husband said she looked a funny color—a bit yellow. This has gradually become more noticeable. She has noticed that her urine has become dark in color. Her bowel motions may be a bit paler than normal. She has not been itching. She is very worried because her sister had yellow jaundice last year and was told she had an infection. Her appetite has been good and she has not lost any weight recently. She has no heartburn, abdominal distension and has not passed any blood in her bowel motions.

Question 1.2: List the risk factors for jaundice.

The patient says she has never been told she has had hepatitis or a liver problem. She does not drink alcohol. She is not taking any pills or medicines and has never used IV drugs. She is in a stable relationship with her husband and has had no casual sex. She has never had a blood transfusion and has had no serious illness that she knows of. She has never been abroad.

Question 1.3: What is your differential diagnosis now?

Question 1.4: Write a summary of this patient's history:

By now you will have an established system or protocol for examining a patient with a GI system complaint.

Question 1.5: Using the protocol list what you will be particularly looking for when you come to examine this patient (based on your differential diagnosis). Answer under the following headings:

General:

Hands

Vital signs

Neck

Chest

Abdomen: I
          P
         A
         P
         PR

These are the clinical findings in this patient:

The patient is alert, conscious and orientated. She is not in any distress. She has not obviously lost any weight. Her sclera are markedly jaundiced. She is not clinically anemic, or dehydrated. There are no abnormalities of the lips or oral cavity and her dentition is good.

Her hands do not show any signs of liver failure. Arms no scratching or bruising.

Her pulse is 80/minute, BP 120/75 and temperature normal, respiration rate = 20.

She has no masses to feel in her neck and no lymph nodes to palpate.

No spider nevi on her chest.

Abdomen is moving normally with respiration. Skin is jaundiced. No scratch marks.

No masses, no distention, no dilated veins. Umbilicus normal and everted.

On palpation, there is mild tenderness in the epigastrium and RUQ. Gallbladder and liver are not palpable. Murphy's sign negative. Spleen not palpable. No ascites.

PR: stool is pale yellow.

Question 1.6: Write the guiding rule for formulating a differential diagnosis.

Question 1.7: With this in mind write down your differential diagnosis for this patient and justify each entry.

Question 1.8: List the investigations you, as the admitting house officer/intern, would order for this patient and why. Start with simple tests first.

Question 1.9: What three features does an ultrasound scan best define in hepatobiliary disease?

Question 1.10: Draw a diagram of normal bilirubin metabolism.

Question 1.11: Make your own table of the changes in the LFTs in hemolytic, hepatocellular and obstructive jaundice.

Question 1.12: List the dipstick urine changes in obstructive and hepatocellular jaundice.

In this patient:

The urine dipstick carried out on the ward shows the presence of bilirubin ++++ and urobilinogen –ve.

Question 1.13: What do you think this indicates?

The LFTs of this patient come back as:

Birubin Total: 40 umol/L (N = 0–24)

Bilirubin direct: Elevated

             indirect: Normal

Alanine aminotransferase (ALT): 26 umol/L (N = 0–42)

Alkaline phosphatase (ALP) : 220 u/L (N = 34–104)

Total protein : 70 g/L (N = 66–87)

S. albumin : 40 g/L (N = 35–52)

A/G ratio : 1.2 (N = 0.9–1.8) (albumin/globulin ratio)

Question 1.14: What do you understand by direct and indirect bilirubin?

Question 1.15: From the liver function tests what type of jaundice does this patient have and what is your likely diagnosis now?

The ultrasound comes back from the radiology department but someone has forgotten to put the report with it.

Question 1.16: A scan picture is shown below (Fig. 2.2). Write your own report of the abnormalities seen.

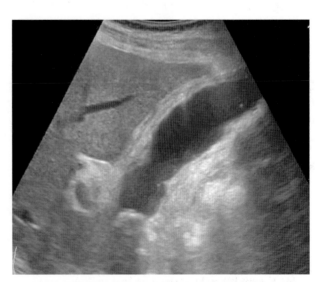

Fig. 2.2 Courtesy of Dr Taco Geertsma

The report comes back confirming the gallstones and thickening and further views suggest that the common bile duct is dilated with contained stones.

Question 1.17: In this lady, what investigation do you think the surgeon will now order?

The surgeon decides to do an ERCP. He asks you to consent the patient.

Question 1.18: What would you say to the patient? Your answer should use non-medical language exactly as, if you were explaining it to the patient.

Question 1.19: What blood investigation would the house officer check before the patient goes for the ERCP?

The results come back and show the patient's INR is raised.

Question 1.20: What would you (the house officer) do?

Question 1.21: This is one of the films from the ERCP (Fig. 2.3). What does it shows:

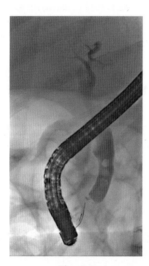

Fig. 2.3

Question 1.22: What procedure will be carried out at the ERCP in this case? What management will the patient then require at a later date?

Question 2: Case scenario

Jaundice and Weight Loss

Mr K is a 71-year-old man who used to be a sailor. He presents with a 2-week history of progressive yellow discoloration of the skin. He has lost 5 kg over the last 3 months.

Question 2.1: What questions will you ask him?

Mr K says his wife noticed he was yellow 2 weeks ago. It has become more noticeable—especially in his eyes. His urine has gone dark. His bowel motions are yellow. He does not have any itching or scratching. He has had a dull pain in the upper abdomen for 3 months which is worse after he eats. The last few weeks he has been vomiting undigested food about 2 hours after he has eaten. He has lost about 5 kg in weight in the last 3 months and his appetite is poor. He has no difficulty in swallowing, no heartburn, and no indigestion in the past. His abdomen is not distended. There has been no change in his bowel habit and he has not passed any blood or slime.

His wife had hepatitis 3 years ago. He has not been abroad recently. He does not drink alcohol. He is not an IV drug user. He has had no blood transfusions. He has no history of blood disorders. He says he had a 'girl in every port' when he was a sailor. He takes a tablet his doctor has given him for anxiety. He started taking these tablets four months ago. PMH, FH, SH, and ROS gave no further relevant facts.

Question 2.2: Write a brief summary of his history (remember this is not just a repeat of the full history—it should not be more than a line or two and requires thought—as it guides you to the next stage of the diagnostic procedure.

Question 2.3: Write below the guideline for making a differential diagnosis.

Question 2.4: In this patient, what do you think the differential diagnosis might be at this stage?

Question 2.5: List the physical signs you would particularly look for in this case when you examine him (using the protocoled examination format).

On examination of Mr K the following is noted:

Mr K is thin and looks unwell. He is orientated and answers questions well. He is not obviously in pain. His sclera are markedly jaundiced and his mucous membranes are pale. He appears a little dehydrated. He has no obvious lesion in his mouth and has dentures.

He has no signs of liver failure in his hands, no scratch marks on arms.

His pulse is 80/min, BP 160/90, RR = 15 and temperature normal.

No neck masses or palpable lymph nodes.

He has no spider nevi on his chest and no gynecomastia.

On abdominal examination, his abdomen is moving normally with respiration. He has evidence of weight loss and yellow discoloration of his skin; his abdomen is not distended, there are no visible scars or masses. His umbilicus appears normal.

On palpation, there is an indiscrete fullness in the epigastrium, his liver is palpable 2 cm below the costal margin and is firm and smooth. His gallbladder is not palpable. There is no evidence of ascites. No groin glands, External genitalia are normal.

On anorectal exam, inspection is normal, PR shows yellow colored stool. No mass. Prostate normal.

Question 2.6: What is your differential diagnosis now?

Question 2.7: List the investigations you, as the house officer, will order for this patient to help you make the diagnosis, justify each one.

These are the results of his tests:

Hb is 9 g/dL

Urea and electrolytes are normal

Liver function tests show a raised alkaline phosphatase and a low serum albumin

Bilirubin is 80 µmol/L

Urine shows bilirubin and no urobilinogen

CA 19-9 is raised. Alpha-fetoprotein normal.

Question 2.8: What do you think about these results?

The chest X-ray comes back reported as normal.

The abdominal film is reported as showing gallstones and possible pancreatic calcification.

Question 2.9: What do you think now?

The ultrasound scan shows the gallbladder to contain stones and to be small and shrunken.

The common bile duct is dilated to 20 mm. No stones seen within common bile duct. Mass in head of pancreas suggested. Liver appears normal.

Question 2.10: What do you think now?

Question 2.11: What investigation would the specialist order now and why?

Please study the X-rays shown below in Figures 2.4 and 2.5. They are to illustrate the type of investigations which are now used. As an undergraduate you are not expected to be able to interpret all the details.

Figures 2.4A and B are part of an MRI-CP showing stones in the gallbladder, cystic duct and common bile duct. The second film is the T2-weighted image.

Figure 2.5 is part of a contrast-enhanced CT scan showing a mass in head of pancreas. This film is the coronal reconstruction.

Back to our patient Mr K:

Mr K has a CT carried out. It shows a cancer of the head of the pancreas with obstruction of the CBD and the second part of the duodenum. He also has liver secondaries.

This explains why he is jaundiced and has been vomiting.

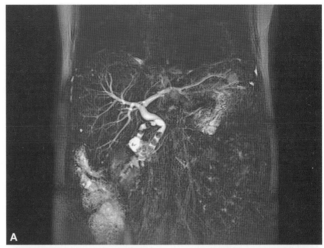
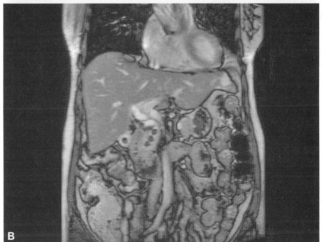

Figs 2.4A and B

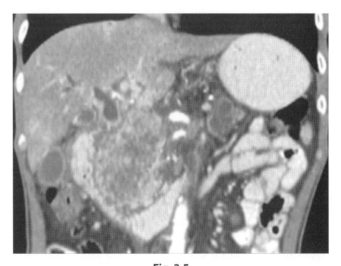

Fig. 2.5

Question 2.12: Is there anything that can be done to help him?

Finally a few revision questions:

Question 2.13: What malignant conditions cause obstructive jaundice?

Question 2.14: Classify tumors of the pancreas.

Question 2.15: A CT reveals a 3 cm lesion in the head of the pancreas with dilated common bile duct.
a. What further investigations and/or procedures are warranted?
b. What sort of CT will be required?
c. What will you look for in the CT to decide operability?
d. How will you stage carcinoma pancreas?
e. What is the prognosis?

TUTORIAL 3: Rectal Bleeding

Question 1: What are the core symptoms and signs of:
a. Cancer of the colon and rectum.
b. Ulcerative colitis.
c. Diverticular disease of the sigmoid colon.
d. An infective colitis.
e. Hemorrhoids.

Remember: These five disease syndromes account for the majority of patients presenting with an alteration of the bowel habit, rectal bleeding or a combination both symptoms. So, some or all of these diagnoses will be in your differential diagnosis for a 65-year-old man presenting with rectal bleeding—so here is his history.

Question 2: Case scenario

Age: 65-years-old
Occupation: Retired mechanic
Complaint of: Bleeding with his bowel motion for
3 months.
Diarrhea for 3 months.
History PC: Noticed bright red blood on his bowel motion 3 months ago. Small in amounts and on the surface and mixed in with bowel motion nearly every time.
His usual bowel habit was once per day but now he is going 3–4 times per day.
He sometimes feels that he has to go again after he has had his bowels work.
He has seen a little slime with his motion.
On direct questioning he has:
• No difficulty in swallowing
• No nausea or vomiting
• No acid regurgitation or heartburn
• No abdominal pain, indigestion or abdominal distention
• No change in his appetite or weight loss.
His PMH, FH, SH and ROS are unremarkable.

Question 2.1: Using the lists of symptoms you gave in Question 1—what are you going to write down as your differential diagnosis?

Question 2.2: When you examine him: What physical signs are you going to particularly look for?
These are the findings on examination of this 65-year-old man: On examination
General: **Well nourished. Not anemic or jaundiced or dehydrated.**
    Tongue/oral cavity: NAD
    Hands: NAD
    Neck: No lymph nodes
Abdominal examination: Inspection: no obvious weight loss, no scars, no distention, no visible mass, no distended veins, no visible pulsations. Umbilicus normal.
Palpation: **No tenderness, no mass, no organomegaly. Hernial orifices, genitalia = normal.**
Percussion, auscultation normal.

Question 2.3: What are you going to do now to help make your diagnosis. Sit and think about this and then list what further physical examination you will do and what basic investigations you will order at the outpatient clinic.

Question 2.4: List what you understand by a full ano rectal examination.

Note: Many medical gastroenterologists do not carry out a rigid sigmoidoscopy—saying they prefer a 'prepped' flexible sigmoidoscopy or colonoscopy. Most colon and rectal surgeons/proctologists would disagree—rigid sigmoidoscopy can be done straightaway, often gives the diagnosis and shows helpful signs (e.g. blood or minimal proctitis). It also allows for immediate biopsy/specimen collection.
    The following are the findings on anorectal examination:
Inspection: Skin tags.
Digital rectal examination: Irregular mass at 8 cm. Left lateral wall bright blood on finger.
Rigid sigmoidoscopy: Ulcerating lesion at 8 cm: Biopsied.

Proctoscopy: 2nd degree hemes.
You arrange for: FBC
                    U and Electrolytes, LFTs
                    Tumor markers
                    Chest X-ray
                    Colonoscopy.

Question 2.5: What does a full blood count (FBC) include and how may it help in this case?

Question 2.6: What indices are measured in 'Urea and Electrolytes? How may they be altered in this case?

Question 2.7: What is included in the liver function tests and how may they help in this case?

Question 2.8: What are tumor markers and which would you choose in this case?

Question 2.9: What is a colonoscopy? Write how you would explain the procedure to the patient.

Question 2.10: You are the house officer. Write below the preparation you would order for the colonoscopy.

Question 2.11: Why do a colonoscopy in this case when you already know he has a CA rectum?

The biopsy histology result comes back as : 'moderately differentiated carcinoma of large bowel origin'. The colonoscopy is negative apart from the lesion at 8 cm.

Question 2.12: What investigations will you carry out to clinically stage this tumor before you operate on the patient?

Chest X-ray is negative
MRI shows a T2 tumor of the mid rectum.

Question 2.13: How do you perform a barium enema?

Question 2.14: Why has colonoscopy largely replaced barium enema?

Question 2.15: What is an MRI? Why is it better for staging a rectal cancer than CT?

This man has a localized cancer of the middle third of his rectum.

Question 2.16: What operation does he require?

Question 2.17: Draw a simple diagram of an anterior resection of the rectum.

Question 2.18: Draw a simple diagram of an abdomino-perineal excision.

BASIC SCIENCE

Question 2.19: Write down Duke's classification for cancer of the colon and rectum and the prognosis for each stage (5 year survival).

Question 2.20: What do you understand by the TNM classification in colorectal cancer?

COMMUNICATION SKILLS

Question 2.21: Write how you would consent the patient for an anterior resection.

ETHICS

Question 2.22: Will this man require a stoma? What are the implications for the patient of a stoma?

Let us consider some other some investigations and a few relevant questions about them.

Question 2.23: What are shown here (Figs 3.3A and B)?

Question 2.24: What is shown here (Fig. 3.4)?

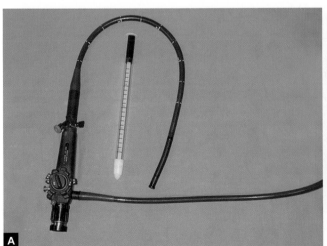

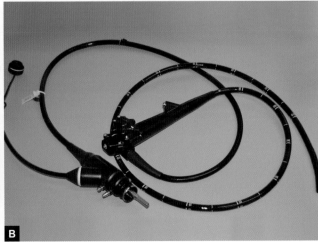

Figs 3.3A and B Copyright RCSI with permission

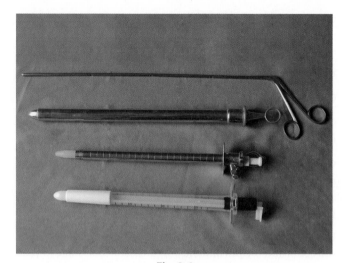

Fig. 3.4

Question 2.25: What investigation is this and what abnormality is shown (Fig. 3.5)?

Question 2.26: What type of investigation is this? What is shown (Fig. 3.6)?

Question 2.27: What investigation is this and what abnormality is shown (Fig. 3.7)?

Question 2.28: What investigation is this and what do the arrows indicate (Fig. 3.8)?

Question 2.29: What investigation is this and what is the basic principle underlying how it works (Fig. 3.9)?

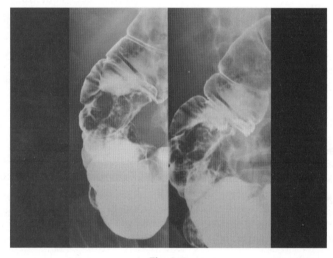

Fig. 3.5

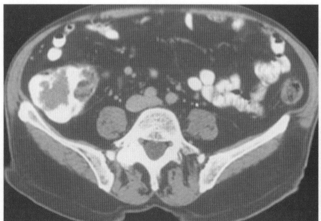
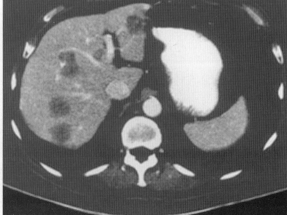

Fig. 3.6

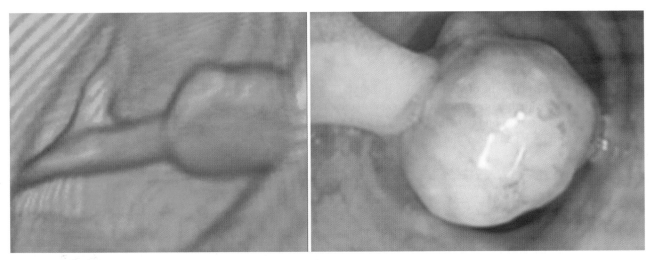

Fig. 3.7

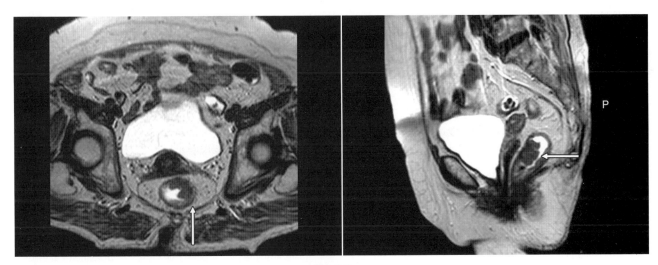

Fig. 3.8

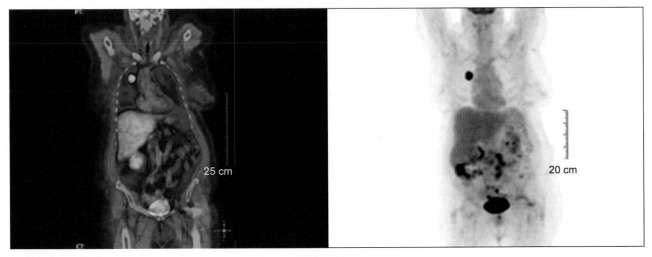

Fig. 3.9

TUTORIAL 4: Abdominal Pain (Acute Abdomen)

Task 1: Reread the chapter on the acute abdomen in your textbook.

Task 2: As we discussed at the end of Module 1 Tutorial 20 you must be very familiar with the core symptoms and signs of the common causes of the acute abdomen. In Module 1, Tutorial 20, you will have prepared a table of the core features of the following conditions:

Acute pancreatitis, acute cholecystitis, ureteric colic, intestinal obstruction, acute appendicitis, perforated peptic ulcer, ruptured abdominal aortic aneurism, ruptured ectopic pregnancy and acute diverticulitis, using the shown in Table 4.1.

Table 4.1 Acute abdominal pain—Core knowledge

Condition	Pain				Other Symptoms	Physical signs	Diagnostic test
	Localization	Character	Aggrevating factors	Relieving factors			

The 'boxes' should be small so that you are forced to just identify the 'core' knowledge and enter these facts only.
Revise this core knowledge and test yourself on it.
The table suggested in Module 1 is shown as Table 4.2.

Table 4.2 Acute abdominal pain—Core knowledge

Condition	Location	Character	Aggravating factors	Relieving factors	Associated symptoms	Physical signs	Diagnostic test
Acute appendicitis	Periumbilical moves to RIF	Initially colicky becomes continuous	Movement coughing	Lies still	Anorexia vomiting 1–2 Xs occasionally diarrhea	Flushed RIF tenderness rebound, guarding	?CT scan
Acute cholecystitis/ biliary colic	Epigastrium, RUQ, may go to back	Sudden or gradual onset usually constant	Movement		Fever previous indigestion, fat intolerance	Tender in RUQ +ve Murphys, sign	Plain X-rays ultrasound
Intestinal obstruction	Small bowel = periumbilical large bowel = lower abdomen	Colicky			SB: Vomiting LB: Vomiting late, absolute constipation	Abdominal distention, visible peristalsis	Erect and supine abdomen films: Distention + airfluid levels CT scan
Ureteric colic	Loin to groin	Severe colicky/severe constant or intermittent		Rolls around	Vomiting, sweating	Usually no abdomen signs sometimes hematuria	KUB CT urogram
Acute pancreatitis	Upper abdomen then moves all over	May start dull and become severe		Usually lie still may sometimes sit forwards	Nausea, vomiting Systemic—fever tachy, BP down	Sometimes local tenderness to start then diffuse tenderness guarding, rebound no bowel sounds	Serum amylase after 4 days urinary amylase
Perforated peptic ulcer	Sudden onset epigastric, then radiates over whole abdomen	Severe	Movement	Lies still	Vomiting	Fever, tachy, hypotension, board like rigidity no bowel sounds	Erect chest X-ray, erect abdomen film may show free gas
Acute diverticulitis	Lower abdomen or LIF	Gradual onset becomes localized in LIF	Coughing moving	Lies still	pH of diverticulosis with abdominal pain, constipation, diarrhea	Local tenderness guarding, rebound, if perforates generalized peritonitis signs	Contrast-enhanced CT

Contd...

Contd...

Condition	Location	Character	Aggravating factors	Relieving factors	Associated symptoms	Physical signs	Diagnostic test
Ruptured abdominal aortic aneurism	Previous back/ loin/lower abdomen then sudden onset lower abdomen pain	Sudden onset severe				Pulsatile mass Tachycardia Hypotension Shut down	Only, if doubt re-diagnosis: CT
Ruptured ectopic pregnancy	Lower abdo/ Shoulder tip/ diffuse abdo	Severe	Movement	Lies still	Sexually active missed period	Tachycardia, hypotension signs of peritonitis	Positive pregnancy test TV ultrasound

Abbreviations: CT, computed tomography; KUB, kidney, ureters and bladder; RUQ, right upper quadrant; RIF, right iliac fossa; abdo, abdominal

We are going to look at a few more case scenarios—as always try to do these without your books. Then look the answers up and correct your document as necessary.

Question 1: Case scenario

A 19-year-old female is admitted to the surgical ward with lower abdominal pain. The pain started 12 hours previously in her lower abdomen and she has had it ever since. It is becoming worse. The pain is constant in nature. It is made worse by moving and is better if she lies still. She is not hungry and has vomited twice since the pain started. Her bowels have not worked since the pain began. She has never had this pain before. Her periods were regular in the past but she has missed her last period. She has a regular boyfriend and does not use contraceptive precautions. Over the last 3 weeks, she has had pain on passing urine and has noticed a slight vaginal discharge.

On examination: She is in pain
        Flushed
        Furred tongue
        Well hydrated
        Pyrexial 39°C
        Pulse 90 BP 120/70.
Abdomen: **I: Abdomen moving with respiration**
        No distention
        Thin
        No scars, mass, distended veins
        Umbilicus normal.
Palpation: **Tender over the whole of lower abdomen, maximal in RIF.**
        Rebound tenderness over lower abdomen with positive cough test, no organomegaly, hernial orifices: Normal.
Auscultation: **Scanty bowel sounds.**
Percussion: **Tenderness in lower abdomen, no free fluid.**
Rectal examination: Negative.
Vaginal examination: Tender when cervix is moved.

Question 1.1: What is your differential diagnosis?

Make a list of these and under each entry justify why you have included each entry.

Question 1.2: Make a list of the investigations you would order as the admitting house officer—starting with blood tests first.

Question 1.3: These are the results—comment on the relevance of each:
a. Hb: 9 g/dL   WCC is: 10,000/mm^3 CRP: normal
b. Urea is 12   Rest of electrolytes are normal.
c. Liver function tests are normal.
d. Amylase is normal.
e. Pregnancy test normal.
f. Urine dipstick shows small amount of blood, moderate amount nitrites.

Question 1.4: The MSU result is awaited: when will it come and what will it contain details of?

Question 1.5: What are the normal values and units of Hb, WCC, amylase?

Question 1.6: Write the details of the pregnancy tests which would be of use in the acute situation.

Question 1.7: What does this chest X-ray show (Fig. 4.1)?

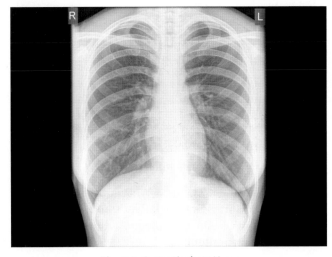

Fig. 4.1 Patient's chest X-ray

It helps to have a protocol for 'reporting' chest and abdominal X-rays.

When you have completed this Module, as a learning exercise, try and make out your own protocols. Do this when you have completed the rest of the module as it will take some time.

Look at the suggested protocols which have been included as an appendix at the end of the book.

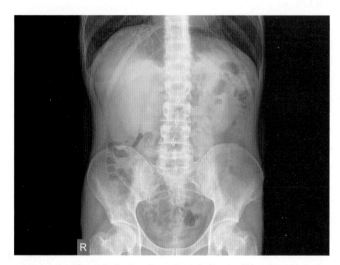

Fig. 4.2 Patient's supine abdominal X-ray

Question 1.8: What does this X-ray show (Fig. 4.2)?

Question 1.9: What types of US scans are used to show pelvic pathology?

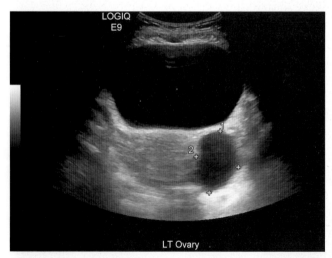

Fig. 4.3 Patient's ultrasound scan

Question 1.10: Look at Figure 4.3. What does it show?

The specialist reviews the patient's investigations and decides he is not certain of the diagnosis but thinks she has lower abdominal peritonitis.

Question 1.11: What will be the correct management of this patient now?

Question 1.12: What should the surgeon do?

Question 2: Case scenario

History: The patient is a 65-year-old man. He presents with a 4-day history of lower abdominal pain. This is colicky in nature. There are periods when the pain just goes down to an ache. He says he has never had pain such as this before but that over the last few months he has had some mild lower abdominal discomfort. His pain is better, if he gets up and moves around. He has vomited greenish fluid 4 times since the pain started. His appetite is very poor and he has only taken a few drinks since the pain started. Over the last 6 months, his bowel habit has changed and sometimes he has to go 3 or more times a day (normal = × 1 per day). Since the pain started, he has noticed that his abdomen is getting bigger and his bowels have not opened nor has he passed any flatus for the last 2 days.

Question 2.1: What is your likely diagnosis from the history?

Question 2.2: List the 4 key symptoms and signs of intestinal obstruction.

Question 2.3: Define these criteria for large bowel obstruction.

Question 2.4: Write the common causes of large bowel obstruction.

Question 2.5: What type of X-ray is this and what does it show (Fig. 4.4)?

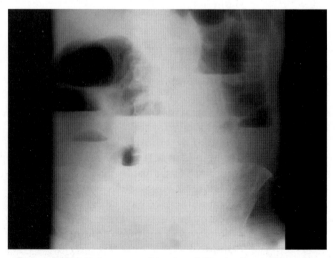

Fig. 4.4 Courtesy of Jon Lund, Nottingham, UK

Question 2.7: What imaging technique would you use to confirm the diagnosis of large bowel obstruction made on these X-rays?

Question 2.8: What type of X-ray is this and what is showing in Figures 4.6A and B?

> **In our patient:**
> **The diagnosis of large bowel obstruction due to a tumor of the rectosigmoid junction is made.**

Question 2.9: How would you manage this patient (In Outline)?

Question 2.10: What is Hartmann's operation (In words)?

Question 2.11: Make a simple drawing of the operation.

Question 2.12: What do these X-rays show (Figs 4.8A and B)?

Question 2.13: What sort of X-ray do you think this is and what does it show (Fig. 4.9)?

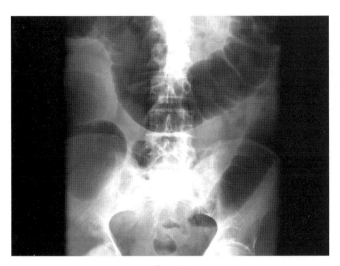

Fig. 4.5

Question 2.6: What type of X-ray is this and what does it show (Fig. 4.5)?

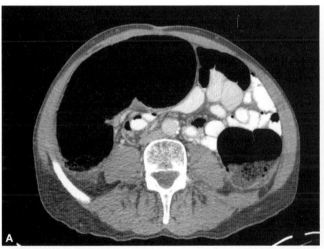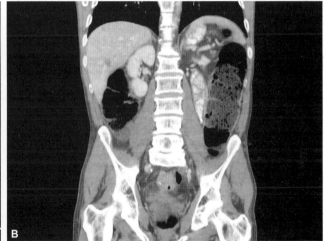

Figs 4.6A and B

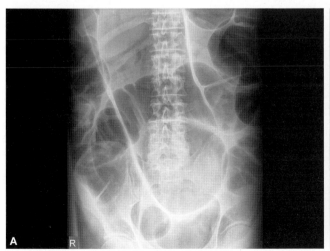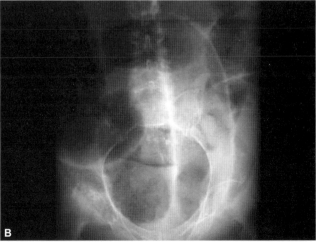

Figs 4.8A and B Courtesy of Scottish Radiology Society

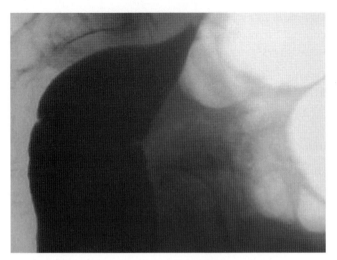

Fig. 4.9 Courtesy of Scottish Radiology Society

Question 2.14: Write a short summary of volvulus of the colon under the headings:

Incidence
Etiology
Pathology
Clinical presentation
Investigation
Treatment
Complications.

Note: If you are asked to discuss a particular condition, then it often helps to use the above headings—you will be surprised how much you can work out, if you use this systematic approach.

TUTORIAL 5: Vascular Disease (Arterial)

Patient 1: Abdominal pain and collapse (arterial disease).
Patient 2: Sudden onset of calf pain.
Patient 3: Sudden onset of leg pain

Question 1: Case scenario

> A 75-year-old man presents to the A and E Department with sudden onset of generalized abdominal pain which radiates into his back. He says he feels dizzy and clammy. For the last year, he has been aware of some lower abdominal and back pain. When he is in bed at night, he sometimes is aware of a pulsating in his abdomen. He has been a heavy smoker for 40 years and 2 years ago had a stroke from which he recovered well. He has been taking aspirin since then. He has no other past medical history. He is retired, financially secure and lives at home with his elderly wife.

Question 1.1: What would be your differential diagnosis at this stage?

Question 1.2: You are the house officer/intern and now examine him. Before you start list here, what clinical signs you would be particularly looking for in this man?

On examination, he is clammy and sweating profusely. He is a little confused. His pulse is of low volume, 100 beats per minute and his blood pressure is 80 systolic. His abdomen is distended, tender all over, and his right femoral pulse is weaker than his left. You think you can feel **an abdominal pulsation and there is an audible bruit in the region of his umbilicus.**

Question 1.3: What is your differential diagnosis?

Question 1.4: You are the surgical house officer and see the patient in the A and E Department. List the exactly what you would do in terms of his practical management?

Question 1.5: List what you would not do and why:

The patient is taken to the operating theater and anesthetized. A laparotomy is performed and the diagnosis of a ruptured aortic aneurysm is confirmed.

Question 1.6: Draw a simple line diagram to show you understand the 'anatomy' of an abdominal aortic aneurysm.

Figure 5.2 shows the typical findings of an aortic aneurysm at operation—in this case, the aneurism is not ruptured.

Question 1.7: Describe what you think the operative findings will be when the aneurysm ruptures as in this current case scenario.

Question 1.8: Describe in simple terms what would be done at the operation for this patient.

Question 1.9: What does this illustration show (Fig. 5.3)?

Question 1.10: What does the illustration show (Fig 5.4)?

Figures 5.6A and B shows two images of an abdominal aortic aneurysm at postmortem (opened and unopen).

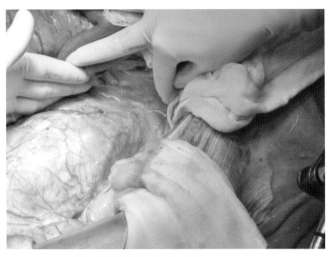

Fig. 5.2 Abdominal aortic aneurysm.
Copyright RCSI with permission

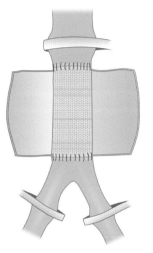

Fig. 5.3

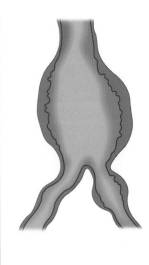

Fig. 5.4

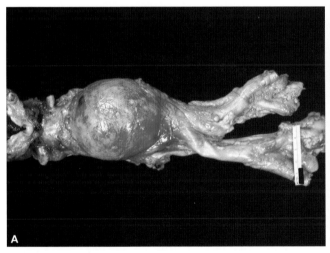

Figs 5.6A and B Abdominal aortic aneurysm seen at postmortem. Courtesy of University of Alabama: Peter Anderson, *peir.net*

Question 1.11: Which of the following statements are true?
a. The aneurysm is more likely to rupture, if greater than 5 cm in diameter
b. Aortic aneurysm is more common in the female
c. The underlying cause is atherosclerosis
d. The patient may have other signs of atherosclerosis.

Question 1.12: Make a list of the other signs of atherosclerosis the patient may have:

Question 1.13: Describe the X-ray (Fig. 5.7).

Question 1.14: Describe this abdominal ultrasound scan (Fig. 5.8).

Question 1.15: Describe this contrast-enhanced CT of the abdomen (Fig. 5.9).

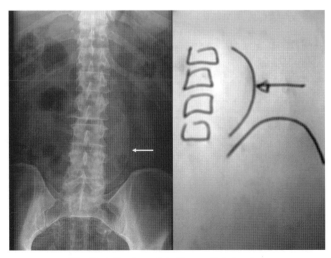

Fig. 5.7 Supine, plain X-ray of abdomen

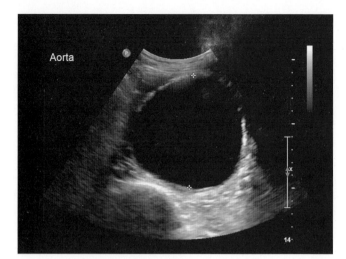

Fig. 5.8 Ultrasound scan of abdomen

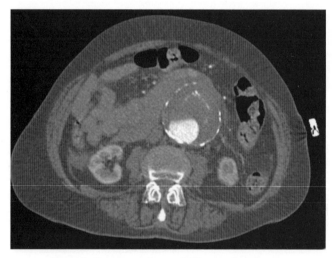

Fig. 5.9 Contrast enhanced CT scan of abdomen

Question 1.16: In relation to the above case (Case scenario 1, ruptured aortic aneurysm) answer the following questions:
a. Why would you not send him for imaging before the operation?
b. Why would you not give him an intravenous fluid load to correct his low BP?
c. What is his chance of surviving the surgery?

Question 1.17: Write a brief synopsis of the symptoms, signs and investigations of a thoracic aortic dissection.

Question 2: Case scenario

Mrs Smith has had her rectal cancer removed at laparotomy 5 days ago. On the evening ward round, she tells you that she slipped and fell in the toilet this morning—she did not hurt herself but now has pain in the back of her leg.

Question 2.1: You are the house officer—what would be your thoughts on the likely diagnosis?

Question 2.2: When you examine her what will you be looking for?

On examination, she has a flicker of pyrexia, her calf is tender to palpation and measures 1.5 cm more than the other side (measured at a fixed point 8 cm below the tibial tuberosity).

Question 2.3: What is your diagnosis?

Question 2.4: What would you do?

Question 2.5: What is Virchow's triad?

Question 2.6: What measures do you take preoperatively to prevent DVT in the patient undergoing surgery, i.e. prophylaxis.

Question 2.7: What anti-DVT measures will you use postoperatively?

Question 2.8: What are the complications of a DVT?

Question 2.9: What is this instrument and what is it used for (Fig. 5.11)?

Question 2.10: What is this investigation (Fig. 5.12)?

Question 2.11: You are called to see Mrs Smith in the early hours of the next morning. She is breathless and complaining of chest pain. What do you think has happened?

Question 2.12: After you have examined Mrs. Smith you think she has had a PE. List in bullet point format exactly how you would manage her.

Question 2.13: How would you confirm your diagnosis?

Question 2.14: What does this X-ray show (Fig. 5.13)?

Question 2.15: What is a VQ scan (Fig. 5.14)?

Question 2.16: What does this CT show (Fig. 5.15)?

Question 2.17: What does this pathology picture show (Fig. 5.16)?

Question 2.18: What is this? When do you use it? How do you insert it (Fig. 5.17)?

Question 3: Case scenario

MR X is known to have atrial fibrillation but he is not anti-coagulated. He is 70 years of age and apart from pain in the right leg which comes on when walking, he is fit and well. He is brought to the A and E Department because of severe pain in his right leg.

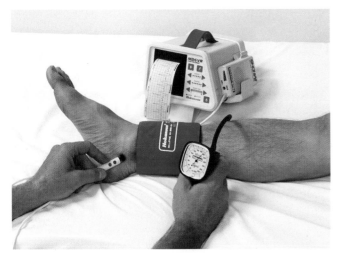

Fig. 5.11 With permission: DE Hokanson, Inc., Bellvue, NA, USA

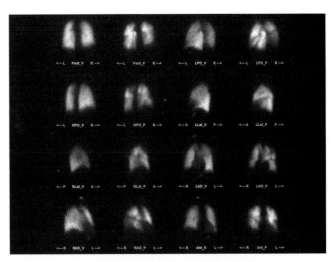

Fig. 5.14 V/Q scan of lungs

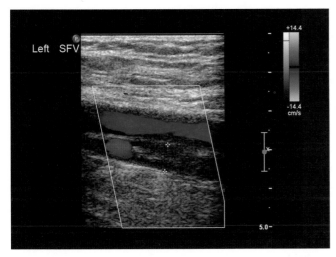

Fig. 5.12

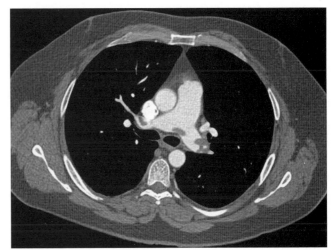

Fig. 5.15

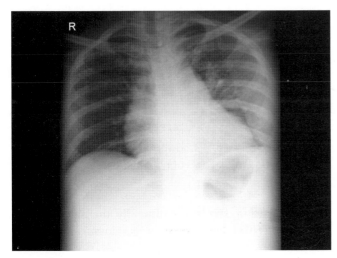

Fig. 5.13

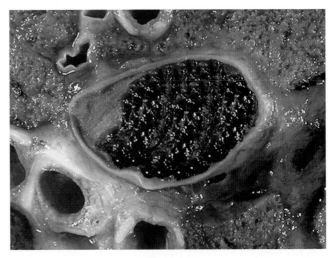

Fig. 5.16

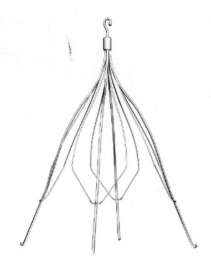

Fig. 5.17 With permission Cook Medical Incorporated, Bloomington, Indiana, USA

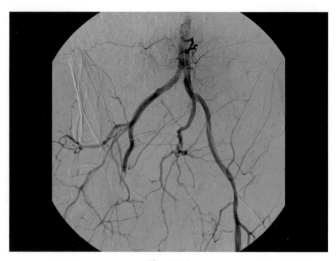

Fig. 5.18

Question 3.1: With this history, what diagnoses will be in your mind?

Question 3.2: List the six symptoms and signs of an acutely ischemic limb (mnemonic).

On examination, the patient's right leg is cold and has no femoral or distal pulses. The appearances are suggestive of acute limb ischemia.

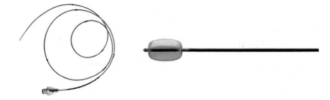

Fig. 5.19 With permission Edwards Life Sciences, Irvine, CA, USA

Question 3.3: What do you think is the likely pathological process?

Question 3.4: If you were the house officer/intern called to see this patient what would be your initial management?

Question 3.5: What other investigations may help?

Question 3.6: What sort of X-ray is this? How do you do it? What does it show (Fig. 5.18)?

Question 3.7: What is shown in Figure 5.19? What is it used for? How do you carry out the procedure?

Question 3.8: If the cause of the acute limb ischemia is due to thrombosis superimposed on long-standing atherosclerosis rather than an embolus and the limb is showing signs of critical ischemia: List in outline, what treatment options are available.

TUTORIAL 6: Lumps in Neck

Patient 1: Solitary thyroid swelling.
Patient 2: Swelling in anterior triangle.

Read up the chapters dealing with conditions of the thyroid and swellings in the neck in your surgical textbook. Look at your lecture notes. Redo Module 1 Tutorial 21.

Try and answer the tutorial questions without your books.

Then read up on the points you cannot answer and redo the tutorial as a top copy.

Question 1: Case scenario

You will remember this patient

The patient is 30-years-old. She has been aware of a swelling in her neck for 3 months. Her husband has also noticed it.

She thinks it has become bigger recently. She is otherwise well. The lump is not painful. She has not lost any weight recently. Her appetite is normal. She has not had any undue sweating or fatigue and has not noticed any change in her voice or appearance. Her bowel habit and periods have not changed. No PMH, FH, SH of note and review of systems is non-contributory.

On examination, she is not clinically anemic. She looks well and there is no evidence of weight loss.

On inspection of neck,

There seems to be a swelling in the R anterior triangle of the neck.

There are no visible scars.

There are no overlying skin changes.

There are no visible distended veins or arterial pulsations.

The swelling appears to move up and down when she swallows.

On palpation from behind:

The swelling is in the R anterior triangle. It is 2 cm in diameter, round in shape, smooth surfaced and firm in consistency.

The edge of the swelling is well defined.

It does not pulsate, is of normal temperature and is non-tender.

The surrounding skin is normal and no lymph nodes were palpable.

The swelling moves up when the patient swallows.

The swelling is not attached to the skin and appears fixed in the thyroid.

The carotid artery is palpable and normal.

Examining from the front,

The trachea is central. Percussion does not suggest any retrosternal extension.

(Please note that the examination findings have been described using a standard look/feel/move protocol. The actual swelling is described using the 4X S, etc. mnemonic. (See Appendix for protocols)

In Module 1, you were asked the clinical features of hyper- and hypothyroidism.

Question 1.1: Write down the clinical examinations you would perform to asses, if this lady is hyperthyroid, hypothyroid or euthyroid. Do this starting with her hands and arms, then the face and finally the legs, i.e. how would you determine her clinical thyroid status?

Clinical examination suggests the lady is euthyroid.

So we have a 30-year-old euthyroid lady with a solitary thyroid swelling.

Questions 1.2: List the 4 most common causes of a solitary thyroid swelling in a lady of this age, i.e. list your differential diagnosis.

Question 1.3: Make out a flow chart for the investigation of a solitary thyroid swelling and add on the 'core' management.

Question 1.4: Pathology: List the histopathological types of thyroid cancer, who they occur in and how they spread, together with the management and prognosis. Do this as a table—so you can use it for revision.

Remember management of thyroid cancer is a complex topic. The above table is a simplified summary and is sufficient for the undergraduate.

If you wish to read more look at Balasubramanian S, Thomas WEG, Surgery (Oxford) 2007;25(11):482-6.

The first investigation we would carry out in a patient with a solitary thyroid nodule would be the thyroid function tests (TFTs).

Question 1.5: Write down what TFTs you would order on this lady.

Question 1.6: Draw a simple diagram to show the regulation of the thyroid hormones—this should show the hypothalamus, anterior pituitary and the thyroid gland.

Question 1.7:
a. What would you expect the TSH, T3 and T4 to be in a euthyroid patient?
b. What would you expect the TSH, T3 and T4 to be in a thyrotoxic patient?
c. A hypothyroid patient?

Question 1.8: What effect do pregnancy and giving estrogens have on the T3 and T4 and what would you do about it to correctly assess a patient's thyroid function in these circumstances?

Question 1.9: What do you understand by the term thyroid antibodies?

Question 1.10: What are the indications for performing thyroid antibody assessment?

Question 1.11: These are the results of this patient's thyroid function studies:

TSH: 2 mIU/L (N = 0.4–4.7)
Free T4: 12 pmol/L (N = 9–24)
Free T3: 3 pmol/L (N = 2.5–5.3)

So what is the patient's biochemical thyroid status?

An ultrasound scan of the thyroid is performed (Fig. 6.2).

Question 1.12: What is seen in Figure 6.2?

The radiologist says there is a large complex solitary swelling in the right lobe of thyroid.

The surgeon sends her for fine needle aspiration cytology (FNAC)—see Figure 6.3.

Question 1.13: Write down how you would explain to the patient what will happen to them when they are sent for an FNAC, i.e. how you would consent them in words the patient will understand.

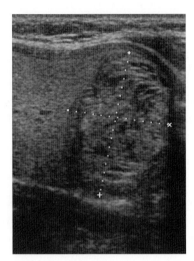

Fig. 6.2 Reproduced from Surgery (Oxford) Simo R and Leslie A Differential Diagnosis and Management of Neck Lumps. 2006;24: 319-22, with permission Elsevier

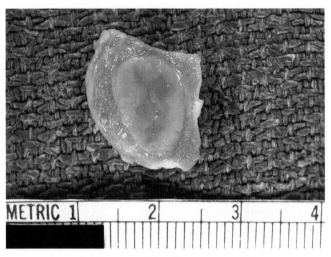

Fig. 6.4 With permission University of Alabama: Peter Anderson, *peir.net*

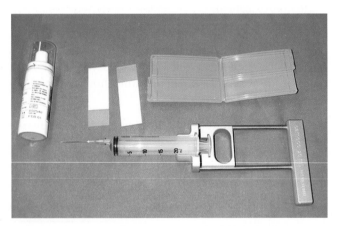

Fig. 6.3 Equipment for FNAC. Copyright RCSI with permission

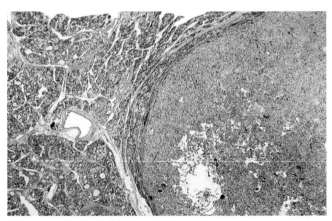

Fig. 6.5 H and E stained slide of benign follicullar adenoma With permission University of Alabama: Peter Anderson, *peir.net*

The pathologist reports the cytology as showing cells compatible with a follicular neoplasm, but he cannot say, if it is benign or malignant.

Question 1.14: What treatment would you advise for the patient?

Question 1.15: Write how you would explain to the patient what needs to be done.

Many hospitals now use formal written consent forms for the surgery. *Google: thyroidectomy patient consent form.*

Have a look at an example of the consent form actually used in hospital. It will give you the correct format to use.

Remember that as the house officer you may be called upon to explain the operation to the patient. By the time you have finished the surgery course you should be able to explain the basics of the common surgical operations.

The patient undergoes a R hemi-thyroidectomy.

The resected specimen is shown in Figure 6.4.

Question 1.16: Describe what do you see?

The histology shows a benign follicular adenoma.

Histology slide is shown in Figure 6.5.

Question 1.17: What will you tell the patient?

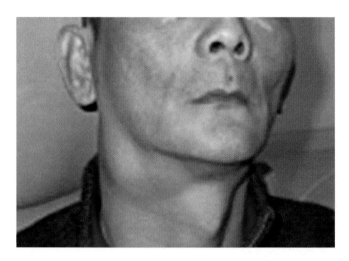

Fig. 6.6 Reprinted from Surgery (Oxford), Simo R and Leslie A, Differential diagnosis and management of neck lumps, 2006;24(9):312-22, with permission Elsevier

Question 2: Case scenario

A 55-year-old farm worker presents at the OP clinic with a swelling in the R side of his neck. He noticed it first about 4 months ago and says it has gradually been getting bigger. He thinks there may be some smaller lumps as well on the same side.

He says he has not been feeling very well recently, in that he has lost his appetite and lost 2 kg of weight in the last 2 months. As regards his past history, he has had no serious illnesses or operations. He is married and says his wife was in hospital last year with what he was told was an infection of the chest—she took a lot of pills and is better now. They live on a farm and have a lot of animals—cats and dogs. He smokes 20 cigarettes per day and he drinks a lot of whisky. The patient's neck is shown here in Figure 6.6.

Question 2.1: As you read this history: make a list of the differential diagnosis you are thinking about.

Question 2.2: Now make a list of the specific additional questions you will ask him—based on the history he has given.

Question 2.3: Make a list of what you will particularly look for on your physical examination.

The findings are as follows:

On examination, he is not cachexic. He has an obvious swelling in the right side of his neck.

His mucous membranes are slightly pale. He is not jaundiced. He has no obvious lesions in his mouth—in particular, he has no visible lesion on his tongue, or his fauces, and there are no obvious ulcers to see.

On examination of his neck, he has an enlarged firm lymph node in the right cervical chain. It is non-tender. He has no supraclavicular nodes. Abdominal examination is negative. Chest auscultation is negative.

Question 2.4: What investigations would you order?

His FBC, biochemical profile and LFTs are all normal.

His chest X-ray is normal.

His Mantoux test is negative.

Question 2.5: Would you ask for any other expert opinion? List here.

An ENT opinion is sought—their examination including direct flexible laryngoscope is negative. The surgeon puts his scope down the esophagus as well and says it is normal. So we have not got a diagnosis!!

Question 2.6: What will you do now?

Question 2.7: What two basic ways are there of getting this?

The fine needle aspiration cytology (FNAC) shows abnormal cells but no specific diagnosis.

Question 2.8: What will you do now?

Question 2.9: How would you stage the disease?

TUTORIAL 7: Nipple Discharge, Breast Lumps and Breast Pain

Patient 1: Blood-stained nipple discharge 1.

Patient 2: Blood-stained nipple discharge 2.

Patient 3: Painful breast swelling.

Patient 4: Young lady with mobile breast lump.

Patient 5: Pain and swelling in breast.

Patient 6: Soreness, retraction of nipple.

Patient 7: Soreness of nipple.

Patient 8: Mother's friend wants to know about breast screening.

This tutorial contains several shorter patient case histories.

Question 1: Before you start and without looking at your notes write out in full exactly how you would proceed with a breast examination. You should have been provided with a protocol for breast examination technique as recommended by your medical school—do it in this way (the sequence and details vary from textbook-to-textbook and doctor-to-doctor).

Question 2: Case scenario

> A 57-year-old lady presents at the breast clinic saying, she has noticed a blood-stained discharge from the nipple.

Question 2.1: What questions will you ask her?

When the lady is examined, gentle pressure on the areola produces the findings shown in Figure 7.1.

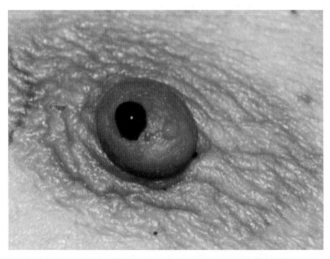

Fig. 7.1 From ABC of Breast Diseases, Dixon JM (Ed), 4th edn, 2012 with permission Wiley

The nipple discharge looks like blood but when dabbed on white gauze was dark green.

Question 2.2: What would you do?

The full breast examination is negative. Dipstick testing is negative for blood.

Question 2.3: What is your diagnosis?

Question 3: Case scenario

> This second patient again presents with a blood-stained discharge from the nipple. When gentle pressure is applied to the areola, a nipple discharge is produced which looks like blood. On this occasion, when dabbed on gauze it is bright red and tests heavily for blood on dipstick.

Question 3.1: What is your differential diagnosis?

Question 3.2: How would you manage this patient?

Question 4: Case scenario

> A 28-year-old girl who is breastfeeding her baby presents to her GP complaining of severe pain in her right breast, fever, and feeling very unwell.

When you examine her, these are the findings (Fig. 7.2).

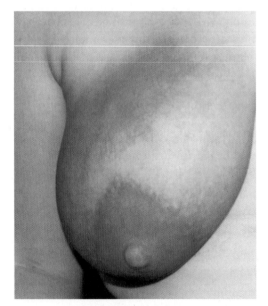

Fig. 7.2 From ABC of Breast Diseases Dixon JM (Ed), 4th edn, 2012 with permission Wiley

The diagnosis is obvious.

Question 4.1: List the clinical signs and symptoms of an abscess (anywhere).

Question 4.2: How would you manage this lady?

Question 5: Case scenario

A 17-year-old girl presents with a solitary, mobile swelling in her left breast.

You will remember this young girl from Module 1, Tutorial 11, Question 2: Case scenario. Look back and see what you have written. Just to make sure you have done that, please answer the questions here.

Question 5.1:
a. What are the clinical features of a fibroadenoma?
b. How would you confirm the diagnosis?
c. Is it acceptable to treat this young girl conservatively?

Question 6: Case scenario
You will recognize this history from Module 1, Tutorial 11, Question 3: Case scenario. Please review your notes. This is a second similar patient but with different clinical findings.

Mrs M is a 35-year-old premenopausal lady who comes complaining of pain in her breasts. She says she has had the pain on and off for 5 years but it is getting worse. It is most severe before her periods and goes away when her periods finish. Her breasts have become very lumpy, especially at period times. Five days ago, she noticed a big lump in her right breast while showering, which she had never felt before. The lump is slightly tender.
When you examine her, her breasts are lumpy throughout with marked thickening of the axillary tail on both sides. In the right breast, there is a discrete 2 cm diameter, smooth swelling which is slightly tender. This, she says, is the lump, she has noticed.

Question 6.1: You are her GP, what will you do with the patient?

The GP refers the patient to the General Surgery Breast Clinic at the hospital, where the surgeon confirms the GP's findings.

Question 6.2: What do you think the surgeon will do?

The surgeon cleans the area with a spirit swab and inserts a green needle into the swelling.

He aspirates 4 mL of green fluid.

Following this, the swelling is no longer palpable.

He reassures the patient—tells her it is a cyst and that the chances of it being anything more serious are very small. He tells her what she needs to have done next.

Question 6.3: What needs to be done?

Look at these mammograms, for practice, describe what you see and you can discuss the results with your tutor. It is NOT suggested you need to be able to read mammograms, we have specialized radiologists who are very good at this. Looking at these films will help you to a better understanding of the problems of benign and malignant breast diseases.

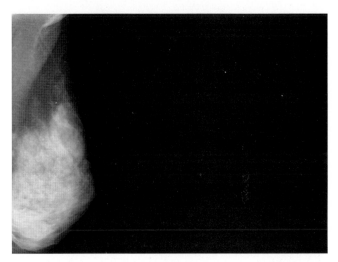

Fig. 7.3

Question 6.4: Describe the above mammogram (Fig. 7.3).

Question 6.5: What is the likely diagnosis in the mammogram in Figure 7.4 here:

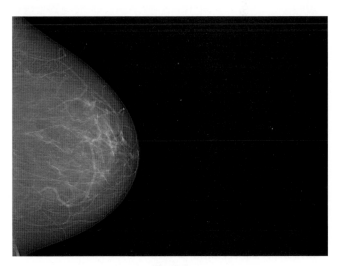

Fig. 7.4

Question 6.6: What is the likely diagnosis in the mammogram shown in Figure 7.5?

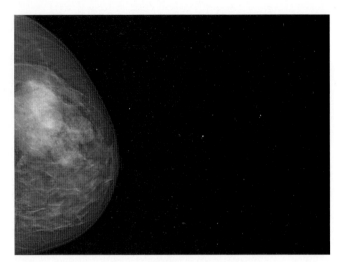

Fig. 7.5

Question 6.7: What is the likely diagnosis in this set of mammograms (Fig. 7.6)?

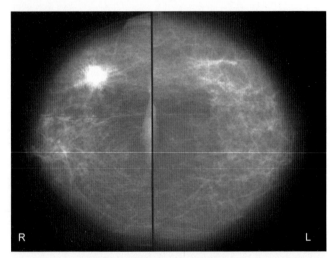

Fig. 7.6 Courtesy Dr Godfrey Geh

As you can see the mammograms are difficult to interpret. This is why we have specialist radiologists to read them. Most breast services have a multidisciplinary meeting where discussion can take place.

Question 6.8: Do you understand the importance of multidisciplinary team meetings (MDTs) in breast cancer management? Write below what you think it means:

Question 7: Case scenario

A 60-year-old lady complains of persistent greenish yellow discharge from her nipple. She has had quite a lot of pain around the nipple which she has noticed has retracted a little. She has noticed an 'opening' has appeared alongside the nipple.

Figure 7.7 shows the findings on breast inspection:

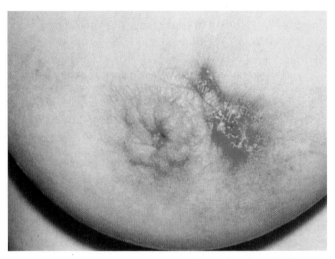

Fig. 7.7 From ABC Breast Diseases editor Dixon JM 4th ed, 2012, with permission Wiley

Question 7.1: Describe what you see.

Question 7.2: What is your diagnosis?

Question 7.3: What is mammary duct ectasia?

Question 8: Case scenario

This is an elderly patient who complains of some soreness of her nipple over the last 6 months.

The appearance of the nipple is shown below in Figure 7.8.

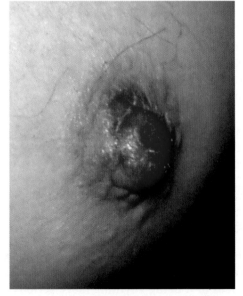

Fig. 7.8

Question 8.1: What is the differential diagnosis?

Question 8.2: If you were the GP what would you do? What would you say to the lady?

Question 9: Case scenario

Your friend's mother has seen on the TV that the Mobile Mammography Screening Van is visiting her town next week. She is 60 years of age and has had no breast problems and there is no FH. She wants to know what to do and because you are a medical student has asked for your advice.

Question 9.1: What will you say to her?

Question 9.2: Write a brief explanation of screening for breast cancer; why it is a suitable vehicle for screening, who is screened and what happens.

Question 9.3: What is shown in Figure 7.9?

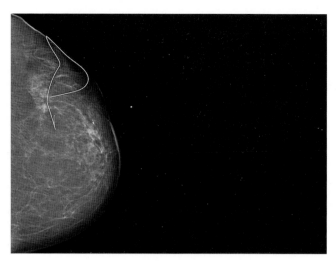

Fig. 7.9

TUTORIAL 8: Difficulty in Passing Urine (Prostate)

Question 1: Case scenario

Mr M is a 70-year-old gentleman who presents to the A and E Department saying that he cannot pass urine.

Question 1.1: What questions will you ask him to evaluate the history?

Question 1.2: In terms of 'urinary tract' symptoms how do you classify the various symptoms? Make a table/box.

Mr M says this is the first time he has been totally unable to pass urine. He had a lot of beer to drink at a party last night and has not passed urine for 6 hours. For the last 2 years, he has had difficulty in starting to pass urine: the flow has become poor. When he finishes, he wants to go again and notices that he leaks a little urine into his underwear. He passes urine every 2 hours in the daytime and has to get up twice at night now to pass urine. On one or two occasions, he has noticed a little dark blood in the urine when he has been straining. He is otherwise fit and well. He has not lost any weight and normally has no pain in his abdomen. At the moment, however, he has a lot of lower abdominal pain and feels as though he wants to pass urine but cannot.

Question 1.3: Based on this history what do you think is wrong with him?

Question 1.4: Define acute urinary retention.

Question 1.5: Define chronic urinary retention.

Question 1.6: List what findings you would expect to find in this man on physical examination.

Question 1.7: How do you do a rectal examination? Write a brief summary of how you would perform a rectal examination.

When Mr M is examined, he is in obvious discomfort but is well orientated. He is well nourished, well hydrated and is not anemic or jaundiced. Examination of his abdomen shows a large swelling in his lower abdomen which is dull to percussion and a little tender.

Question 1.8: What would you expect to find on rectal examination?

Pathology Revisited

Question 1.9: Draw a line drawing of the prostate and its zones.

Question 1.10: Which zone is affected in benign prostatic hypertrophy? Which zone is affected in prostatic cancer?

In Mr M's case the prostate feels large in both lobes, the median groove is palpable and the gland feels rubbery.

Question 1.11: So, what is your diagnosis?

Question 1.12: You are the house officer: describe how you would manage this patient with acute urinary retention.

Question 1.13: Describe how you would explain 'catheterization' to the patient. Answer in bullet points describing the exact practical steps you would take, in the sequence you would carry them out.

Question 1.14: What sorts of catheters are available—types, size, and material.

Question 1.15: You are going to catheterize this man. What type and size of catheter will you use?

Question 1.16: What will you do, if you cannot pass the catheter?

You get the catheter in successfully and proceed to decompress the bladder slowly.

Question 1.17: How and why do you do this?

The patient is now very comfortable and is very grateful to you.

Question 1.18: What will you tell the nurses to do?

Question 1.19: What investigations are you now going to order on this patient and why?

Question 1.20: Draw a diagram of the late anatomical consequences of prostatic obstruction.

Question 1.21: Make a bullet point list of how benign prostatic hypertrophy may be treated (in outline only).

Question 1.22: How would you manage the patient we have been considering here?

Question 2: Case scenario

A second patient presents to his GP with poor stream, frequency and nocturia. On examination of his prostate, the GP thinks it is malignant.

Question 2.1: List here the rectal findings suggestive of prostate cancer.

In patient 2, the GP describes the prostate as small and hard with irregular nodules in one lobe. He is referred to the OP clinic and you are the House Officer taking the presenting history. In addition to his urinary tract symptoms, he says he has felt unwell for months, has lost weight and has an ache in his back.

Question 2.2: What does this suggest to you?

Question 2.3: What investigations would you order? List here.

These are his investigation results: (Question 2.4 deals with the interpretation of the results of these investigations).

Full Blood Count:

Hb	8 g/dL	
PCV	50%	(n = 45–52%, M, 37–48%, F)
MCH	26	(n = 27–31pg)
MCV	70	(n = >80 fL)
MCHC	26	(n = 32–36%)
WCC	$10,000 \times 10^9$/L	
Platelets	300,000	(n = 150,000–400,000/cmm)

Question 2.4a: What do these FBC results indicate?

Urea and electrolytes:

Urea	20	n = 3–9.2 mmol/L
Na	128	n = 136–145 mmol/L
K^+	3.5	n = 3.5–5.0 mmol/L
Cl	98	n = 98–107 mmol/L
Creatinine	180	n = 53–115 umol/L

Question 2.4b: What do these electrolyte changes suggest?

LFTs		
Bilirubin	10 umol/L	n = 3–21
ALT	30 umol/L	n = 6–55
ALP	10 umol/L	n = 45
Total protein	70 g/L	n = 66–82
Albumin	40 g/L	n = 35–50
Globulin	30 g/L	n = 20–36
Calcium (total)	2.25 mmol/L	n = 2.12–2.65 mmol/L

Question 2.4c: What do you think of these LFTs and calcium results?

MSU: micro: >3 FBCs per high powered field. No growth on culture

PSA	56	(n = 0–4 ng/mL)

Question 2.4d: What does the MSU result suggest? What does this PSA indicate?

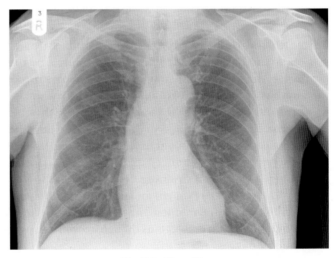

Fig. 8.3 Chest X-ray

Question 2.4e: Describe this X-ray (Fig. 8.3).

Lumbar spine and pelvis X-ray (see Fig 8.4).

Question 2.4f: Describe this X-ray (Fig. 8.4).

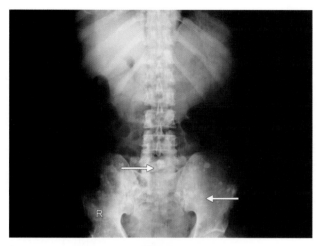

Fig. 8.4

Question 2.5: A trans-rectal US scan is performed on the patient. How is this scan done?

A trans-rectal ultrasound of a patient with a prostatic neoplasm is shown in Figure 8.5.

Multiple biopsies are taken.

Question 2.6: Discuss the histopathology of cancer of the prostate.

Question 2.7: What type of investigation is this and what does it show (Fig. 8.7)?

Finally, we are going to look at 2 further urological investigations (not belonging to Patient 2).

Question 2.8: What type of X-ray is this and how is it performed (Fig. 8.8)?

Question 2.9: Before the procedure is carried out what is a very important question that you ask the patient?

Question 2.10: What X-ray is this and what does it show? (Fig. 8.9)

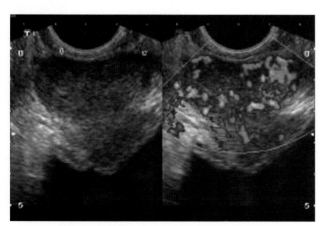

Fig. 8.5 Courtesy of Dr. Joe Anthony, India

LT

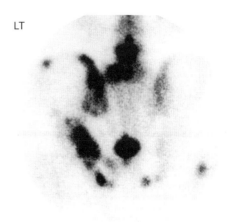

Posterior pelvis

Fig. 8.7 Reprinted from Surgery (Oxford) Prostate Cancer Kirby R and Madhaven S, 2010; 28(12):594-8, with permission from Elsevier

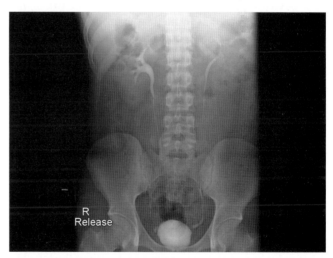

Fig. 8.8

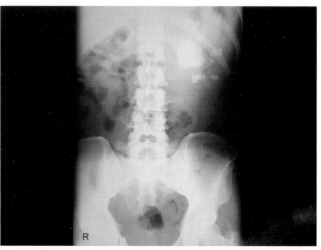

Fig. 8.9

TUTORIAL 9: Scrotal Swellings

Patient 1: Child with scrotal pain
Patient 2: Adult with scrotal pain
Patient 3: Adult with scrotal swelling

Question 1: Case scenario

> You are the houseman/intern on duty and are called to A and E to see a 14-year-old boy who is complaining of a pain in his right scrotum.

Question 1.1: What questions will you ask him?

The patient complains of the sudden onset 2 hours ago of severe pain in his scrotum. When questioned, he says it is on the right side. It is the worst pain he has ever had. It is severe, constant and makes him feel sick. He has vomited on 2 occasions. He says he also has pain in his lower abdomen. He says that in the last year, he has had pain in his scrotum on 2 occasions after he had been playing football, it was not as severe as this episode and went away after an hour. There is no history of trauma. He has had a feeling of wanting to pass urine frequently, since the pain started.

Question 1.2: At this stage, what is your differential diagnosis?

Question 1.3: What examination will you carry out?

Question 1.4: In the case, what specific signs will you be looking for?

On examination, the boy is in obvious pain. He is a little flushed and has a tachycardia of 100/min. He is tender in the right iliac fossa. On examination of the right scrotum, the skin looks red; the testis seems higher than the left side and on gentle palpation is very tender but has a horizontal lie. The left testis and scrotum are normal. Penis is normal.

Figure 9.1 shows a picture of the genitalia.

Question 1.5: What is your diagnosis now?

Question 1.6: You are the house officer, what will you do now?

Question 1.7: Will any investigations be necessary in this case?

Question 1.8: What will the surgical resident/medical officer do now?

Figure 9.2A is a picture of the findings at operation in a similar patient with left scrotal pain.

Question 1.9: What is the diagnosis?

Question 1.10: In this case, what will the surgeon do?

Question 1.11: What will he have to do in this case shown in Figure 9.3?

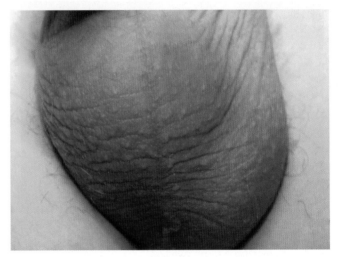

Fig. 9.1

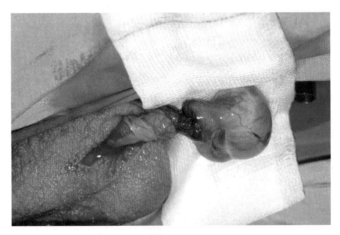

Fig. 9.2A

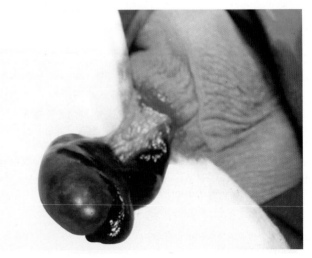

Fig. 9.3

Question 1.12: How much time do you have to get the patient to surgery?

A few relevant questions and facts:

Question 1.13a: Is there any place for attempted untwisting on the ward by manual detorsion?

Question 1.13b: Draw the testis and appendages in a normal anatomical situation.

Question 1.13c: Draw the anatomical arrangements when torsion is more likely to occur.

Question 2: Case scenario

You will remember this patient from Module 1, Tutorial 11, Question 2.

> A 58-year-old man presents at the surgical clinic saying that he has noticed his scrotum is becoming bigger. He first became aware of this about one year ago, although it may have been longer. The swelling has gradually increased in size and seems to affect only the left side. The swelling sometimes aches but there is no bad pain. He says he has come to the hospital because it is starting to get in the way when he rides his bicycle.
>
> The patient says the swelling never goes away and he cannot push it back. He has to get up in the night to pass urine in the last year which he did not do before. There is no history of trauma. His appetite is good and he has not lost any weight recently. He continues to work as a gardener, has had no serious illness and never been in hospital.

Question 2.1: What differential diagnosis is going through your mind before you examine him?

General, abdominal and inguino-scrotal examination is carried out.

Question 2.2: You made out a protocol for scrotal examination in Module 1: write this out again without looking back.

Figure 9.6 is a picture of the patient's scrotum.

On examination, inspection shows that there is swelling of the left scrotum which appears to extend up to the inguinal area. The right scrotum appears normal and there do not appear to be any inguinal or lower abdominal swellings. On palpation, it is possible to get above the swelling and define a normal spermatic chord above the swelling. The swelling measures 12 by 12 cm and is smooth; the shape is round. It is tense and not fluctuant. It is none tender. The testis is not palpable. It transilluminates.

The right scrotum is normal with a normal feeling testis and chord. There is no evidence of a hernia on either side and no palpable lymph nodes.

Question 2.3: What is your diagnosis now?

Question 2.4: (Anatomy—Basic science)

Draw the anatomy of a hydrocele and explain below the drawing what you understand by the term hydrocele.

Question 2.5: Do hydroceles occur at any other age than in adults?

Question 2.6: Draw a diagram of an infant hydrocele. Using *bullet points* only say how they present and their management.

Now back to Question 2: Case scenario

Question 2.7: Make a list here of the causes of a hydrocele in the adult.

Question 2.8: In this case, what is the likely diagnosis and why?

Question 2.9: If you are in doubt what investigation would you order to confirm the diagnosis?

Question 2.10: This is an ultrasound of the scrotum, what does it show (Fig. 9.9)?

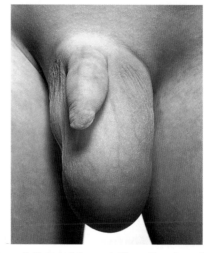

Fig. 9.6 From Bailey and Love, A Short Practice of Surgery, Ed. Williams N. Hodder, 2008. Reproduced by permission of Taylor and Francis Books, UK

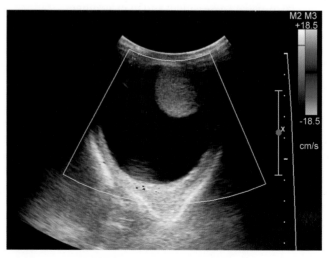

Fig. 9.9 Ultrasound scan of scrotum

Question 2.11: What treatment will you offer this patient?

Question 2.12: Name one operation used and make an outline drawing of the operation.

Question 2.13: The patient says he does not want surgery. Is there anything else you can offer?

Question 2.14: If you aspirate the fluid, then what will you do with it?

Question 2.15: Will you perform any other investigations in this patient?

Question 3: Case scenario

A 28-year-old man presents at the surgical clinic and says he has had a dull ache in his testis for about 3 months. It is getting worse. He has seen a notice in his GP's surgery about well-man screening, including feeling your own testes. He thinks his right testis is bigger and harder.

Question 3.1: What is Well Man Screening?

Back to our patient:

On examination, the right testis is firm, bigger than the left side and measures about 4 × 4 cm. There appears to be a small soft hydrocele. There are no nodes in the groins.

Question 3.2: What investigation will be the next step?

Look at the ultrasound in Figure 9.11.

The scan show a tumor of the right testis

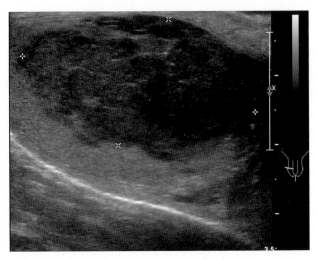

Fig. 9.11 Ultrasound scan of right tesis

Question 3.3: What other investigations will you perform?

Revision basic science

Question 3.4: Where do testicular tumors spread to?

Question 3.5: Write a simple staging system for testicular cancer:

Question 3.6: Write down the main histopathological types of testicular tumor (Pathology).

Question 3.7: Finally, write a short note on the tumor markers used to help diagnose the different types of testicular tumor.

TUTORIAL 10: Burns

Several short case studies of common burn scenarios are provided to help you with 'first aid' management as well as hospital in-patient assessment and management.

Question 1: Case scenario

A housewife, Mrs M, upset a pan of boiling water over her arm.

The injury is shown in Figure 10.1.

You are at home on holiday and your mother says you must come next door quickly and help Mrs M.

Question 1.1: What First Aid will you offer to Mrs M?

Mrs M then asks you to take her to the Accident Department of the hospital. She is quickly seen thereby the A and E doctor.

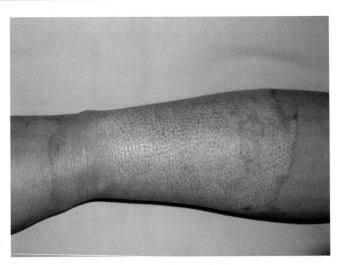

Fig. 10.1 Thermal burn of right arm

Question 1.2: What questions will the doctor ask Mrs M?

Mrs M says she was cooking some potatoes and upset the pan of boiling water over her right arm. She says she called for her next door neighbor who is a medical student, they ran cold water from the tap over the burn straight away. The medical student wrapped the arm loosely in a clean dry table cloth and brought her to hospital. She says the arm is very painful and throbs. Mrs M says that she is fit and healthy and has had no serious illnesses. She is not on any drugs.

Question 1.3: What will the doctor look for when she examines the patient?

Here is the burn again. Look at it (Fig. 10.2).

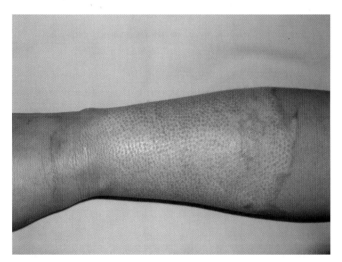

Fig. 10.2

Question 1.4: How do you assess the extent of a burn?

Question 1.5: What do you think is the extent of the burn in this case (Fig. 10.2)?

Question 1.6: How do you classify the depth of a burn?

Question 1.7: What is the depth of the burn in this case (Fig. 10.2)?

Question 1.8: Draw a diagram of the structures of the skin and burn-depth involved.

Question 1.9: Now make out a simple table to help you with deciding clinically the depth of a burn.

Illustrations are given below, to help you with this: [After Rawlins: Surgery, Oxford: 2011;29(10):523]

Superficial (epidermal): Red such as sunburn. Do not blister and have normal capillary refill and normal sensation. Heal normally and do not scar. Not included when calculating size of burn (*see* Fig. 10.5).

Partial thickness—superficial: Involve the epidermis and superficial part of dermis, very painful, capillary return is

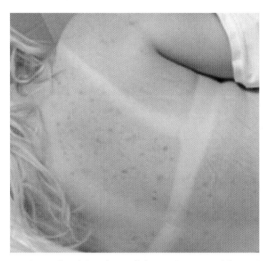

Fig. 10.5 Superficial (epidermal) burn. Reprinted from Surgery (Oxford), Rawlins JM, Management of burns, 2011:29(10):523-8, with permission from Elsevier

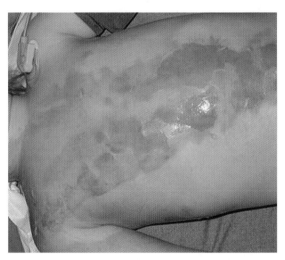

Fig. 10.6 Partial thickness—superficial burn. Reprinted from Surgery (Oxford), Rawlins JM, Management of burns, 2011:29(10): 523-8, with permission from Elsevier

brisk, characteristic is blistering—when this bursts or is separated the exposed papillary dermis is pink (*see* Fig. 10.6).

Partial thickness—deep: Extensive blistering which ruptures early exposing the deep damaged reticular dermis, may be pale white due to damaged blood vessels or red due to RBC extravasations—hence blotchy appearance, hallmark is diminished, capillary return with sluggish blanching (*see* Fig. 10.7).

Full thickness: White or black, leathery to touch. No capillary blanching and nontender (*see* Fig. 10.8).

Question 1.10: Write the reason why we assess the depth and area of the burns.

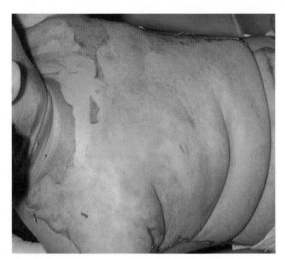

Fig. 10.7 Partial thickness—deep burn. Reprinted from Surgery (Oxford), Rawlins JM, Management of burns, 2011:29(10):523-8, with permission from Elsevier

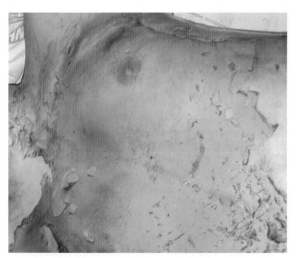

Fig. 10.8 Full thickness burn. Reprinted from Surgery (Oxford), Rawlins JM, Management of burns, 2011:29(10):523-8, with permission from Elsevier

Question 1.11: What treatment and follow-up will the doctor arrange for Mrs M?

Question 2: Case scenario

A 60-year-old man is brought by ambulance to the A and E Department, having been badly burned in a house fire. He was found unconscious in his bedroom and was thought to have been smoking in bed.
When examined in the A and E Department he is unconscious—he does not react to verbal commands but reacts to painful stimuli. He has no accompanying relatives.

His pulse is 140/min, BP 140/90, RR 25 per minute and O_2 saturation 90%. He has burns involving his back, buttocks and both his arms. There are burns involving all his face with blackening of the skin and charring of his hair and nasal hairs. Examination of his oropharynx with a laryngoscope shows redness and edema.

You are the Casualty Officer in A and E Department.

Question 2.1: In this patient, what will you do first? Describe in detail.

On inspection, the burns involve the whole of his face and back of his head, half of his back, and the whole of his right arm and leg.

Question 2.2: What is the estimated area of his burn?

The burns on his face are blistered and red.
The burns on his arms and legs are similar.

Question 2.3: What is the likely depth of these burns?

The burns on his back and buttocks show red and blistered areas but also defined white areas and also some areas of black skin.

Question 2.4: What is the likely depth of these burns?

Question 2.5: How does the surface area of the burn relate to the seriousness of the burn?

Question 2.6: While you are resuscitating the patient would you leave the burns open?

You are the doctor assigned to look after the patient in the ICU.

Question 2.7: How would you calculate his fluid requirements and what fluid would you give?

Question 2.8: What local treatment would you advise for the burns?

Question 2.9: You continue to look after this patient—list the likely complications which may occur:

Question 3: Case scenario

This 40-year-old burned his hand and arm on boiling fat (see Fig. 10.9).

Question 3.1: What is the depth of the burn and why?

Question 3.2: How would you treat it?

Question 4: Case scenario

This patient received this burn while plugging a hair dryer into a faulty socket (see Fig. 10.10).

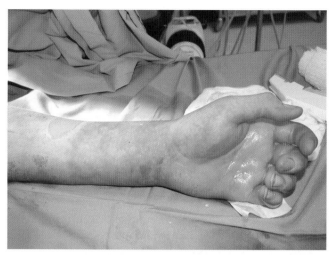

Fig. 10.9 Thermal burn of left hand and arm. With permission of Alfred Health Burns Unit, Melbourne, Australia

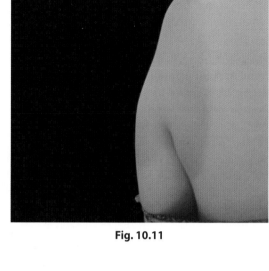

Fig. 10.11

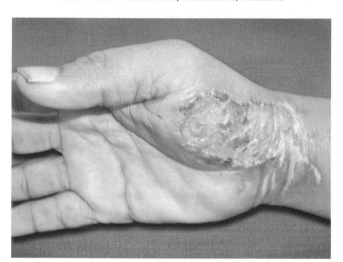

Fig. 10.10

Question 4.1: What classification of burn will it be? What will be the depth?

Question 5: Case scenario

Question 5.1: What sort of burn do you think this is and how would you treat it (Fig. 10.11)?

If you want to read more about burns and their management, I suggest you download the Victorian State Burns Clinical Guidelines from the Alfred Health Burns Unit in Melbourne, Australia *(www.alfred.org.au/burns_unit/)*.

Question 5.2: Finally, because it may be very helpful, make out a box containing *bullet points* summarizing the first aid treatment of a patient with burns.

TUTORIAL 11: Fluid and Electrolyte Balance

Most medical students and many postgraduates (juniors and seniors) have a fear of fluid and electrolyte balance because they never really understood the teaching they received. I think it would be true to say that the chapters in the standard textbooks are not a great deal of help, mainly because they are too complicated.

The Directed Self-learning Tutorials on Fluid and Electrolyte Balance in Module 2 and Module 3 are aimed at providing the knowledge and understanding for the house surgeon to be able to competently and confidently handle the common fluid and electrolyte problems he or she will come across. They are not aimed at enabling them to either understand or deal with complex electrolyte or acid-base problems.

Before you start this tutorial you must put time aside to carefully study and understand 4 articles which will provide you with the necessary core knowledge.

It is suggested that you put all your time and energy into these articles rather than devoting time to the textbooks.

It will be good practice for you to search these articles yourself via the internet. If you are having problems do approach your medical school librarian who will be glad to help.

First read and evaluate:

1. Roe P. *Peri-operative Fluid Management: Surgery 1998;16(7):165-8* [*Note:* This is from the British Journal 'The Medicine Publishing Company', sometimes listed as Surgery (Oxford) not the US Surgery journal].

2. Davidson T. ***Essentials of fluid balance 1***. Assessing patients' requirements. sBMJ. 1994;2:317-9 (sBMJ is the Student British Medical Journal)

3. Davidson T. ***Essentials of fluid balance 2***. Surgical patients. sBMJ. 1994;2:364-6.

Then read the publication:

4. ***British Consensus Guidelines on Intravenous Fluid Therapy for Adult Surgical patients***
   Powell Tuck J et al 2008: BAPEN Medical, 2008
   www.bapen.org.uk/pdfs/bapen_pubs/giftasup.pdf
   (omit pages 2-9, 27-39 for the purposes of this tutorial)

This looks a daunting article but it is very well written. Spend 2 hours reading and understanding the content and then make a list of the main conclusion/recommendations of the document.

Note: The recommendations in some cases are different to the conventional teaching and practice of 'surgical' fluid and electrolyte management but will mean you are up-to-date—even though some 'older doctors' you encounter may not be!!

Question 1: Make a list of your own main recommendations from the British Consensus Guidelines—do not immediately copy out those listed in the article—think and make your own.

Finally, in preparation for the tutorial, read this author's summary of the 4 articles which follows:

FLUID AND ELECTROLYTE BALANCE IN THE PERIOPERATIVE PATIENT

Basic Physiology

70 kg man = 60% body water = 42 liters—distributed in three compartments
   1. Intracellular
   2. Interstitial ⎤
   3. Intravascular (plasma) ⎦ extracellular

In Health

ECF compartment size is controlled by homeostatic control of tonicity (effective osmotic pressure) (*see* Fig 11.1).

Total amount of Na ions determines ECF volume, so the volume and volume control is via mechanisms controlling retention or excretion of Na (volume receptors in circulation and renal mechanisms). Tonicity is controlled by osmo receptors which affect thirst and AVP (argentine vasopressin).

The interstitial compartment is separated from the intravascular compartment by the capillary membrane (microvascular endothelium). Flow across here is decided by hydrostatic (colloids) and osmotic pressures. There is free flow of water and electrolytes but the membrane is relatively impermeable to proteins.

The Intracellular compartment: The principle ion of the ICF is the potassium ion (K^+). Fluid flux at cell membrane depends on osmotic forces generated by the ions. ICF volume is sensitive to the Na concentration of ECF, hypernatremia causes cell shrinkage and hyponatremia cell swelling.

WHY DO WE NEED TO KNOW THESE FACTS?

Because the compartments may be altered by surgery and anesthesia as follows:

1. *Capillary (microvascular) membrane:* Surgery and illness make the membrane 'leaky'; histamine, bradykinins, leukotrienes, platelet factors, endotoxins and tumor necrosis factors are involved. The leaky capillaries result in passage of colloid into the interstitial space (hydrostatic pressure becomes more important than oncotic pressure). The interstitial compartment has 2 subcompartments, parenchymal and loose CT, fluid overflows into this normally dry compartment. The lymphatics cannot deal with its removal and it accumulates as edema (3rd space).

2. *Cell membrane:* Abnormal concentrations of Na in ECF will alter the size of the ICF by osmosis. Also the Na/K pump which controls the ionic gradient at the cell membrane is affected by sepsis/shock (sick cell syndrome).

3. Alteration in size of compartments by anesthesia. General and epidurals cause vasodilation, so the intravascular space is underfilled (hypovolemia).
   Vasodilation occurs when patient warms up after anesthesia—require extra fluid in intravascular space.

4. Third space sequestration causes increase in ECF but with depletion of intravascular space.
   Alteration in intake and output cause overall fluid deficits:

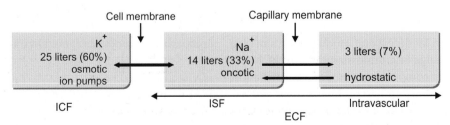

Fig. 11.1 Body fluid compartments

Fluid is lost from the intravascular compartment in

- Hemorrhage
- Burns.

Fluid is also lost by:

- Vomiting
- Diarrhea (fluid that would normally have been reabsorbed)
- Fistulae
- Ileus (large volumes of fluid stay in intestinal lumen).

Consequences:

1. Loss of plasma volume results in net move from ISF into plasma.
2. Tissue damage results in 3rd space loss and into sick cells with net loss of intravascular and ISF volume.
3. Loss of Na and water from gastrointestinal and renal causes results in a reduced intravascular volume and ISF and, because Na levels in ECF are raised, cause a reduction in ICF volume.

The concept of the 3rd space is not well explained in most textbooks but an understanding of the concept is necessary for the management of fluid and electrolyte balance—what follows may be an over-simplification of a complex physiological situation but, hopefully suffices from the practical point of view.

THE THIRD SPACE: A WORKING EXPLANATION

The third space is a 'physiological compartment' which lies within the interstitial fluid compartment. When the blood vessel walls become damaged by surgical trauma and handling, inflammation (bacterial and viral), sepsis or burns the capillary membrane is damaged and fluid 'leaks' into the interstitial space—entering the so-called 'third space', i.e. it is a consequence of increased capillary permeability.

The fluid enters the normally dry loose connective tissue between the cells causing edema of the tissues, or it may enter the normally nearly dry cavities of the peritoneum or pleura. In intestinal obstruction or gut inflammation large volumes of fluid enter the intestinal lumen and this is also regarded as a "third space" loss. The distinguishing feature of a third space loss is that the fluid is sequestrated away from the normal intravascular-interstitial-intracellular ionically driven fluid exchange. The fluid does not pass back into the intravascular compartment until the underlying pathological cause or 'illness' is recovering. In the case of surgical trauma this is usually over the course of two or three days.

WHAT TO DO ABOUT IT?

Because the extent of 'third spacing' is not known or accurately quantifiable, it is not possible to give a figure for the fluid volume needed to replete the loss. However, as the effect of third spacing is to pull fluid out of the intravascular space and cause hypovolemia, replacement in the intravascular compartment with crystalloid/colloid will help in the short-term. The real treatment for 'third spacing' is to treat the underlying pathological process. Note that although the patient may be edematous and therefore appear fluid overloaded, they may still be 'dehydrated' in the intravascular space due to the 'third spacing', so aggressive diuresis should be avoided.

Look at ***Overview: Third spacing*** *http://www.wikidoc. org/index.php/Third_spacing_of_fluids.*

APPLIED PHARMACOLOGY

The aim of fluid and electrolyte balance is to make sure the volume and components of the three body compartments are kept 'normal.'

Different types of fluids will distribute in the ECF and ICF in different ways. You must know the basics of which fluids to use to replete the three body compartments:

Colloids stay in the intravascular space, exert an oncotic pressure at the microvascular membrane and pull ISF into the plasma. This effect is temporary and varies with different colloid preparations.

Crystalloids are solutions of ions (e.g. 0.9N saline) or small sugars (5% dextrose) that are iso-osmotic with plasma. They pass freely through the microvascular membrane. After IV administration, their distribution depends on their Na concentration-isotonic solutions of Na stay in the ECF space (plasma 20%, ISF 80%). If Na content is less than isotonic they have 'free water' that can also pass into the ICF, e.g. 4% glucose/0.18N saline is 20% normal saline and 80% water. 5% dextrose has no sodium content; its osmotic pressure is maintained by the sugar. It acts as 'free water' and distributes through all three compartments (plasma 8%, ISF 32% and ICF 60%).

Table 11.1 lists the contents of some of the most commonly used intravenous solutions you will be prescribing as a house surgeon:

What does all this really mean in practical terms?

1. If the acute loss is from the intravascular compartment (e.g. bleeding) you can give a crystalloid solution but it will not stay in the intravascular compartment for long, so you need to use a colloid and then, if necessary, blood or blood components.
2. The other fluid replacements will depend on what has been lost, i.e. you should try and replace like with like e.g. sweating and other insensible loss is 'water' so replace with dextrose 5%, gastrointestinal losses are mainly

Table 11.1 Most commonly used intravenous solutions							
Type of fluid	Water (mmol)	Na (mmol)	K (mmol)	Cl (mmol)	Ca (mmol)	HCO₃ (mmol)	Sugar
1 liter							
0.9 saline	1 L	153	—	153	—	—	—
5% dextrose	1 L	—	—	—	—	—	50 g
Hartmann's sol	1 L	130	5	111	2	29	—
Haemaccel	1 L	145	5	145	6	(+ polygeline 35 g)	
PPF	500 mL	70	0.1	70	—	(+ protein 25 g 95% albumin)	

replaced by 'balanced' electrolyte solutions which contain Na ions and free water and distribute accordingly. For 3rd space losses use same 'balanced' solutions.

So let us look at what you will be doing as a house surgeon:

In all situations, i.e. preoperatively, during the operation and postoperatively:

1. Correct pre-existing deficits
2. Continue maintainance requirements
3. Replace on going losses

Look first at the pre-operation situation: the patient may present with a fluid deficit because of:

Decreased intake, i.e. not drinking

Increased output: Vomiting

Diarrhea

Bowel preparation

Loss into peritoneal cavity and gut (e.g. obstruction/ peritonitis)

Hemorrhage.

HOW DO YOU DECIDE IF THEY ARE FLUID DEPLETED?

- History and clinical examination
- Circulating volume measurement, e.g. CVP/esophageal US
- Fluid balance charts.

Table 11.2 summarizes how to estimate the type of loss and its likely amount.

Note: This table, you will remember, comes from the 'consensus document'.

WHAT TO GIVE?

Should try and replace the loss with a rehydration fluid similar to the fluid lost, e.g. use Hartmann's solution in isotonic and hyponatremic dehydration where both Na and water have been lost, e.g. small bowel content vomiting/diarrhea, or use 0.9% saline to replace gastric content vomiting or aspiration.

For blood loss, use colloid initially and then, if necessary blood products.

Table 11.3 is a useful table from the consensus document. Use as a reference, do not try and remember any more than the guidelines given immediately above.

Note: In elderly, cardiac and renal cases do not give fluids very quickly (up to 48 hours, if possible).

HOW MUCH?

This will depend on your estimate of the amount of fluid lost, using clinical parameters, volume measurements and the fluid balance chart. If the deficit is severe, e.g. peritonitis/ obstruction, the patient will benefit from being in a high dependency situation or ICU. They may need:

- CVP
- Urinary catheter
- Esophageal US
- Arterial line.

As advised in the consensus document, the 'fluid bolus' technique is used for replacement. Provided, there is no obvious cardiac/renal problem—give a 250 mL bolus of Hartmann's, see what effect this has on general condition, CVP and urine output and continue with 250 mL boluses until clinical signs of dehydration/volume measurements/urine output are corrected.

If after giving the fluid bolus, the CVP rises and then shortly after falls again the patient is still fluid depleted. If CVP rises and stays high the patient is overfilled. If CVP rises and then falls gradually to target level the patient is likely rehydrated.

Clearly, as an inexperienced house officer/intern, you will seek help from the more senior surgeon/anesthetist/ intensivist in a situation like this.

THE POSTOPERATIVE SITUATION

The patient is going to require MAINTENANCE fluids, and if indicated REPLACEMENT fluids.

Postoperatively, the patient may need rehydration, if he has been in theater for a long time and has not had adequate MAINTENANCE/REPLACEMENT.

Table 11.2 Assessment and monitoring of fluid balance—from perioperative intravenous fluid guidelines. British Consensus Guidelines (Bapen) with permission

Parameter	Significance
History	Alerts to likelihood of fluid deficit (e.g. vomiting/diarrhea/hemorrhage) or excess (e.g. from intraoperative fluids)
Weighing	24-hour change in wight (performed under similar conditions)—best measure of change in water balance. Simple to carry out by bedside.
Fluid balance charts	Inherent inaccuracies in measurement and recording. Does not measure insensible loss. Large cumulative error over several days. Good measure of changes in urine output, fistula loss, gastric aspirate, etc.
Urine output	<30 mL/hour is commonly used as indication for fluid infusion, but in the absence of other features of intravascular hyovolemia is usually due to the normal oliguric response to surgery. Urine quality (e.g. urine: plasma urea or osmolality ratio) is just as important, particularly in the complicated patient.
Blood pressure	Cuff measurements may not always correlate with intra-arterial monitoring. Does not necessarily correlate with flow. Affected by drugs, etc. Nonetheless, a fall is compatible with intravascular hypovolemia, particularly, when it correlates with other parameters such as pulse rate, urine output, etc.
Capillary refill	Slow refill compatible with, but not diagnostic of volume deficit. Can be influenced by temperature and peripheral vascular disease.
Autonomic responses	Pallor and sweating, particularly, when combined with tachycardia, hypotension and oliguria are suggestive of intravascular volume deficit, but can also be caused by other complications, e.g. pulmonary embolus or myocardial infarction.
Skin turgor	Diminished in salt and water depletion, but also caused by aging, cold and wasting.
Dry mouth	Usually, due to mouth-breathing, but compatible with salt and water depletion.
Shunken facies	May be due to starvation or wasting from disease, but compatible with salt and water depletion.
Serum biochemistry	Indicates ratio of electrolytes to water in the extracellular fluid and is a poor indicator of whole body sodium status. Hyponatremia most commonly caused by water excess. If change in water balance over 24 hours is known, then change in serum sodium concentration can guide sodium balance. Hypokalemia nearly always indicates the need for potassium supplementation. Blood bicarbonate and chloride concentrations measured on point of care blood gas machines are useful in patients with acid-base problems including iatrogenic hyperchloremia.
Urine biochemistry	Urine sodium concentration reflects renal perfusion and a low value (<20 mmol/L) indicates renal hypoperfusion. Measurement of urine sodium allows assessment of postoperative sodium mobilization. Urine potassium measurement is helpful in assessing the cause of refractory hypokalemia. Urine urea exation increases several fold in catabolic states (e.g. sepsis) and is an indication for provision of additional free water to avoid hypernatremia and uremia.

Table 11.3 Composition of some bodily secretions. From British Consensus Guidelines (Bapen) with permission

Body secretion	Na^+ (mmol/L)	K^+ (mmol/L)	Cl^- (mmol/L)	HCO_3^- (mmol/L)	Volume (L/24 hr)
Saliva	2–85	0–20	16–23	14	0.5–15
Gastric juice	20–60	14	140	0–15	2–3
Pancreatic juice	125–138	8	56	85	0.7–2.5
Bile	145	5	105	30	0.6
Jejunal juice	140	5	135	8	—
Ileal juice	140	5	125	30	—
Ileostomy (adapted)	50	4	25	—	0.5
Colostomy	60	15	40	—	0.1–0.2
Diarrhea	30–140	30–70	—	20–80	Variable
Normal stool	20–40	30	—	—	0.1–0.25
Sweat (pilocarpine)	47–60	9	30–40	0–35	0.5 + variable
Visible sweat	58	10	45	—	0.5

How are you going to judge the degree of fluid replacement necessary?

You will need to access the following data:

1. Fluid loss in theater and the replacement in theater and the recovery room (from the surgeon's operation note and the anesthetic records).

2. Clinical signs—pulse/BP/skin turgor (see Table 11.2)—Assessment and monitoring of fluid and electrolyte balance plus also CVP and urine output.
   (*Note:* Which may be altered by cardiac status and the metabolic response to surgery).

3. The input-output charts from recovery and those started when the patient returns to the ward.

4. If required, and available, more sophisticated methods of estimating circulating fluid volume—Esophageal Doppler (usually used preoperatively), arterial pressure lines and Swan Ganz catheter (now rarely used).

5. Daily weight (a weight gain of greater than 1 kg a day almost certainly indicates fluid retention).

POSTOPERATIVE MAINTENANCE REQUIREMENTS

Average 70 kg man in temperate climate: normal daily water loss is:

Urine	1500 mL	
From skin	600 mL	insensible loss
Lungs	400 mL	
Feces	100 mL	
	= 2,600 mL water per day	

Note: The insensible loss from the skin is water and should be replaced as such. Sweating is a different loss (which most people do not appreciate)—it can increase fluid loss by up to 1 liter per hour and contains a significant amount of sodium (20–70 mmol/L) and potassium (10 mmol/L).

He also loses electrolytes with this water:

Sodium 70–110 mmol per day

Potassium 60–80 mmol per day

He normally replaces these losses by eating/thirst mechanisms as:

Fluids	1300	
Solids	1000	
Metabolism	300	= total 2,600

But, if he is on nil-by-mouth (NBM) he will need daily maintenance replaced intravenously:

2600 water

70–110 mmol of Na and 60–80 mmol of K

You may remember this by the simple mnemonic:

2:1:1

2 liters water + 1 mmol/kg Na + 1 mmol/kg K

The consensus guidelines suggest 1.5–2·5 liters maintenance fluid. 2.5 liters would be for a healthy 70 kg man—most patients are less than 70 kg and are not healthy. It is therefore suggested that you use 2 liters as the basic maintenance requirement.

BUT REMEMBER THIS

1. If ambient temperature is high, or the patient has a fever or is tachypneic or hypermetabolic, he/she will lose more water, which will need replacing:

   Fever : Add 10% of total insensible loss for each degree above 37°C

   Sweating : Add 10–15 %

   Hyperventilating : Add 25–50%

   Hypermetabolic : Add 25–75%

   Less fluid needed, if patient is humidified or ventilated.

2. The patient's MAINTENANCE requirements are altered by the metabolic response to surgery: catabolic phase 3–5 days: Involves adrenaline/noradrenaline/cortisol/adrenocorticotrophic hormones, aldosterone and antidiuretic hormones.

   Net result is Na and water retention and potassium excretion (by aldosterone). The antidiuretic hormone (ADH) prevents water excretion by the kidney but K is released by cell injury and damage.

   This means that in the first 3–5 days postoperative you do not need to give the full maintenance amounts of water, sodium and potassium.

   More patients suffer from inappropriate overload than dehydration.

   May only need to give: 500 mL Hartmann's (60 mmol Na; 2.5 mmol K) 1000 mL Dextrose 5% or even just 'water' alone

   As has been highlighted in the 'consensus document', the big danger is in giving too much water and sodium, i.e. 'drowning in salt water.'

   This may happen, if you employ the much used conventional 1 liter 0.9N saline and 2 liters dextrose 5% 8 hourly bottles.

   This has now led to 0.9N saline being replaced by Hartmann's solution as the maintenance/replacement fluid of choice in most situations.

REPLACEMENT LOSSES

Postoperatively, some patients will require much more than the 2–2.5 liters of fluid for maintenance. Any additional fluid is regarded as 'replacement'. The additional loss may be because of any of following:

1. So-called 3rd space losses = fluid loss at site of injury in major abdominal surgery/trauma – discussed previously (usually use Hartmann's solution).
2. Vomiting of gastric contents or gastric aspirate from nasogastric tube (use 0.9 N saline).
3. Small bowel content aspiration in obstruction/ileus (use Hartmann's).
4. Diarrhea or high ileostomy output (use Hartmann's).
5. Fistulae—gastric/small bowel/biliary/pancreatic/fecal (usually Hartmann's).

Remember that replacement losses may need additional electrolytes depending on the type of fluid loss, e.g. vomiting/aspiration of gastric juice: potassium supplementation diarrhea/ileostomy effluent: potassium supplementation.

HOW DO YOU DECIDE HOW MUCH REPLACEMENT THE PATIENT NEEDS?

By assessing:

1. Clinical condition
2. Input/output chart
3. Urine output
4. Daily electroytes
5. Sometimes urine osmolarity

An additional helpful Figure and Table from Concensus Document are shown in Figure 11.2 and Table 11.4.

In the next section, we are going to consider some practical examples of dealing with fluid and electrolyte balance which you will encounter as a house officer/intern.

DO THE FOLLOWING

- Obtain a copy of the FBC and bioprofile request form from your hospital and note the normal values.
- Obtain a copy of the input/output chart from the hospital where you are working and familiarize yourself with it—it is going to be an important part of your life.
- Look at the IV fluid/drug prescription chart so that you know where to write-up the fluid balance instructions.
- Please remember, these should be written legibly and without abbreviations and that crystalloid solutions are given in 500 mL/liter bags not pints.

Familiarize yourself with the crystalloid/colloid solutions which are used in the hospital attachment where you are. In this tutorial, we are going to use only Hartmann's solution (Ringer lactate), 5% dextrose and 0.9 N saline—there are good reasons for this—it means you are using the solutions recommended by the new guidelines, it simplifies matters and can prevent fatal errors of mismanagement. If on the rare occasions you need a different, more complex solution, it means you have to ask for it (and it is not just lying around to be given in error).

Now try and answer the tutorial as far as possible without looking up the answers, then redo it after doing the necessary reading.

Question 2: Write down the parameters measured in:
a. Urea and electrolytes
b. A chemical bioprofile—used in most UK hospitals
c. Blood gases.

Include the normal values, because although these are usually provided you should have a working knowledge of the common parameters without having to look at the normal values each time. Remember that normal values will differ slightly from laboratory to laboratory.

Table 11.4 Typical properties of commonly used intravenous solutions (British Consensus Guidelines (Bapen) with permission)

Type of fluid	Sodium (mmol/L)	Potassium (mmol/L)	Chloride (mmol/L)	Osmolarity (mOsm/L)	Weight average (Mol Wt kD)	Plasma volume expansion duration (hrs)
Plasma	136–145	3.5–5.0	98–105	280–300	—	—
5% dextrose	0	0	0	278	—	—
Dextrose 4% saline 0.18%	30	0	30	283		
0.9% 'normal' saline	154	0	154	308	—	0.2
0.45% 'half normal' saline	77	0	77	154	—	
Ringer's lactate	130	4	109	273	—	0.2
Hartmann's	131	5	111	275	—	0.2
Gelatine 4%	145	0	145	290	30,000	1–2
5% albumin	150	0	150	300	68,000	2–4
20% albumin	—	—	—	—	68,000	2–4
HES 6% 130/0.4	154	0	154	308	130,000	4–8
HES 10% 200/0.5	154	0	154	308	200,000	6–12
HES 6% 450/0.6	154	0	154	308	450,000	24–36

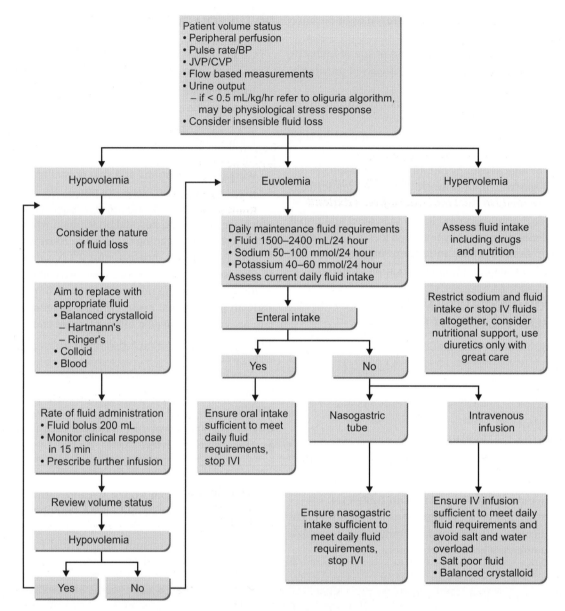

Fig. 11.2 Guidelines for fluid therapy: with permission Bapen
Abbreviations: JVP, jugular venous pressure; CVP, central venous pressure; IVI, intravenous infusion

Question 3: Write down below the water and electrolyte composition of:
a. Hartmann's solution (Ringer lactate): 1 liter
b. 0.9 N saline: 1 liter
c. 5% dextrose: 1 liter
d. Haemaccel: 1 liter
e. PPF: 1 liter

Question 4: Write down exactly how you would give a patient the following supplements: both orally and IV.

Note: These medications are from the British National Formulary (BNF) and may be different from the names and

preparations in other countries, you must always check the local formulary.
a. Potassium
b. Calcium
c. Magnesium
d. Bicarbonate

Question 5: Write the normal body fluid and electrolyte losses for a 70-kg man over a 24-hour period and how you would replace them (*Note:* This is MAINTENANCE), if the patient was on no oral intake.

How would this alter, if the patient was fevered/sweating/hyperventilating (hypermetabolic).

Question 6: What urine output do you want to achieve?

Remember that the urine output is not the major source of fluid output in the normal situation.

About 7 liters per day are excreted into the GI tract and all but about 100 mL are reabsorbed.

Question 7: In vomiting and diarrhea what will you replace the loss with?

Question 8: In pyloric stenosis, is it any different?

Question 9: What about small bowel and biliary fistulae?

We are now ready to start the house officer's duties!!!

Question 10: Case scenario

Mr Mann comes back to the high dependency unit after a routine anterior resection of his rectum for cancer. He has a covering loop ileostomy. He has an IV line in place in his left cubital fossa and a jugular CVP line. He has a urinary catheter in place and is on oxygen. No nasogastric tube. He is drowsy but is responding to verbal commands. The nurses have put him on a 'dinamap'—continuous monitoring of pulse/BP/CVP/ECG/oxygen saturation.

The anesthetist was called to ICU and has not written up his postoperative fluids and the nurses ask you, the house officer, to write them up.

Question 10.1: Describe in detail the practical process that you would go through in assessing his fluid requirements:

His pulse is 90/minute
BP 120/80
CVP + 5
Temperature 38°C
He has received 2 liters of Hartmann's solution in theater and the recovery bay and 500 mL haemaccel in theater. He has not received any blood. Total losses in theater = 400 mL blood.

Urine output from recovery 50 mL per hour.
OP note: 1. **Routine anterior resection with covering ileostomy**
2. **Pelvic corrugated drain (now used less and less)**
3. **IV fluids and medications as charted**
4. **Full operative note dictated**

Question 10.2: What readings and charts will the nurses have put him on?

Question 10.3: What instructions will you write-up for him, including IV fluids? Use Chart 11.1 Daily intravenous fluid-order chart seen on page 144.

(If you are using the text in hard back format, you can scan the charts and print them off or draw them onto a separate piece of paper. If you are using e-version, you can download and print off. *Note:* This applies to all the charts which appear in this tutorial and in Module 3, Tutorial 13. Remember this is what you will be doing as a house officer so take the trouble to do it as instructed.)

The same patient is reviewed by you and the Specialist Registrar on the next morning ward round, i.e. the patient is now postoperative day 1.
You look at the patient's
Input/output chart: Chart 11.3 (shown on page 145)
Routine readings chart
Last nights' U and Es and FBC

Hb	**9 g/dL**
WCC	**11000 ($\times 10^3$ u/L)**
Urea	**14 mmol/L**
Na	**132 mmol/L**
K	**3.9 mmol/L**
Cl	**100 mmol/L**

Question 10.4: Write up his fluids—exactly as you would on the IV fluid order chart (Chart 11.1) for the next 24 hours, give your reasons for the chosen regime below:

You have seen the fluid balance chart, know what the operation was done and the associated bloodloss. You have also seen his Hb level on the morning of Day 1.

Question 10.5: Would you transfuse him? Give your reasons.

Regarding the same patient:
At 6 pm, the nurse pages you and says she would like you to look at Mr Mann. She says he has been vomiting a lot and his pulse rate has gone up and he is not passing much urine.

You go to see him. He says he is feeling very sick and has been vomiting. He says he is not had any pain since his last injection.

On examination, his tongue is very dry, and skin turgor non-elastic. His pulse is 100/min and BP is 100/60. His CVP is +1, his temperature 38°C, RR 14/min. His hands and feet are cool. His urine bag contains very little urine. His abdomen is not distended and there is only a 20 mL of blood in his drainage bag.

You look at his input/output Chart 11.5 (shown below on page 146).

Question 10.6: What do you think is the problem?

Question 10.7: What will you do about it as the house officer/intern?

The Registrar suggests you give him an IV bolus of 250 mL of Hartmann's solution as quickly as possible

Chart 11.1 Daily intravenous fluid-order chart

Name				
First Name				
Reg. No.				
Ward				
Bag/Bottle Order	State infusion fluid/blood, volume to be given period of infusion and drip site, if applicable	State drug and dosage to be added	Doctor's initials	Blood bottle/bag no. infusion batch no. to be confirmed by nurse
1				
2				
3				
4				
5				
6				
7				
8				

and then reassess his clinical condition, urine output and CVP.

He asks you to send off an FBC and a bioprofile so you can check his urea and K^+ (he is vomiting gastric contents) and to let him know the result of the 'bolus'.

The 1st fluid bolus does not change his general condition, or his pulse, CVP or urine output. The Registrar comes to look at him and orders a second fluid bolus of 500 mL of Hartmann's. Following this, the patient's pulse falls to 80 beats per minute, his peripheries are warm, his CVP rises to 7 and then drops down to 5 and remains at this level. His urine output goes up to 50 mL per hour. The Registrar who has stayed on the ward says he is happy that the patient was volume depleted, probably due to an ileus. He says to continue with Hartmann's solution 1 liter 8 hourly and to add 20 mmols potassium to each bag, if the K = comes back < 3.5 mmol/L.

He will come and review the patient with you in 4 hours.

Finally, two common fluid and electrolyte scenarios you will come across as a surgical HO.

Question 11: Case scenario 2

75-year-old man who is admitted as an emergency with colicky abdominal pain, vomiting and abdominal distension. His X-rays show small bowel obstruction and the specialist has decided he needs surgery. Clinically he looks dehydrated, has a tachycardia, a blood pressure of 120/80. His peripheries are cool and he has not passed urine for 4 hours.

His emergency U+Es come back as below:

Urea	17 mmol/L
Na	130 mmol/L
K	2.9 mmol/L
Cl	95 mmol/L
HCO_3	21 mmol/L

Question 11.1: What is the problem with his fluid and electrolyte status?

Question 12: Case scenario

A postoperative patient with peritonitis due to perforated duodenal ulcer. He is 24 hours postoperatively and you look at his U +Es on the evening ward round: the patient is well with no raised JVP or signs of dehydration and his urine output is adequate.

Urea	3 mmol/L
Na	128 mmol/L
K	3 mmol/L
Cl	96 mmol/L
HCO_3	26 mmol/L

You look at his fluid balance charts and find he has been given 3 liters of 5% dextrose since theater.

Question 12.1: What has happened? What will you do about it?

Note: Hyponatremia is seen in two situations on the general surgical ward:

1. Water overload hyponatraemia (as illustrated earlier), when the patient has been given too much 'water' and

Chart 11.3 Daily input and output chart

Fluid Chart
University Hospital

Day	Input (mL)						Output (mL)				
	Intravenous		Oral		Others		Urine	Feces	Vomit	Nasogastric	Others (Drain)
Time	Type	Volume	Type	Volume	Type	Volume					
7.00 am											
8.00 am											
9.00 am											
10.00 am											
11.00 am											
12.00 pm											
1.00 pm											
2.00 pm											
AM											
2.00 pm	HARTMANN		Ice	30 mL							
3.00 pm		500					30				
4.00 pm			Ice	30 mL			30				
5.00 pm							40				
6.00 pm			Ice	30 mL			40				
7.00 pm							30				100
8.00 pm	DEXT	5%	Ice	30 mL			30				
9.00 pm		500					30				
PM											
10.00 pm							50				
11.00 pm							50				
12.00 pm							45				50
1.00 am							50				
2.00 am	DEXT	5%					50				
3.00 am		500					50				
4.00 am							45				
5.00 am							20				
6.00 am			Ice	30 mL			50				
7.00 am			Ice	30 mL			50				50
ON		1400		180			690				200

Name:	Mr Mann, R		Total Intake:	1580 mL
Consultant/Ward:	Mr X Gen Surg		Total Output:	890 mL
Unit No.:			Balance:	+ 690 mL

Chart 11.5 Daily input and output (Postoperative of day 1)

Fluid Chart
University Hospital

Day	Input (mL)						Output (mL)				
	Intravenous		Oral		Others		Urine	Feces	Vomit	Nasogastric	Others (Drain)
Time	Type	Volume	Type	Volume	Type	Volume					
7.00 am	Dextrose	5%	Ice	30 mL							
8.00 am		100	Ice	30 mL			40				
9.00 am	Dextrose	5%	Ice	30 mL			30				
10.00 am		500	Ice	30 mL			30				
11.00 am			Ice	30 mL			20				
12.00 pm							20				
1.00 pm							20		400		
2.00 pm							20				
AM			NBM								
2.00 pm	Dextrose	5%					30		200		50
3.00 pm		500					10				
4.00 pm							10				
5.00 pm							10		200		
6.00 pm											
7.00 pm											
8.00 pm											
9.00 pm											
PM											
10.00 pm											
11.00 pm											
12.00 pm											
1.00 am											
2.00 am											
3.00 am											
4.00 am											
5.00 am											
6.00 am											
7.00 am											
ON											

Name: Mr Mann, R	Total Intake:
Consultant/Ward: Mr X Gen Surg	Total Output:
Unit No.:	Balance:

2. Hypovolemic hyponatremia when the patient has lost water and sodium—usually from a GI fistula or, say, from ileostomy diarrhea.

The investigation which differentiates these extrarenal causes from a renal cause is the urine osmolarity of sodium (as opposed to urinary electrolytes).

If urine Na osmolarity is > 30, then the cause is renal

is < 30, then it is extrarenal.

TUTORIAL 12: Patient 1 Varicose Veins
Patient 2 Ulcer on Leg

Question 1: Case scenario

The patient goes to see her general practitioner (Dr S) and gives the following history:

Mrs P is 50 years of age and works as a shop assistant. For the last year she has noticed that her legs have started to ache at the end of the day and that her ankles are swollen as well. Her mother had varicose veins and Mrs P was very upset when her mother said to her last week that her veins were worse than her own! She has come to Dr S to ask his advice.

Question 1.1: What questions will Dr S ask Mrs P?

Mrs P tells Dr S that she has been aware of the veins standing out on her legs—both sides for nearly 20 years. She first noticed them after the birth of her first child and they were much worse during the latter stages of her subsequent 2 pregnancies. She does not intend to have any more children but she is now ashamed of how her legs look when she is in her bathing suit. Also, over the last year they have become much more noticeable and extensive. It is only in the last few months that her legs have started to ache and swell. When she gets home at night, she sits down for 20 minutes with her feet up and the ache and swelling get better. Her husband has told her she is getting lazy and does not like waiting for his supper!

On direct questioning Mrs P tells Dr S that she is currently fit and well. He checks her records and sees that she has not had any serious illnesses or hospital admissions. He notes that she is slightly overweight, is not on the contraceptive pill and is not currently taking any other medications.

Question 1.2: What is the etiopathology of primary varicose veins, i.e. why do they occur (basic science)?

Question 1.3: Draw a diagram of the normal venous return of the leg.

Question 1.4: Draw a further diagram of the leg showing the major sites of venous incompetence.

You should now be in the position to be able to answer the next question:

Question 1.5: What will Dr S look for when he examines Mrs P?

First of all Dr S asks Mrs P to undress in the examination room and sends his nurse in, to help (the nurse remains in the room at all times). The nurse asks Mrs P to remove sufficient clothing so that the doctor can examine her abdomen, see both her groins and the full extent of both her legs. The doctor asks Mrs P to stand by the bed and notes that she has full length varicosities affecting the long saphenous vein on both legs. He does not see any ulcer or skin pigmentation. **(Professional Conduct)**

Question 1.6: What advice does he give to Mrs P?

Mrs P says she has to stand at work a lot; does not like how her legs look and she wants something done about them if possible. Dr S says 'fine'—he will arrange for her to see a surgeon and in the meantime gives her a diet sheet and arranges for her to obtain graduated (compression) stockings.

Mrs P comes to Professor O's OP clinic.

He asks you, the house officer/intern to take a history and examine Mrs P and to record your findings in the notes.

Question 1.7: Describe in detail how you will examine her legs—including how you will define which of her venous systems are incompetent and where the major sites of incompetence are.

Your answer should include:

a. The anatomy of the long and short saphenous veins.

b. The anatomical location of the common perforators and how you decide if there is incompetence.

c. What clinical tests you will use.

d. Whether there is any evidence of venous hypertension and how you would know this.

e. Whether you would examine her abdomen and why.

Professor O comes and checks your findings. He agrees that she has bilateral saphenofemoral incompetence with a saphena varix on the R side (This is shown by the Trendelenberg Test). The tourniquet test then shows incompetence at both mid thigh perforators and that she has below the knee perforators in three places along the medial aspect of her leg below the knee, with demonstrable defects in the deep fascia.

Question 1.8: What is a saphena varix?

Question 1.9: What is the differential diagnosis in a patient presenting with a soft swelling of diameter 2 × 2 cm in the right groin? List 6 causes.

Note: If you are having difficulty answering this—revert to basic principles:

What are the structures in right groin—skin, subcutaneous fat, femoral canal, femoral vein, artery and nerve. What in these structures will give you a swelling?

Question 1.10: What operation do you think Professor O will advise Mrs P to have done?

Question 2: Case scenario

Mrs N is a 60-year-old diabetic lady who has had varicose veins for years. Her diabetes has been well controlled with oral hypoglycemics. For 3 months now, she has had an ulcer on her leg and comes to the OP clinic because she is worried about it. When she is seen at the clinic, she says it is getting bigger. It does not hurt her and as far as she is aware she has not fallen on or injured her leg. Her past history is non-contributory except for the diabetes and she says she was in hospital with a swollen leg after the birth of her child.

Question 2.1: What is the relevance of the swollen leg after childbirth?

Below is a picture of the her leg (Fig. 12.6).

Question 2.2: Describe what you see.

Question 2.3: What is your protocol for describing an ulcer?

Question 2.4: List the differential diagnosis for any ulcer of the leg.

Question 2.5: Make a list of the features of the three main ulcers you see on the wards and how you differentiate between them.

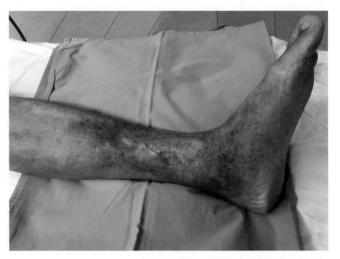

Fig. 12.6

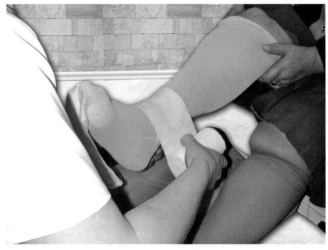

Fig. 12.7 Copyright RCSI with permission

Now back to Mrs N:

The ulcer measures about 3.5 × 2.5 cm and is on the gaiter area. It is circular in shape with a slightly irregular and sloping edge. It is 2 mm deep and had red granulation tissue in its base. No discharge is seen. The surrounding skin is pigmented and thickened. No obvious varicose veins are seen.

The temperature of the leg is normal and the same as the other side. The peripheral pulses are all present and there are no local clinical signs of limb ischemia.

Question 2.6: What would these clinical signs of limb ischemia be?

There is no muscle wasting. Sensation of the lower limbs is normal.

Question 2.7: What is your diagnosis?

Question 2.8: What is lipodermatosclerosis and how does it occur?

Question 2.9: List the investigations you would carry out on Mrs N.

Question 2.10: There are three steps which form the basis of the treatment of a varicose ulcer. Please list them.

Question 2.11: What form of management is illustrated in Figure 12.7?

TUTORIAL 13: Loin Pain (Renal)

Question 1: Case scenario 1

Mr S is 35 years of age and is admitted to the surgical ward with the sudden onset of right loin pain which started 8 hours ago. It is the first time, he has had it and it is the worst pain, he has ever had in his life. He has been rolling around the bed with the pain.

Question 1.1: When you take his history what specific questions will you ask in the history of presenting complaint?

The patient says the pain is in his right side and points to his loin. It is colicky in nature and he gets periods of up to 5–10 minutes' pain, then it goes away completely. The pain radiates down to the right lower quadrant of his abdomen. It does not go into his scrotum. He says he has had to pass urine a little more often than usual but has not had any pain on micturition or noticed any blood in the urine. He has not had any urinary problems in the past.

He does not admit to any fever, he has no pain elsewhere in his abdomen, his appetite is good and he has not lost weight recently. He does not feel like eating or drinking at the moment because of the pain. He has vomited once when the pain was really bad. He has had no recent change in his bowel habit.

Question 1.2: What differential diagnosis are you formulating in your mind from the history you have taken?

Question 1.3: When you examine him, list what physical signs you will be looking?

On examination:	He is in obvious distress and says he has the pain at the moment.
	He is a little pale.
	He is not anemic or jaundiced.
	He is clinically well hydrated.
	His temperature is 37.4°C.
	Pulse 90 per minute.
	BP 120/80.
	Peripheries well perfused.

Abdomen examination:	I	Well nourished.
		Abdomen moving normally with respiration.
		No scars. No distension. No mass.
		No skin discoloration.
		No dilated veins or pulsations.
		Umbilicus normal.
	P	No tenderness guarding or rigidity.
		No organomegally as far as could be felt with him moving.
		No ascites.
		No groin hernia.
		Scrotum and penis normal.
	A	Normal bowel sounds.
		PR not done.
		Legs = N

Question 1.4: What is your diagnosis now?

Question 1.5: You are the house officer/intern: What investigations will you arrange on this patient?

Question 1.6: You obtain the results because you know there is a consultant ward round in the evening. Please look at the results below and give your interpretation of them— in particular what they mean to your diagnosis/differential diagnosis.

FBC:	Hb	14
	WCC	11,000
	Platelets	300,000

Note: Normal values should be inserted by you in your answer to question 1.6.

While you are looking for the blood results the nurse comes up and says she does not know what charts to put Mr S on.

Question 1.7: What will you say?

Question 1.8: Have you any other instructions to the nurse?

The nurse comes back 5 minutes later and says Mr S is in a lot of pain and is vomiting.

Question 1.9: What will you do?

We will continue to look at his results:

Question 1.10: Comment on the following:

Urea	9 mmol/L
Na	140 mmol/L
K	4.0 mmol/L
Cl	111 mmol/L
HCO_3	24 mmol/L
Creatinine	80 umol/L

Question 1.11: Urine dipstick. List below what parameters are tested and briefly explain their clinical relevance.

Question 1.12: These are the patient's dipstick results—how do you interpret them and what action will you take?

pH: Normal

Glucose +++

Nitrites +

protein +

Blood ++

Bilirubin +

Urobilinogen ++

Question 1.13: The MSU result is shown below. What is its relevance?

MSU - microscopy:

A few red blood cells and many WCCs are seen

Gram –ve rods present

Culture and sensitivity to follow.

Question 1.14: The patient's 'KUB' is shown in Figure 13.1. What does KUB stand for and how does it differ from a plain abdominal X-ray?

Study the X-ray.

Question 1.15: What are you particularly looking for in reference to this case?

You show this film to the consultant, he asks the X-ray department to perform a urological CT.

Here is one film from the series (Fig. 13.2).

Question 1.16: What do you see?

Question 1.17: Write here in bullet point only, how you will manage this patient.

Now here is a bit of basic anatomy and science revision. Try and answer these questions without the books and then check them. Make the answer short and succinct, so, they will be useful for revision.

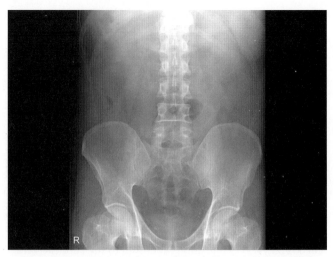

Fig. 13.1 The patient's KUB X-Ray

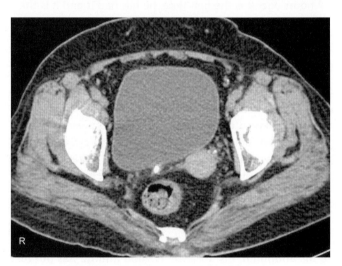

Fig. 13.2 The patient's urological CT scan

Question 1.18: What is the anatomical course of the ureter?

Question 1.19: What are the chemical compositions of the common renal stones?

Question 1.20: What are the risk factors for renal stones?

To finish with here are some relevant X rays.

Question 1.21: Describe the abnormality shown on this X-ray (Fig. 13.3).

Question 1.22: What is your diagnosis?

Question 1.23: What is it made of?

Study the X-ray (Fig. 13.4).

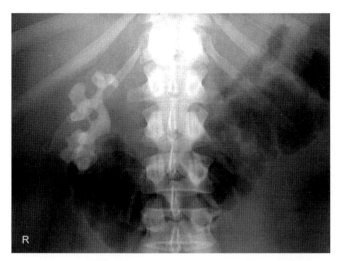

Fig. 13.3 Plain abdominal X-ray

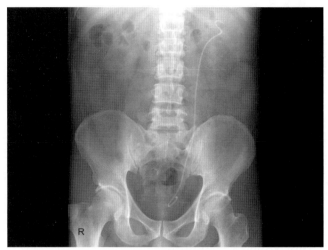

Fig. 13.5

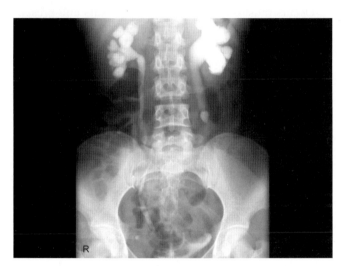

Fig. 13.4

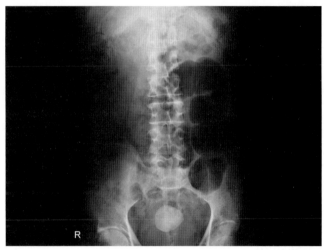

Fig. 13.6 KUB X-ray

Question 1.24: What type of X-ray is shown in Figure 13.4 and what does it show?

Question 1.25: What is seen on the plain abdominal X-ray (Fig. 13.5)?

Question 1.26: What is the diagnosis to be made from the X-ray shown in Figure 13.6?

Answers

TUTORIAL 1: Upper Gastrointestinal

CASE SCENARIOS

Answer 1.1:
1. Cancer of the esophagus or
2. A high cancer of the stomach or
3. Just possibly a reflux stricture.

The main causes of dysphagia, you will encounter are:
- Ca esophagus
- Fibrous narrowing from reflux disease
- Ingestion of caustic agents.

Achalasia is rare but you must be familiar with this condition.

Pharyngeal pouch (Zenker Diverticulum) is relatively uncommon (2 per 100,000 per year in UK).

Answer 1.2:
CA *esophagus:*
- Gradual onset of dysphagia
- Difficulty with solids to start and then may progress to intolerance of liquids as well
- Progresses quite rapidly over weeks to 2–3 months
- Marked loss of weight.

Benign structure:
- Gradual onset over months or years
- Solid intolerance first
- Progressive slowly
- May have heartburn
- Slow weight loss.

Achalasia:
- Gradual increasing dysphagia over years
- Solids and liquids from the start
- May eat standing up
- Regurgitation of old food
- Last to finish meal
- If advanced—weight loss, bad breath, aspirate at night—chest infection
- May become malignant.

Ingestion of caustic agent:
- Accidental ingestion in children
- Intentional in adults (suicidal)
- Note that acid ingestion (more injurious to stomach than esophagus) may not have oropharyngeal burns
- Solid alkali gives burns of mouth and pharynx
- Liquid alkali burns esophagus
- Get immediate symptoms of ingestion (pain)—edema, ulceration and inflammation giving obstruction and may lead to perforation/stricture later on—all depends on severity.

Pharyngeal pouch:
- Occurs most often in males over 70 years and present with chronic symptoms of regurgitation of undigested food particularly when lying flat and dysphagia (>90%), coughing and spluttering during a meal (due to aspiration). Symptoms are slowly progressive and rarely related to types of food eaten.

Answer 1.3:
- Cachexia and weight loss
- Pale (anemic)
- Jaundice
- Dehydrated
- Changes in voice (hoarse)
- Enlarged supraclavicular nodes
- Chest signs on auscultation, if aspirating/fistula
- Abdomen: Enlarged liver.

Answer 1.4:
- FBC—? anemia
- U and Es—? dehydration
- LFTs—nutritional status (albumin) and metastases
- Clotting screen, if jaundiced
- Imaging: Chest X-ray
          CT neck, thorax, abdomen
- Upper GI endoscopy + biopsy
- Ba swallow, if suspect fistula
- Bronchoscopy, if chest symptoms.

Answer 1.5: Opacification R lower zone probably due to aspiration.

Answer 1.6: Fiber optic upper GI endoscope.

Answer 1.7:
- Patient takes no solids for 6 hours before procedure. Clear fluids permitted until 2 hours before

- Make sure aware of patient's past medical history and medications and act accordingly
- Usually takes 20 minutes to do + 3–4 hours recovery
- Usually done under LA throat spray +/– IV sedation
- Patient on side
- Asked to swallow as the endoscope touches back of throat
- Scope passed down under direct vision
- Note the condition of esophageal mucosa. Identify esophagogastric junction. Note gastric mucosa, D_1 and D_2 (1st and 2nd parts of duodenum). Reverse the scope and look at fundus
- Biopsy as necessary (HP and formal histology).

Answer 1.8:
- Explain that the doctor in charge wants you (the patient) to have an examination to look at the esophagus which is the tube down which your food goes when you swallow. The stomach and its outlet will be seen at the same time.
- The test is done by putting a narrow tube down the throat—pictures of the esophagus and stomach will be looked at on a television screen by the doctor as he goes along.
- The test will be done as an outpatient. Although, it takes only approximately 20 minutes you will be at the hospital for about 4 hours—to make sure you have recovered satisfactorily.
- You must not have anything to eat 6 hours before the test and drink clear fluids (water) up until 2 hours before—this is very important.
- Please tell the doctor, if you have any serious illnesses such as diabetes or heart trouble, and if you are on tablets, injections or pills.
- When the test is carried out you will be given a local anesthetic throat spray so the tube does not hurt you. You may also be given a mild sedative through a vein.
- A bit of tissue may be taken during the test, if anything abnormal is found, called a biopsy.
- Afterwards you must remain in the recovery ward until you have recovered. You must have someone to take you home. If you have been given sedation you should not drive a car or motorcycle or use machinery for 24 hours. You should not be alone that night.
- The doctor will tell you what he found straight after the test or arrange for you to come to the clinic for the results.
- This is a very safe test and has been used for many years. You may have a bit of a sore throat afterwards. Complications are rare but include perforation—a tear of the stomach wall which would need repair, and bleeding which may need transfusion.

Answer 1.9:
- There is an irregular, polypoid lesion with ulceration.
- This is suggestive of a malignant lesion.

Answer 1.10: 25 cm long—it extends from the cricoid cartilage at level of C6 to the esophagogastric junction. It is divided into cervical/thoracic and abdominal portions—the final 2–4 cm lie in the peritoneal cavity.

Answer 1.11: Measure from the lower incisors using markings on the endoscope, the esophagogastric junction is approximately 40 cm from lower incisor teeth.

Answer 1.12: The mucosa consists of stratified squamous epithelium except for the distal 1–2 cm which is lined with columnar epithelium.

In Barrett's esophagus, the columnar epithelium undergoes metaplasia due to damage from acid and bile reflux. The risk of cancer is increased by 40–90%.

Answer 1.13: This is based on the TNM classification:

T = How far the tumor is into the wall of esophagus.

N = Whether nodes are involved.

M = Distal metastases (any involved nodes distal to L gastric nodes are considered M).

Answer 1.14: Must know from basic pathology how a cancer of esophagus spreads, then you can work the answer out:

Spread is by: Local Lymphatic Blood

Local (T) and mediastinal node spread (N) best assessed with endoscopic ultrasound—if not available use CT.

Metastatic spread (M): Chest X-ray (lung metastases)

CT chest: Local extension, lymph nodes

CT abdomen (liver metastases, distal lymphadenopathy)

Laparoscopy (peritoneal metastases)

Answer 1.15: Advanced tumor and any treatment will be palliative.

Answer 1.16:

Stage of the tumor

Fitness of the patient (mainly CVS and RS).

Answer 1.17:
- Chemoradiotherapy
- Laser debulking
- Stenting
- Analgesia and palliative care.

Any or all of these may be used depending on the individual tumor and patient.

Answer 1.18: See Figures 1.5 to 1.7.

Answer 2.1: Gastroesophageal reflux disease (GERD).

Answer 2.2:
1. Hiatus hernia with reflux
2. Reflux with normal anatomy.

Answer 2.3a: Sliding hiatus hernia.

Answer 2.3b: Paraesophageal or rolling hiatus hernia.

Answer 2.4: An air-filled cavity in the thorax—this is a hiatus hernia—confirm with CT.

Answer 2.5: Upper GI endoscopy showing a hiatus hernia and esophagitis.

Answer 2.6: Full blood count, biochemical profile and an upper GI endoscopy.

Answer 2.7: The changes of severe esophagitis—inflammation and ulceration.

Answer 2.8:
- General—lose weight, sleep sat up on pillows at night avoid late night eating—especially chocolate, spirits.
- H_2 receptor antagonists or proton pump inhibitors to reduce gastric acid production.
- Alginates to coat the esophagus, e.g. Gaviscon.
- Prokinetics, e.g. Maxalon to promote better lower esophageal muscle tone and gatsric emptying.

Answer 2.9: pH manometry records the level of acidity in the lower esophagus and is carried out over a 24-hour period. An electrode is placed 4–5 cm above the gastroesophageal junction. The patient keeps a diary of their symptoms to correlate with the recorded changes.

Answer 2.10: Yes—it is regarded as the investigation of choice for the diagnosis and should always be carried out, if surgery is being contemplated.

Answer 2.11: Those patients with established reflux in whom medical management has failed (but only with careful assessment of likely benefit!).

Answer 2.12:
Fundoplication—gastric fundus is wrapped around the abdominal part of the esophagus. Can be done at open laparotomy but is now usually done by laparoscopy (Fig. 1.13).

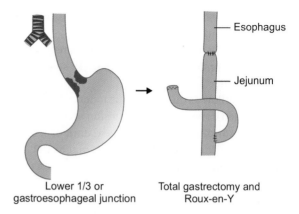

Lower 1/3 or gastroesophageal junction — Total gastrectomy and Roux-en-Y

Fig. 1.5 Total gastrectomy and Roux-en-Y for cancer of lower third esophagus or at gastroesophageal junction

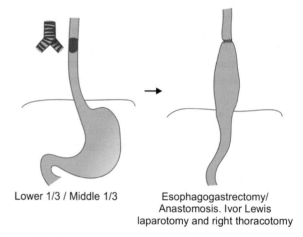

Lower 1/3 / Middle 1/3 — Esophagogastrectomy/Anastomosis. Ivor Lewis laparotomy and right thoracotomy

Fig. 1.6 Esophagogastrectomy and esophagogastric anastomosis for cancer of lower third of esophagus esophagectomy and esophageal gastric anastomosis performed-called an Ivor Lewis Operation using a laparotomy and right thoracotomy

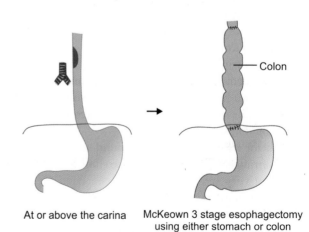

At or above the carina — McKeown 3 stage esophagectomy using either stomach or colon

Fig. 1.7 Cancer of esophagus at or above the carina. Three stage McKeown esophagectomy with stomach or colon transposition

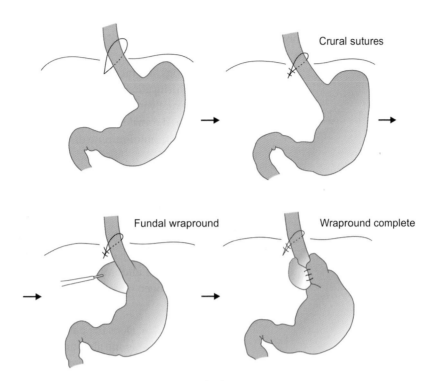

Fig. 1.13 Fundoplication operation

Answer 3.1: Upper GI endoscopy.

Answer 3.2: The esophagus is very dilated and there is a narrowing at its lower end (called 'birds beak' or rat's tail appearance).

Answer 3.3: Esophageal manometry will show incomplete relaxation of the lower sphincter in response to swallowing, if the diagnosis is correct.

Answer 3.4: A fine perforated tube connected to a pressure transducer is put into the stomach. Recordings are taken in the stomach and then the tube is withdrawn with readings taken at the gastroesophageal junction and in the esophagus between swallowing. This is really the test of choice for diagnosing achalasia.

Answer 3.5: Treatment may be by:
• Forceful dilatation of the cardia with pneumatic dilators (may perforate).
• Heller's myotomy—dividing the lower esophageal sphincter.

Answer 4.1:
Upper GI malignancy— stomach
pancreas
possibly liver metastases.

Answer 4.2:
• FBC
• U and Es
• Tumor markers
• Chest X-ray
• CT of abdomen
• Upper GI endoscopy.

Answer 4.3: There is a large irregular ulcerated lesion in the antrum consistent with a gastric neoplasm.

Answer 4.4: Barium meal. Large irregular filling defect just below cardia consistent with a carcinoma of stomach.

Answer 4.5: Biopsy and brushings.

Answer 4.6: See Table 1.1
TNM classification or
UICC (Union International Contre Cancer) classification

Table 1.1 Staging and prognosis of gastric cancer			
UICC	*TNM*	*Treatment*	*5-year survival*
1	T1 N0 M0	Radical resection	70%
2	T2 N0 M0	Radical resection	30%
3	T0-4 N1-3 M0	Radical resection	10%
4	T4 N 3 M0-1	Palliation	1–2%

As an undergraduate, you would not be expected to remember the details of these classifications, only that most gastric cancers present late, and therefore have a very poor survival rate.

Answer 4.7: See Figure 1.17

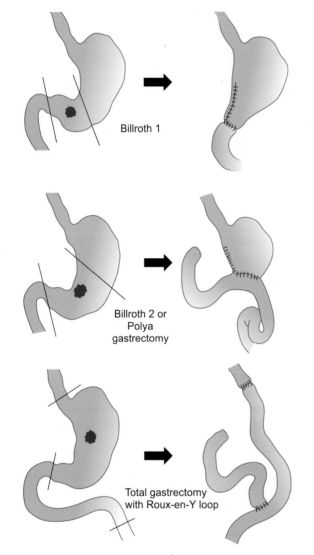

Fig. 1.17 Operations for gastric cancer

TUTORIAL 2: Hepatobiliary and Pancreas

CASE SCENARIOS

Jaundice and Abdominal Pain

Answer 1.1: With this information, it would be difficult to say anything more than either hepatocellular or obstructive jaundice.

Answer 1.2:
- Hepatitis
- Alcohol
- Drugs and medications
- IV drug abuse
- Sexually transmitted diseases
- Blood transfusion
- Blood/autoimmune disorders
- Travel.

Answer 1.3: Either obstructive jaundice or hepatocellular jaundice specifically, gallstones (painful jaundice) or hepatitis.

Answer 1.4: This is a 35-year-old female presenting with abdominal pain, jaundice and dark urine against a background of long-term abdominal discomfort and flatulence. She has probably been in contact with infective hepatitis.

Answer 1.5:

General	• Does the patient look in any distress?
	• Is she alert and orientated?
	• Is she cachexic?
	• Is she dehydrated?
	• Scleral icterus?
	• Clinically anemic?
	• Oral signs and dental hygiene?
Hands	• Any signs of liver failure?
	• Palmar crease pallor? Arms-any scratch marks, bruising
	• Pulse/BP/temperature/RR
Neck	• Any thyroid swelling?
	• Any enlarged lymph nodes?
Chest	• Gynecomastia?
	• Spider nevi?

Abdomen

I
- Moving normally with respiration
- Evidence of weight loss
- Evidence of jaundice
- Distention
- Abdominal mass
- Distended veins
- Arterial pulsation
- Normal and everted umbilicus

P Tenderness, guarding, rebound mass/query gallbladder palpable/Murphy's sign
Organomegaly—particularly liver/spleen groin glands

A Normal bowel sounds

P Ascites

PR Color of stool

Answer 1.6:

No entry must be made into the differential diagnosis unless the patient has the symptoms and signs suggestive of that disease.

Every time you formulate a differential diagnosis, apply this simple rule.

Answer 1.7:

1. Gallstone disease with stone(s) in common bile duct (history suggestive of gallstones, history suggestive of episode of biliary colic, jaundice, dark urine).
2. Hepatitis—query infective (contact, jaundice, upper abdominal discomfort, yellow stools).

Answer 1.8:

1. FBC—query anemia, raised WCC—suggests infection.
2. U and Es—query dehydration.
3. Liver function tests—will suggest type of jaundice.
4. Full clotting screen—jaundice will affect liver function and hence clotting.
5. Full hepatitis screen—try and rule out viral hepatitis. Viral serology includes screening for hepatitis B and C, cytomegalovirus (CMV) Epstein-Barr virus.
6. Urine dipstick test—will help to differentiate obstructive and hepatocellular jaundice.
7. Chest X-ray (exclude obvious chest disease) and plain X-ray abdomen—may show gallstones.
8. Ultrasound of abdomen—initial imaging investigation of choice for hepatobiliary disease.

Answer 1.9:

1. Presence of gallstones in gallbladder.
2. Thickened gallbladder wall.
3. Dilated ducts.

Answer 1.10: Bilirubin comes from the hemoglobin of broken down red blood cells. Most of this breakdown occurs in the spleen. This gives unconjugated bilirubin (water insoluble) which is bound to albumin in the blood and carried to the liver (Fig. 2.1).

In the liver, it is conjugated with sugar residues to form conjugated bilirubin which is water soluble. Most of the conjugated bilirubin passes down the CBD into the duodenum. The rest is reabsorbed back into blood and excreted in the urine.

In the gut, the intestinal flora hydrolize and reduce the conjugated bilirubin to form urobilinogen, which is colorless and water soluble. Most of the urobilinogen is oxidized by intestinal flora to form stercobilinogen, which is excreted in the feces and turns them dark. Some urobilinogen is

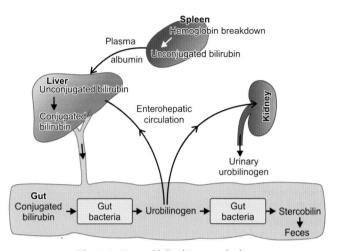

Fig. 2.1 Normal bilirubin metabolism

reabsorbed from the gut via the portal system—some of this is recycled through the liver and some excreted in the urine.

Look at ***Jaundice for Beginners*** Student BMJ Oct 1998.

Answer 1.11: See Table 2.1.

Note: γ-GT is γ-glutamyltransferase usually abbreviated as GCT. Alkaline phosphatase (ALP) is high in cholestasis. The transaminases used are aspartate aminotransferase (ASP) and alanine aminotransferase (ALT). These are raised in hepatocellular damage.

ALT is more liver cell specific as ASP is also found in cardiac and skeletal muscle cells.

Answer 1.12:

Obstructive jaundice: Urine contains bilirubin but no urobilinogen.

Early hepatocellular jaundice: Contains urobilinogen but no bilirubin.

Easy to remember as follows:

- In obstructive jaundice, the urine is dark because bilirubin is in it. There is no urobilinogen.
- In early hepatocellular, it is the opposite, i.e. no bilirubin but urobilinogen positive.
- In late hepatocellular same as obstructive jaundice because the cholestatic element predominates.

Answer 1.13: Obstructive jaundice.

Answer 1.14:

Direct = Conjugated (water soluble)
Indirect = Unconjugated (water insoluble).

Only really necessary to have this test when you suspect a hemolytic cause because the total bilirubin is raised but by an increase of unconjugated bilirubin.

The direct bilirubin is raised in obstructive and hepatocellular jaundice.

Table 2.1 Biochemical features of different types of jaundice

	Hemolytic	Early hepatocellular	Late hepatocellular	Obstructive
Unconjugated bilirubin	↑	N/↑	N/↑	N
Conjugated bilirubin	N	N	↑	↑↑
Urinary bilirubin	N/↑	↑	↑	↑↑
Urobilinogen	N/↑	N	↓	↓↓
Alkaline phosphatase	N	N	↑	↑↑
γ-GT transaminases	N	↑	↑	↑↑
Transaminases	N	↑	↑↑	N/↑
Lactate deydrogenase	N	↑	↑↑	N/↑
Reticulocytes	> 2%	N	N	N

Abbreviation: N, normal

Answer 1.15:

Obstructive jaundice

Gallstone disease.

Answer 1.16:

The gallbladder wall is thickened.

The gallbladder contains echogenic material consistent with gallstones and biliary sludge.

There is a large gallstone impacted in Hartmann's pouch

The CBD is not visualized on this picture.

Answer 1.17: An ERCP (endoscopic retrograde cholangio-pancreatography).

Note: If the diagnosis was in doubt (i.e. not sure if due to stones), then the investigation of choice would be an MRI with 3D reconstruction.

Answer 1.18: ERCP is an examination which lets the doctor examine the small tubes (called ducts) that drain your liver, gallbladder and pancreas.

In your case, we think you have gallstones and some of these are blocking the main tube coming from your liver and causing your jaundice.

You will be given sedation through a vein to make you relaxed and sleepy—so you will only feel mild discomfort at the most.

The doctor will use a thin, black, flexible tube called an endoscope and views what he sees on a television monitor. The tube is put down your throat but he will spray your throat with a local anesthetic so it does not upset you.

The doctor will pass a fine tube through the endoscope and inject dye into your ducts and take some X-rays.

If he sees the stones, he will try and remove these either with a little basket or by widening the opening at the bottom of the main duct (called a sphincterotomy).

Before the operation:

- You must not have anything to eat or drink for 6–8 hours.
- Take your usual drugs but tell the doctor if you are on aspirin or arthritis medications, anticoagulants, have a pacemaker or are diabetic.
- You may be given an antibiotic before the test—please tell the doctor if you are allergic to any antibiotics.

After the ERCP, you will be able to go home once the effects of the sedation have worn off, and if the procedure has been straight forward. You will need someone to accompany you home and stay with you overnight. Do not drive or operate machinery for 24 hours.

The complications of ERCP are infrequent and depend on why the test is done, what is found and what treatment is carried out. Sometimes infection can occur and sometimes inflammation of the pancreas gland. Sometimes bleeding occurs, if a sphincterotomy has been done. Very rarely, a perforation of the bowel or bile duct can occur.

After the ERCP when you have gone home contact your doctor, if you feel generally ill with headache, chills and fever, have a high temperature, have black bowel motions, feel dizzy, faint or short of breath, have pains in the stomach or start vomiting.

Answer 1.19: Full clotting screen.

Answer 1.20: Tell the surgeon, he will either:

1. Cancel the ERCP or
2. Advise giving vitamin K_1 (Phytomenadione, Konakion).

Answer 1.21: The common bile duct is dilated with several hypodense filling defects likely to be gallstones. The gallbladder does not fill.

Answer 1.22:
1. Remove the stones from the CBD (using a basket and sphincterotomy).
2. Readmit the lady for a laparoscopic cholecystectomy when jaundice has settled.

Jaundice and Weight Loss

Answer 2.1:
- How did he notice he had become yellow?
- When was it noticed?
- Has it become worse?
- Does he have any pain? (+ full description)
- Has his urine changed color?
- Have his bowel motions changed color?
- Any itching?
- Risk factors for jaundice?
- Rest of GI tract protocol questions.

Answer 2.2: The patient is a 71-year-old ex-sailor with a 3-month history of abdominal pain and weight loss, a month's history of vomiting and a 2-week history of jaundice. His wife had hepatitis 3 years ago and he takes an anxiolytic drug.

Answer 2.3:

> No entry into the differential diagnosis must be made unless, the patient has the symptoms and signs suggestive of that disease.

Answer 2.4:
1. Obstructive jaundice—more likely malignant cause than gallstone disease—query cancer head of pancreas with duodenal obstruction.
2. Obstructive jaundice—GI primary with metastases to liver.
3. Query hepatitis.
4. Query drug-induced jaundice.

Answer 2.5:
Ex: Look at general condition—start with face
          Alert, conscious and orientated
          In pain?
          Cachexic?
          Jaundiced?
          Anemic?
          Dehydrated?
          Any signs in mouth/oral hygiene/dentition
Look at hands + arms—Signs of liver failure
          Scratches
Feel neck for enlarged nodes
Look at chest—spiders nevi or gynecomastia
Axillae—nodes/acanthosis nigricans

Abdomen examination—as in protocol, particularly:
Inspection: Evidence of weight loss/jaundice
          Distension
          Mass
          Dilated veins
          Umbilicus eversion
Palpation: Upper abdominal mass, gallbladder palpable
          Liver and spleen query palpable
          Query ascites present
          Groin nodes/genitalia (ex-sailor)
          PR—stool color, mass in pouch of Douglas
          (Kruckenberg—transcelomic spread)

Answer 2.6: Same as before but the malignant diagnosis seems more likely.

Answer 2.7:
- FBC query anemic
- U and E query dehydrated/renal function (very important in jaundiced patient)
- LFTs—will suggest type of jaundice
- Urine dipstick for bile/urobilinogen—suggests type
- *Clotting screen:* May be deranged—very important with likelihood of invasive tests and operation
- Tumor markers; CA199 for pancreas + alpha-fetoproteins for HCC
- Hepatitis screen—helps with diagnosis. Note, may be carrier
- Serum amylase—just in case
- Chest X-ray—query metastases
- Plain film of abdomen query gallstones/pancreatic calcification
- Abdominal ultrasound—first investigation of choice in hepatobiliary disease: gallstones/thickness of gallbladder wall/obstructed ducts. May show metastases.

Answer 2.8: Would suggest a malignant lesion of the pancreas.

Answer 2.9: Still more likely to be pancreatic malignancy.

Answer 2.10: Likely neoplasm of head of pancreas.

Answer 2.11: If available, the investigation of choice would be magnetic resonance cholangiopancreatography (MRCP). This is noninvasive and will give better images than a CT in the jaundiced patient. If an MR angiogram is possible this will help to decide, if the lesion is resectable, i.e. involvement of portal vein/lymph nodes/metastases.

If MRI not available, perform a CT, but remember the IV contrast is not well excreted, if liver function is reduced because of the jaundice.

Answer 2.12: Clearly, any treatment will be palliative: his CBD could be stented but this will not help the duodenal obstruction. Some specialist units can now stent the duodenum endoscopically. If this is not available and he is fit for anesthesia, probably the better option is to stent the common bile duct and perform a gastroenterostomy, i.e. bypass duodenum at laparotomy.

Answer 2.13:
- Pancreatic
- Ampullary
- Bile duct—cholangiocarcinoma
- Liver—primary or secondary.

Answer 2.14:
- Pancreas:
  - Adenocarcinoma—head/body or tail
  - Adenocarcinoma—ampullary
  - Cystadenocarcinoma
  - Rare endocrine tumors.

Answer 2.15:
a. Investigations—need to try and make tissue diagnosis, hence:
   CT-guided biopsy, if skill available
   ERCP—brushing for cytology
   ERCP—biopsy, if ampullary or invading the DU.
b. Multislice CT, contrast-enhanced, with arterial and venous phase.
c. *Look for:* • Demographics of mass
   • Enlarged lymph nodes
   • Involvement of portal vein
   • Extra pancreatic spread, e.g. metastases
   • Laparoscopy may help in deciding, if operable.
d. **Staging:** Undergraduates do not need to know this in detail, other than:
   • Localized—may be resectable
   • Tumor with extrapancreatic disease—lymph nodes, peritoneal cavity deposits or distal metastases usually not considered for resection.
e. **Prognosis:** Only about 10% of all pancreatic cancers are suitable for resection. Cancer of periampullary region/distal CBD has 20–40% 5 year survival.
   Pancreas: < 5% still alive at 5 years overall median survival from diagnosis < 6 months.
   For those undergoing resection, median survival = 12–19 months with 5-year survival of 15–20%.

> Want to read more about Liver *Function tests* ? Look at *www.patient.co.uk/doctor/Abnormal-Liver-Function-Testshtm* Excellent detailed review.

TUTORIAL 3: Rectal Bleeding

Answer 1a: Rectal bleeding—bright red from rectum/sigmoid; dark red (purple) from colon.

Alteration in bowel habit, the textbooks say alternating diarrhea and constipation but more often, it is increased frequency.

Symptoms and signs of advanced disease: anemia, weight loss, abdominal mass, abdominal pain and jaundice.

20% present obstructed: Pain/vomiting/distension/absolute constipation.

Answer 1b:
- Depends on the extent of the disease:
- *Proctitis:* Blood/mucus/pus-stained diarrhea
- *L sided:* Bloody diarrhea + abdomen pain + some systemic disturbances
- *Total colitis:* As above but more pronounced
- *Toxic dilatation:* Systemically ill, frequent blood-stained bowel motions, abdominal tenderness and abdominal distension.

Answer 1c:
Diverticulosis: Lower or L-sided abdominal pain/diarrhea/constipation.

Acute diverticulitis: Pain—lower abdomen or LIF plus systemic signs of infection, constipation or diarrhea; signs of localized peritonitis.

Perforated diverticular disease: Symptoms and signs of peritonitis.

Note: Diverticular disease rarely presents with rectal bleeding except in the elderly patient as a cause of 'massive' rectal bleeding.

Answer 1d: Diarrhea/blood in stools/vomiting/abdominal pain, source of infection, e.g. food or travel.

Answer 1e:

Uncomplicated: Painless bright red bleeding—intermittent on defecation, pruritis ani, lumps on anus.

Complicated: Thrombosed prolapsed piles—severe perianal pain irreducible perianal swellings.

CASE SCENARIO

Answer 2.1: Most likely neoplasm of colon or rectum.

Answer 2.2:
- Anemia
- Jaundice
- Cachexia and weight loss.

Abdomen: ***I*** Weight loss/mass/distension
P Mass/ascites/hepatomegaly
P Mass/liver/ascites
A Obstructed BS
A/R examination: Mass/blood on finger.

Answer 2.3:
- Full anorectal examination
- FBC/bioprofile (Including LFTs)/Tumor markers/stool specimen for microscopy and culture
- Chest X-ray
- Colonoscopy.

Answer 2.4:
- Inspection
- Digital rectal examination
- Rigid sigmoidoscopy
- Proctoscopy.
  Carried out in that order.

Answer 2.5: An automated full blood count will include:

Red cells: Hemoglobin (g/dL)
Hematocrit/PCV (fraction of whole blood volume that consists of red blood cells)
Mean corpuscular volume (MCV): Average volume of RBC measured in femtoliters micro- or macrocytic depending on whether low or high
Mean corpuscular hemoglobin concentration (MCHC): Average concentration of Hb in the cells.
In this case: Hb—may be low
MCHC/MCV may indicate
Fe-deficiency anemia.

White cells: Total white cell count
Differential WCC *Neutrophils*—raised in bacterial infection
Lymphocytes—raised in viral infections/leukemias
Monocytes—raised in chronic infections, autoimmune disease, IBD
Eosinophils—raised in parasitic infections/asthma
Basophils—leukemias/ lymphoma

Platelets: Total platelet count.
In this case, the WCC and platelets will likely be normal.

Answer 2.6:
- Urea/Na/K/Cl/HCO$_3$
- May indicate dehydration and give guide line to renal function.

Answer 2.7:
- Bilirubin
- Alkaline phosphatase
- ALT/AST
- Total proteins/serum albumin
- Raised bilirubin/alkaline phosphatase may indicate metastases
- Low albumin—sensitive marker of liver function and may indicate malnutrition.

Answer 2.8: Tumor markers are glycoproteins found in the blood, urine or body tissues that can be elevated in cancers. They can be cancer specific, e.g. CA19-9 or tissue specific, e.g. PSA.

In this case, you would perform a CEA level (carcinogenic embryonic antigen) which may be raised in colorectal cancer.

(Look at *www.patient.co.uk/Tumor-Markerhtm* for further details)

Answer 2.9: Colonoscopy is the direct examination of the colon and rectum using a flexible fiber optic instrument.

To the patient:

"We think that because of the bleeding you have had need the bowel examined with a long telescope. This lets the doctor look at the lining of the bowel to see if there are any abnormalities. We can also take tissue samples to look at under the microscope, if we find anything wrong. The day before the test—which is called a colonoscopy—you will have to take some medications to empty the bowel out. You will then come to the endoscopy department at the hospital and you must have not had anything to eat for 8 hours or drink for 2–3 hours. You will be given some sedation and painkillers by injection so that the examination does not upset you. It takes about 30 minutes to do. Afterwards you must stay in the recovery area for an hour or two. You should have someone accompany you home and should not drive or use machinery for 24 hours. The doctor who performs the examination will talk to you about the results when you have recovered from the investigation.

The endoscopy department will give you a booklet describing a colonoscopy in detail together with any problems which might occur from the procedure. You must read this carefully before signing the consent form.

Answer 2.10: The most commonly used preparation is:
Picolax (sodium pico sulfate) 2 sachets to be taken.

The patient should be on a low fiber diet for 3 days before the examination and drink copious clear fluids. Nothing to eat for 8 hours or to drink for 2 hours before the colonoscopy.

Other regimes, you will encounter are 'Golightly' and 'Fleet'. Whole Gut Irrigation is rarely used nowadays.

The patient instruction leaflet from Nottingham University Hospitals NHS Trust, shown here, will help both you and the patient to understand the preparation better.

Preparation for Colonscopy (*Courtesy:* Nottingham University Hospitals NHS Trust)

Nottingham University Hospitals **NHS**

**Bowel preparation for patients
using Picolax**

Instructions for patients

This information can be provided in different languages
and formats. For more information, please contact the
Radiology Department at City Hospitals Campus on
0115 9627703 or the Radiology Department at QMC
Campus on 0115 9709159

Page 1

The day before the procedure

Not later than 8 am
Drink plenty of clear fluids throughout the day. This should preferably
be water, but you can also have tea or coffee without milk, soft drinks
(not fizzy), clear soups with no bits in it, or Bovril.

Breakfast (7 am–8 am)
Choose one of the following:
• 30 g crisped rice cereal or comflakes with up to 100 mL of milk.
• Two slices of white bread/toast with a this spread of butter or
  margarine and honey (if desired).
• Boiled or poached egg, with one slice of white bread and thin spread
  of butter or margarine.
• 50 g cottage or cream cheese with one slice of white bread with a thin
  spread of butter or margarine.

PLUS
• Tea or coffee, without milk.
• Soft drinks (not fizzy), or water.

Mid morning
Tea or coffee without milk.

Page 2

10 am
Stir one sachet of Picolax in a cup of cold water. Stir for two to three
minutes and drink the mixture. The water may become hot. If this
happens, wait until it is cool enough to drink.

  You should expect frequent bowel motions and eventually diarrhea,
starting within three hours of the first dose of Picolax. Some stomach
discomfort is normal. Please use a barrier cream, if your bottom
becomes sore and stay within easy reach of the toilet.

Lunch (1 pm–2 pm)
Choose one of the following:
• 75 g minced or well-cooked tender, lean meat/fish (beef, lamb, ham,
  veal, pork, chicken, fish or shelfish or Quom for vegetarians). You can
  have gravy made from stock cubes—while flour or comflour may be
  used to thicken.
• Two boiled or poached eggs.
• 100 g cream or cottage cheese or cheese sauce.

PLUS one of the following:
• Two tablespoons plain white rice or pasta (not wholemeal), or two
  slices of white bread with thin spread of butter or margarine, or two
  egg-sized potatoes without the skin.
• Unlimited tea or coffee without milk, soft drinks (not fizzy) and meat
  extract drinks.

**No further solid food, milk and diary products are allowed until
after the examination.**

Continue to take plenty of sugar-free clear fluids (at least one 150 mL
glass every hour).

Page 3

4 pm
Stir the second sachet of Picolax in a cup of cold water. Stir for two to
three minutes and drink the mixture. The water may become hot. If this
happens, wait until it is cool enough to drink.

Evening meal
• Clear soup (i.e. soup without milk and any solids) or a meat extract
  drink.
• Clear jelly may be taken for dessert.
• Tea or coffee, without milk.
• Clear fluids.

You should continue to drink plenty of clear fluids—preferably water—
through the day (at least one 150 mL) glass every hour whilst awake
and to satisfy your thirst). You can continue to drink up until two hours
before the procedure.

Bedtime
Tea or coffee without milk.

Page 4

Fluid chart

Please use this chart to help you record the glasses (150 mL) of fluid taken each hour you are awake. You must stop drinking two hours before your procedure.

(Pleas tick against the hour each time you have a glass/cup of fluid)

Time		Time	
7 am	✓	3 pm	
8 am		4 pm	
9 am		5 pm	
10 am		6 pm	
11 am		7 pm	
12.00		8 pm	
1 pm		9 pm	
2 pm		10 pm	

Examples of clear fluids that you may have:
• Water
• Tea (without milk)
• Coffee (without milk)
• Bovril
• Tonic water
• Squash (No fizzy drinks)

After the procedure

You may eat normally once the examination is over. A high fiber diet (e.g. wholemeal bread, all bran, etc.) will help you restore your normal bowel pattern, which will usually return within a day or two.

Page 5

Answer 2.11: To make sure, there are no synchronous bowel cancers (1–4%).

To identify any additional polyps—need a 'clear' colon before operation.

(Definitions: synchronous—2 or more bowel cancers identified in the patient at the same time. Metachronous-further bowel cancer detected at an interval after the initial lesion(s)—considered to be a 'new' lesion.)

Answer 2.12:

Chest X-ray (better CT of chest, abdomen, if available)

MRI of rectum (+MRI liver if doubt on CT).

Answer 2.13: Patient takes same picolax prep regime as for a colonoscopy.

Patient lies on X-ray table and a small amount of barium is put into the rectum via an enema tube. This is then spread over the surface of the mucosa by pumping air into the bowel and rotating the patient. X-rays are taken to show all parts of bowel up to the terminal ileum. Further X-rays are taken when the patient has emptied the barium out.

This is a double contrast barium enema. Single contrast enemas using barium alone are rarely used now.

Answer 2.14: Colonoscopy is now the gold-standard investigation for the large bowel because it allows a direct view of the mucosa, will show very small lesions, allows biopsies to be taken and simultanously may be used therapeutically (e.g. to remove polyps/small cancers).

Answer 2.15: Magnetic resonance imaging—combines a powerful magnet and radiowaves with a computer to produce images of the particular area under study.

Better than US or CT for rectal cancer because the wall of the rectum is better imaged and a T-staging of the tumor can be accurately performed (See later).

Answer 2.16: Anterior resection of the rectum—this may be performed by open surgery or laparoscopically.

(The tumor with adequate clearance is resected and the descending colon anastomosed to the remaining rectum—usually by a stapling technique.)

For a middle third tumor, a TME (total mesorectal excision) is performed and a covering loop ileostomy is usually necessary.

Answer 2.17: See Figure 3.1.

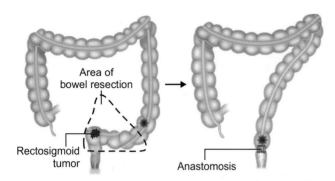

Fig. 3.1 Anterior resection of rectum (AR)

Answer 2.18: See Figure 3.2.

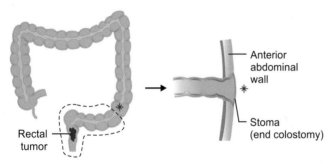

Fig. 3.2 Abdominoperineal resection of rectum (APER)

Answer 2.19: See Table 3.1.

Table 3.1 Duke's classification of colon and rectal cancer	
Duke's	*5-year survival*
A – Limited to bowel wall	90%
B – Through the bowel wall or through serosa into extra-rectal tissue	70%
C1 – Lymph nodes involved with tumor but not up to mesenteric ligation	
C2 – Lymph nodes involved to high tie (apical nodes)	30%
D – Distal metastases (prognosis 6 month–1 year—without resection/chemo)	

Note: Some would say the Dukes classification is now out of date and has been replaced by the TNM classification. However, it is simple and gives a good guide to prognosis.

Answer 2.20:

T = Tumor depth in relation to bowel wall, e.g.

    T1 = Into submucosa

    T4 = Directly involving another organ

N = Nodal involvement, e.g.

    N0 = No involved nodes

    N1 = 1–3 nodes involved

M = Presence of metastases, e.g.

    M0 = No distal metastases

    M1 = Distant metastases.

Note: It is important to have an accurate T-staging in rectal cancer, because it may indicate the need for neoadjuvant therapy. In colon cancer, a CT is usually used for staging.

Answer 2.21: First of all ask the patient if he would like his immediate relatives present—this helps because then everyone knows what is going on. If he says no you should do as he wants—if this happens, you should ask how much, he wants his relatives to know.

Start off with something like, "Do you know what is wrong with you?" If he says yes, 'I have cancer', then you can proceed—if not, then you must first explain to him that he has cancer, in simple terms and trying to give as much support as possible, e.g. if there is no evidence of spread tell him this and that we would hope to be able to cure him. Tell him that he will be given preparation to empty his bowel and that he will not be able to eat for 4–6 hours before the operation. He will also be given an injection preoperatively to cut down the risks of leg thrombosis and antibiotics to reduce the risk of infection. The operation will be done under a general anesthetic—so he will be asleep and not feel anything. The operation takes about 3 hours and he will wake up in the recovery area. He will have an IV line in his arm and a tube in his bladder—these are routine and do not mean the operation has gone wrong.

The details of the operation, you need to explain will depend, if it is done laparoscopically or open. In this case, we will describe an 'open' operation.

Tell him that he will have a cut down the middle of his abdomen which will be sown up at the end with stitches or clips. The bit of bowel with the cancer in it will be taken out and the ends joined back together. It will probably be necessary for him to have a temporary ileostomy so you should explain this in simple terms, unless, it has already been done by the stoma nurse.

Tell him that after the operation, he will probably be in the high dependency unit for 24 hours so his progress can be closely monitored. He will be given painkillers, when he needs them and fed through the drip in his arm. He will be able to drink small amounts of fluid after a few hours and then these amounts will be increased depending on how he is doing. Most bowel resection patients these days are eating and drinking in 48 hours (fast-track surgery).

He will be in hospital for 3–7 days and then will be at home with his general practitioner taking care of him. An appointment will be made for him to be seen at the surgical clinic about 1–2 weeks after he has been discharged and he will then be told the results of the tests done on the piece of bowel taken out and whether or not he needs any further treatment.

You will need to explain the common complications and how often these occur, namely, wound infection/ileus/leak/DVT.

Then you ask if he has understood and has he any questions. You are then in the position to ask him to sign the consent form.

Most hospitals now have a booklet with all these details in it for the patients—helps a lot and is good medicolegal practice.

You should only consent the patient, if you know what is planned and feel competent to explain this. If you are unhappy to take the consent approach a more senior member of the staff.

Answer 2.22: If the anastomosis is in the lower third of the rectum (i.e. below 6 cm from the anal verge), then a temporary covering loop ileostomy is performed. This is to allow the join up to heal safely. Although the ileostomy does not cut down the number of leaks, it reduces the incidence and severity of the complications.

The implications to the patient of a stoma are very important:

1. Patients are terrified of having 'a bag'—because they think, it will disrupt their lifestyle and make them a social 'outcast'.

2. This is why it is essential that the patient has access to a stoma nurse both before and after the operation. She will explain why the stoma needs to be done, where it will be and how the patient will manage it after the operation. She will also make sure the proposed site is correctly marked preoperation. Clearly, the patient will be told if the stoma is temporary—how long they will have if and how long they will be in hospital for the reversal.

Please remember that different religions have differing views on the acceptability of a stoma. These views must always be heeded.

Answer 2.23:

60 cm flexible sigmoidoscope + rigid sigmoidoscope
120 cm colonoscope.

Answer 2.24:

Rigid sigmoidoscope—disposable and nondisposable
Biopsy forceps.

Answer 2.25: Barium enema showing a carcinoma of colon (apple-core lesion).

Answer 2.26:

- CT scan of abdomen (with contrast).
- Shows a cancer of caecum and multiple liver metastases.

Answer 2.27:

- Polyp on VR colonoscopy (CT colonoscopy)—picture on left.
- Same polyp shown at colonoscopy—picture on right.

Answer 2.28: MRI of rectum showing a T2 tumor.

Answer 2.29:

- PET/CT scan (positive emission tomography).
- PET scanning usually uses an FDG—a glucose analog. Concentrations of this tracer are imaged.

Changes depend on the degree of metabolic activity in terms of glucose uptake—higher in malignant tissue.

PET scanning is now usually combined with CT, adding the benefit of anatomical localization to functional imaging. (Look at *www.en.wikipedia.org/wiki/PET-CT*)

TUTORIAL 4: Abdominal Pain (Acute Abdomen)

CASE SCENARIOS

Answer 1.1:

1. Acute appendicitis—because she has had lower abdominal pain + vomiting with history of peritonism and her signs are maximal in RIF. Also common things are common.

2. Pelvic inflammatory disease—history of pain, missed period, vaginal discharge, is sexually active. Lower abdominal peritonism at least and cervical excitation.

3. Ectopic pregnancy—missed period with lower abdominal signs.

Answer 1.2:

- Full blood count
- Bioprofile
- C-reactive protein (CRP) (inflammatory marker)
- Liver function tests
- Amylase
- Pregnancy test
- Urine—dipstick and MSU
- Chest X-ray
- US of pelvis rather than plain X-rays of abdomen.

Answer 1.3a:

Hb: Below lower limit of normal—may indicate bleeding.
WCC: Upper limit of normal—may indicate infection.
CRP: Normal CRP does not exclude inflammatory cause.

Answer 1.3b: Above upper limit of normal—patient may be dehydrated.

Answer 1.3c: Usually come as part of bioprofile—probably not relevant in this case.

Answer 1.3d: Pancreatitis has a myriad of ways of presenting—good to exclude in any undiagnosed acute abdomen.

Answer 1.3e: Need to know, she is not pregnant—ectopic pregnancy.

Answer 1.3f: Could indicate UTI, could be inflamed appendix pressing on ureter.

Answer 1.4: The report will not be available for 24 hours (except for microscopy). It will contain details of:
- Urine microscopy
- Culture
- Sensitivity.

Answer 1.5:

Hb = male = 13–18 g/dL female 12–16 g/dL

WCC = 4,300–10,800/mm^3

Serum amylase = 0–200 IU.

Answer 1.6: All depend on detection of human chorionic gonadotropin (hCG).

Urine hCG can be detected at the bedside using a chemical strip or sent to laboratory.

Serum hCG can be qualitative or quantitative—need to send blood to lab—result can be available in hours.

Serum hCG –ve = Not pregnant (98%) accurate.

Note that raised with some drugs, e.g. anticonvulsants, phenothiazines, promethazine and in some testicular tumors.

Answer 1.7: Normal

Answer 1.8: Normal

Answer 1.9: Transabdominal or transvaginal.

Answer 1.10: L-sided ovarian cyst.

Answer 1.11: Laparoscopy is carried out and shows a normal L sided luteal ovarian cyst and an inflamed appendix.

Answer 1.12: If the surgeon has the necessary training and experience, then he may choose to remove the appendix laparoscopically. If not, then he should convert to open operation and remove the appendix.

Answer 2.1: He probably has intestinal obstruction.

Answer 2.2:
- Abdominal pain
- Vomiting
- Abdominal distension
- Constipation.

Answer 2.3: Remember that the 4 criteria above may vary with the level of the obstruction. Thus, an obstructing cancer of the cecum may mimic a small bowel obstruction with early onset of pain and vomiting.

A cancer of the distal colon may present with persistent lower abdominal pain becoming worse when the degree of obstruction increases. Vomiting is usually late in onset and abdominal distension occurs late when the obstruction becomes complete. The history of increased frequency of defecation over a period of months may turn to absolute constipation as the degree of obstruction becomes complete.

Answer 2.4:
- Large bowel cancer
- Large bowel obstructed in a hernia
- Volvulus
- Stricture—diverticular.

Answer 2.5:
- Erect abdominal X-ray
- Shows air-fluid levels in R and L colon with no gas below mid descending colon
- Indicative of large bowel obstruction.

Answer 2.6:
- Supine plain abdominal X-ray
- Shows dilated cecum and colon dilated up to pelvic brim.

Answer 2.7:
- Contrast-enhanced CT
- If immediate CT is available, then this is now the investigation of choice in a patient with the above history: the 'scout' films alone will often indicate the diagnosis.

Answer 2.8:
- Contrast-enhanced CT abdomen
- Dilated large bowel
- Sigmoid tumor.

Answer 2.9:
1. Assess the patient's clinical and biochemical hydration status.
2. Start IV infusion with appropriate fluids (usually Hartmann's solution).
3. Insert urinary catheter (and nasogastric tube if indicated).
4. Administer pain relief, if required.
5. Start subcutaneous heparin and prophylactic antibiotics.
6. Obtain informed consent (including discussion of stoma).
7. Perform open laparotomy via midline incision.
8. Depending on findings, patient's condition and experience of operator performing the operation—perform a Hartmann's operation or total colectomy and ileorectal anastomosis or on table lavage + primary resection and anastomosis.

Answer 2.10:

Sigmoid colon (+/– rectosigmoid junction) is resected.

Descending colon is brought out as end-LIF colostomy.

Rectum closed over.

Answer 2.11: See Figure 4.7.

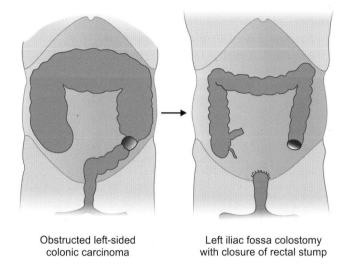

Obstructed left-sided
colonic carcinoma

Left iliac fossa colostomy
with closure of rectal stump

Fig. 4.7 Hartmann's operation

Answer 2.12:

Figure 4.8A shows a very distended gas-filled loop with other gas dilated loops in the background.

Figure 4.8B shows a central distended loop—the 'coffee bean' sign of sigmoid volvulus.

Answer 2.13:
- Gastrografin enema
- Shows hold up of contrast at rectosigmoid junction indicative of sigmoid volvulus of colon.

Answer 2.14:

Incidence:	Accounts for some 5% of all large bowel obstruction: more common in elderly and in Africa. Sigmoid volvulus much more common than cecalvolvulus.
Etiology:	Predisposing factor is a long colon. The underlying cause being chronic constipation. Therefore, occurs in elderly patients with underlying neurological conditions (e.g. Chaga's disease) and in patients in nursing homes or mental health hospitals.
Pathology:	Sigmoid colon twists around mesenteric axis, cecal volvulus around a long mesentry. Sequence of events is twist, obstruct, ischemia, perforation, peritonitis.
Presentation:	Will depend on 'pathological stage' Hence, uncomplicated = abdominal pain/distension/absolute constipation. Complicated will be signs of local or diffuse peritonitis.
Investigation:	Plain abdominal X-rays CT scanning Gastrografin enema.
Treatment:	*Uncomplicated:* Decompression with rectal tube or endoscopy (sigmoid) *Uncomplicated recurrent:* Surgery. Usually resection and anastomosis for sigmoid volvulus (rather than fixation). *Complicated:* Laparotomy

- If bowel viable—Resection + Anastomosis
- If gangrenous—Hartmann's operation

Complications: Gangrene, perforation, peritonitis.

TUTORIAL 5: Vascular Disease (Arterial)

CASE SCENARIOS

Answer 1.1:
- Ruptured abdominal aortic aneurysm
- Perforated viscus with peritonitis
- Acute pancreatitis.

Answer 1.2:
- Does he look pale and sweaty? Is he in pain? Moving about or lying still?
- What is his mental status? Is he tachypneic?
- What is his circulatory status—pulse/BP/peripherally shut down?

Abdominal examination:

I Moving normally with respiration
Visible mass or pulsation
Any bruising visible on abdominal wall/flanks
Any scars
Evidence of weight loss.

P Tenderness/guarding/rebound
Palpable mass/expansible swelling
Organomegaly
Free fluid
Bowel sounds/bruit
Femoral pulses.

Answer 1.3:
- Most likely a ruptured aortic aneurysm
- Pancreatitis and peritonitis from another cause remain a possibility.

Answer 1.4:
1. Put him on an oxygen mask—facemask 100% flow.
2. Put up wide bore IV line.
3. Take off blood and send urgently for FBC, bioprofile, amylase, group and X match.

4. Ask nurse to contact Senior Surgical Registrar/Specialist/ Vascular Consultant and tell them, you think the patient has a ruptured AAA and could he/she come and see urgently.
5. Start continuous monitoring—pulse, BP, ECG.
6. Put in a urinary catheter.
7. Write-up a fluid balance chart.
8. Warn the emergency anesthetist and operating suite that there may be a ruptured AAA requiring surgery.

Answer 1.5:
• Do not fluid overload—this may precipitate more bleeding.
• Do not send-off to X-ray until reviewed by senior.

Answer 1.6: See Figure 5.1.

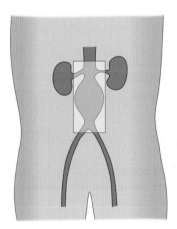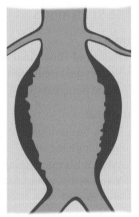

Fig. 5.1 Infrarenal abdominal aortic aneurysm

Answer 1.7: There will be a tense swelling in the left retroperitoneum with evidence of hematoma formation. This will be pulsatile and always seems higher up than you would think. The intestinal contents may be pushed upwards or sideways.

Answer 1.8: The first move is to define the upper limit of aneurysm and its relation to the renal arteries. The surgeon has to obtain proximal control—usually putting a vascular clamp around the neck of the aneurysm. He then gets distal control of either the common iliacs or the internal and external iliacs (depending on how far distally the aneurysm extends).

Once the surgeon has control, the aneurysm is split open, clot evacuated and an onlay graft put in place— either a straight graft or a Y graft (*Note:* The aneurysm is not resected).

Answer 1.9: This shows an infrarenal AAA which has been controlled (see clamps) and an onlay straight graft inserted.

Answer 1.10:
This shows an AAA also involving the left common iliac artery
This would need a Y-graft reconstruction.
A synthetic Y-graft is shown in Figure 5.5.

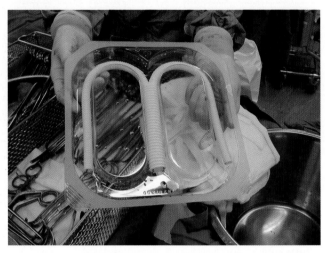

Fig. 5.5 Aortic prosthetic Y graft

Answer 1.11: a, c and d are correct. (review this topic at *www. patient.info/doctor/Abdominal-Aortic-Aneurysms*)

Answer 1.12: When you take the history you will be seeking evidence of cardiac problems and stroke.
When you examine the patient you will be looking for:
• Abnormal radial pulse rhythm
• High blood pressure
• Carotid bruit
• Any aneurysm of other palpable pulses
• Evidence of peripheral vascular disease in the legs— dystrophic changes, ulcers on pressure points, gangrene, absent or diminished pulses
• Evidence of a stroke.

Answer 1.13: This is a plain X-ray of the abdomen almost certainly taken in the supine position. There is irregular, linear calcification to the L of the Lumbar vertebrae in the line of the abdominal aorta consistent with an aortic aneurysm.

Answer 1.14: This ultrasound examination shows a hypoechoic vascular structure measuring about 9 cm in diameter consistent with an aortic aneurysm.

Answer 1.15: Contrast is seen in the aorta. There is a large hematoma surrounding the aorta consistent with a ruptured aortic aneurysm.

Answer 1.16a: His condition will be very unstable. If the diagnosis is reasonably certain, it is safer to take him straight to the operating theater (see addendum re EVAR).

Answer 1.16b: Rapid refilling of his intravascular space may raise his blood pressure and extend the rupture leading to collapse and death.

Answer 1.16c: As many as 2 out of 3 patients with a ruptured AAA die before reaching hospital. Of those who reach hospital about one-fifth die before reaching operation. Overall, mortality rate is about 50%.

Answer 1.17: Thoracic aortic dissection is the most common catastrophe of the aorta (2–3 times more than ruptured AAA). Untreated, one third of patients die within 24 hours.
- Type A involves ascending aorta and needs surgery.
- Type B involves the descending aorta and may be managed medically.

Note: Distinguish dissection from thoracic aortic aneurysm and aortic transection (RTA).

Symptoms:	Severe ripping or tearing chest pain of acute sudden onset Anterior chest pain—suggests ascending aortic dissection. Neck or jaw pain—suggests aortic arch.
Signs:	• BP may be raised or decreased. • The patient frequently faints or is mentally confused. • Other diagnostic clues are a pulse deficit and asymmetrical radial BP measurements.
Investigation:	• In 80% of cases, the CXR is abnormal—mediastinal widening of > 8 cm on AP CXR. • CT angiography has now replaced catheter angiography as the primary imaging modality of choice. (For more detail look at *www.patient.co.uk/aortic-dissection*)

Look at the image (Fig. 5.10).

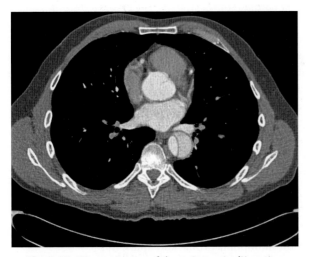

Fig. 5.10 CT scan image of thoracic aortic dissection

Answer 2.1: First of all you will have to make sure that she does not have evidence of soft tissue or bony trauma. Then you must remember that the 'fall' may be a 'red herring' and that because she is at risk, she may have a DVT.

Answer 2.2: First of all, you will look for bruising, grazing, bony tenderness and lack of movement.
In the absence of these you must look for the signs of DVT:
- Calf tenderness
- Calf swelling
- Flicker of temperature on chart
- Much less common—increased warmth in affected leg red blue limb (extensive DVT)
- Always check the leg pulses—just possible the cause may be an arterial problem.

Answer 2.3: Deep venous thrombosis of the calf (DVT).

Answer 2.4:
1. Confirm the diagnosis by sending her for an immediate Doppler US scan.
2. Obtain the result as soon as possible.
3. If the diagnosis is confirmed—inform your specialist and discuss and institute treatment.
   If the DVT is below the popliteal fossa, treatment will probably involve increasing the dose of subcutaneous heparin to twice daily [Low Molecular Weight Heparin (LMWH)].
   If the clot extends above the popliteal fossa, provided there are no contraindications, the patient will need full anticoagulation with either IV heparin (then oral anticoagulants—warfarin) or therapeutic LMWH.

Answer 2.5:
1. Alteration in blood flow (stasis).
2. Injury to vascular endothelium (trauma).
3. Alteration in the constituents of the blood (hypercoagulability).

Answer 2.6:
1. Keep as mobile and well hydrated as possible.
2. Anti-thrombotic (TED) stockings.
3. Low dose prophylactic subcutaneous heparin—either low molecular weight heparin (LMWH) or conventional fractionated heparin.
4. In theater—use calf pumps, if indicated.

Answer 2.7:
- Continue calf pumps until fully mobilized or use TED stockings.
- Continue subcutaneous heparin.
- Physiotherapy and mobilize as quickly as possible.
   House officer/intern checks patient's calves each day on ward rounds.

Answer 2.8:

1. Extension of clot to give 'phlegmasia carulea dolens'—blue leg or phlegmasia alba dolens—white leg.
   Note: In phlegmasia alba dolens, the clot involves only the major deep venous channels and spares the collateral veins.
   In phlegmasia carulea dolens, the clot extends into the collateral veins as well.
2. Clot breaks-off and causes pulmonary embolus.
3. Long-term complications of varicose veins and post-phlebitic limb.

Answer 2.9: Doppler US probe.

Used for:

a. Imaging the deep and superficial venous system and flow within it.
b. Identifying sites of venous incompetence.
c. Identifying peripheral pulses and performing A/B ratios.

In Figure 5.11, it is being used for ABI measurement.

Answer 2.10: Color Doppler—showing the artery (orange) and clot in vein.

Answer 2.11: She may have had a pulmonary embolus, but do not forget there are other causes of chest pain and breathlessness in a postoperation patient.

The classic triad for PE is hemoptysis, dypsnea and pleuritic chest pain, but these are neither sensitive or specific (occur in < 20% patients).

Remember that the signs in patients with massive PE can include:

Tachypnea (RR > 16/min)	95%
Added noises on auscultation (wheezes and crackles)	(50%)
Accentuated 2nd HS	(50%)
Tachycardia	(40%)
Fever	(40%)
S3 S4 gallop	(30%)
Cardiac murmur	(20%)
Cyanosis	(20%)

Answer 2.12:

1. Administer oxygen via facemask or nasal prongs.
2. If hypotensive, try small bolus of IV fluid.
3. Perform ECG and blood gases.
4. If possible arrange for immediate spiral CT to confirm diagnosis.
5. *If delay:* Start on IV heparin immediately.

Answer 2.13: CT scan has largely replaced VQ scanning.

Answer 2.14: Marked oligemia in R lung due to large PE in R main pulmonary artery.

Remember: In PE the early, CXR may be normal. After 24–48 hours the classic changes of PE—atelectasis, raised diaphragm and pleural effusion are indistinguishable from the signs of pneumonia.

Answer 2.15:

- Ventilation/Perfusion scan.
- Indicated now only when CT not available.
- Compares and correlates perfusion with ventilation.
- For the ventilation scan the patient inhales a small amount of radioisotope gas and for the perfusion scan radioisotope is given IV.

Areas of under perfusion matching with normal ventilation are indicative of PE.

Answer 2.16: Shows clot in both R and L main pulmonary arteries with obliteration of distal flow.

Answer 2.17: Shows clot in pulmonary artery.

Answer 2.18: This is a caval filter or umbrella.

Its use is in patients throwing off repeated leg or pelvic emboli despite adequate anticoagulation.

Sometimes used prophylactively in high-risk patients prior to surgery who cannot be anticoagulated.

Inserted under radiographic screening via femoral vein into lower IVC.

Answer 3.1: A thromboembolic episode, but do not forget it may be due to other disorders, e.g. Musculoskeletal trauma, neurological cause.

Answer 3.2:

- Pain
- Paresthesia
- Paralysis
- Pallor
- Pulseless
- Perishing cold.

Answer 3.3: Thrombosis on pre-existing PVD (60%) or embolus (AF or cardiac source) (30%).

In this patient, because of the sudden onset and AF, the most likely cause is an embolus (remember there are other causes of acute limb ischemia: trauma, iatrogenic injury, thrombosed popliteal aneurysm, extreme cold, IV drug administration, venous gangrene, prothrombotic states).

Answer 3.4: Full history and examination with attention to pre-existing coronary, cerebrovascular and renovascular abnormalities, then:

1. Give 100% oxygen via facemask.
2. Obtain IV access and start slow infusion with Hartmann's solution.
3. Withdraw blood for FBC, U and E's, glucose, cardiac enzymes, clotting screen group and X match, thrombophilia profile and lipids.
4. Call for senior help.

5. Arrange for chest X-ray and ECG.
6. Insert a urinary catheter and commence an input and output chart.
7. Opiate analgesia, if indicated.

Answer 3.5: Color Doppler or angiogram.

Answer 3.6: Arteriogram showing a cut-off in the right common femoral artery, consistent with an acute embolus. Angiography used to be performed percutaneously via the aorta or femoral artery. This has now been largely replaced by CT angiograms or MRI angiogram.

Answer 3.7: Fogarty catheter used for extracting emboli from femoral and distal vessels. Open surgery with femoral vessels exposed and catheter, inserted via arteriotomy.

Answer 3.8: Management depends on the severity of ischemic process:
1. Irreversible with nonsalvageable limb = Amputation.
2. Complete with acutely threatened limb = Thrombolysis, angiography, angioplasty, embolectomy, or urgent bypass surgery depending on circumstance.
3. Incomplete with viable limb = IV heparin (IV bolus 5000 units and 1000 units per hour), then arrange angiograms to plan management.

Note: All of these situations require urgent senior surgeon input, so if you are the house surgeon make contact straightaway.

TUTORIAL 6: Lumps in Neck

Patient 1: Solitary thyroid swelling
Patient 2: Swelling in anterior triangle

CASE SCENARIOS

Answer 1.1:
1. Look at hands • Nails – leukonychia (hyper)
       – clubbing
         (thyroid achopachy—hyper)
     • Feel hands for excess sweating/warmth (hyper)
     • Hold out hands—tremor (hyper)
     • Feel pulse—tachycardia/ bradycardia/AF (hyper)
2. On way 'up' • Test for proximal myopathy (hyper)
3. Look at face • Exophthalmos – hyper
     • Staring gaze – lid retraction (hyper)
     • Lid lag – hyper
     • Diplopia + pupil divergence (hyper)
Look at face—peaches and cream of myxedema/thin fine hair.

Note: Thyroid eye disease is usually associated with Graves' disease.
4. Pretibial myxedema—hyper
5. Test tendon reflexes—quick = hyper
          slow = hypo

Answer 1.2:
1. Dominant nodule (solid or cystic swelling) as part of a multinodular goiter.
2. Solitary thyroid cyst.
3. Benign follicular adenoma.
4. Malignant swelling.
(Localized Hashimoto's and metastasis are very uncommon)

Answer 1.3: Algorithm for solitary thyroid nodule is shown in Flow chart 6.1 (page 172).

Answer 1.4: Table 6.1.

Answer 1.5:
• TSH (thyroid stimulating hormone)
• T3
• T4
• Thyroid antibodies.

Answer 1.6: See Figure 6.1 (page 173).
• The thyroid is made up of follicles containing colloid.
• Follicles are lined by cuboidal epithelium (thyrocytes) which secrete
    – Tri-iodothyronine (T3) and
    – Thyroxine (T4)
• T3 is the active hormone and T4 is converted into this in the periphery.
• T3 and T4 are bound to thyroglobulin and are stored in the follicles and when released circulate either free or bound to plasma protein.
• T3 and T4 secretion is controlled by TSH (thyroid stimulating hormone) which is released from the anterior pituitary by the stimulus of thyrotrophic releasing hormone from the hypothalamus (TRH).
• Circulating levels of T3 and T4 act as negative feedback on the pituitary and hypothalamus.
• TSH is low in the thyrotoxic patient and high in hypothyroidism. T3 and T4 are raised in the toxic patient and low in hypothyroidism.
• Graves' disease is an autoimmune disease with high thyroid stimulating immunoglobulin in the blood which releases T3 and T4.
• Remember total T3 and T4 are not accurate in the pregnant woman because there is more thyroid binding globulin.
• Free T3 and T4 are unchanged.

Flow chart 6.1 Algorithm for management of a solitary thyroid nodule

Abbreviations: TFTs, thyroid function tests; RA, radioactive scintiscan; FNAC, fine needle aspiration cytology; FU, follow-up; MNG, multinodular goiter; TSH, thyroid stimulating hormone

Table 6.1 Thyroid cancer summarized				
Type	*Incidence*	*Spread*	*Management*	*Survival 5-year*
Papillary	• 80% all thyroid cancers • <40 years • >Females x3	• Locally to neck • Lymph nodes	If >1 cm, total thyroidectomy + remove palpable nodes +TSH suppression radioactive iodine ablation	>50%
Follicular	• 10% of all • 30–50 years • >Females x3	Via bloodstream	If >1 cm, total thyroidectomy + involved nodes + radioactive iodine + TSH suppression	>50%
Anaplastic	Older	Local Blood to lungs	Surgery or DXR + chemotherapy for local control	Most die in <1 year
Medullary (secrete calcitonin)	Sporadic or Familial—MEN2	Usually solitary May be bilobar	Total thyroidectomy + palpable node removal	Poor Good, if detected early

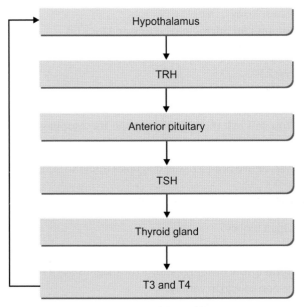

Fig. 6.1 Regulation of thyroid hormones

Answer 1.7a: Normal.

Answer 1.7b:
  TSH = Low
  T3 and T4 high.

Answer 1.7c:
  TSH = High
  T3 and T4 low.

Answer 1.8:
- Both pregnancy and estrogen supplements give false levels because of excess thyroid binding globulin (total T3 and T4).
- Measure free T3 and T4.

Answer 1.9: Consists of:
- Thyroid peroxidase antibodies
- Thyroglobulin antibodies
- Thyroid stimulating hormone receptor antibodies.

Answer 1.10: Used to help diagnose an autoimmune thyroid disease and help distinguish it from other forms of thyroiditis.

Answer 1.11: Normal (euthyroid).

Answer 1.12: Swelling in R lobe of thyroid.

Answer 1.13: Explain to the patient that the scan has shown a swelling in one lobe of the thyroid gland. The doctor needs to get a sample of tissue from this to tell him, if it is abnormal. This test is quite simple and is done at the OP clinic. It takes a few minutes and you will be able to go home almost straight after the test. It involves a pinprick, does not need anesthesia and is not really painful. Some doctors use a local anesthetic.

You will be asked to lie on the couch. The doctor will clean the skin over the lump and then put a needle into the swelling and draw off some cells which will be sent to the laboratory. The complication rate is very low—sometimes you can get a bit of bruising. If pain or swelling of the neck occurs after the procedure you should come back to the hospital clinic straight away.

The results will be ready in a few days and the clinic doctor will make you an appointment to be seen to discuss the results.

Answer 1.14: This is a problem with follicular adenomas. The FNAC often cannot distinguish between a benign follicular adenoma and a malignant one. So to start with, the patient should be advised to have that lobe of the thyroid removed.

Answer 1.15: Explain to the patient that the cells are abnormal but it is not possible to tell, if the swelling is a cancer or not. The swelling needs to be removed to be on the safe side. This will involve the patient having an operation on her neck under a general anesthetic. Half of the thyroid gland will be removed to include the swelling. The operation is not dangerous and she will need to be in hospital for a day or two. The thyroid tissue removed will be looked at under the microscope, if it is benign nothing more will need doing, if it is cancerous the surgeon will probably advise that the rest of the thyroid gland be removed.

Tell her that the operation is usually straight forward. Explain she will have a scar across her neck and show her where this will be. Complications are uncommon but she may have bruising of the neck. Very occasionally a nerve might be damaged but this is uncommon.

Answer 1.16: There is a well-defined, homogeneous, whitish/pink swelling in the center of the lobe, measuring about 2×2 cm. It has a smooth cut surface and appears encapsulated. Rest of the lobe appears normal.

Answer 1.17: That she is cured of the problem and does not require any further surgery.

Answer 2.1:

Malignant lymph node:	From skin of head and neck
	From oropharynx
	Metastatic
	Primary reticuloses: Lymphoma, lymphosarcoma, reticulosarcoma.
Infective:	Tuberculosis
	Toxoplasmosis
	Cat scratch fever
	(tonsillitis, glandular fever).
Others:	Sarcoidosis.

Answer 2.2:

Need to know more about his general malaise
- Has he had fever or rigors?
- Why has he lost weight?
- Has he had skin irritation (lymphoma)?

Need to know more about his wife's illness
- What was diagnosis?
- What treatment did she have including the medications?

Need to know more about specific head and neck symptoms:
- Pain in mouth
- Sore throat
- Nasal discharge
- Pain in throat
- Dysphagia
- Voice change
- Difficulty with breathing
- Lumps or ulcers of the skin or head that have changed in size or bled.

In addition to this, the routine questions of the review of systems may give valuable information, e.g. has he any symptoms of cough/hemoptysis/breathing problems (CA lung, tuberculosis, sarcoid).

Also symptoms suggestive of GI malignancy.

Lumps elsewhere—groin/axillary glands/abdomen mass or pain.

Answer 2.3:

Define the site of the swelling(s)—anterior or posterior triangle.

Define the characteristics of the swellings:

Look Any skin changes: Skin lesions
Sinuses/fistulae
Signs of infection—redness/edema.

Feel Use the 4X S/C/T/P mnemonic (see appendix at end of book) particularly interested in what they feel like (e.g. hard, rubbery) tenderness/fluctuant/irregular.

Move Are the lumps fixed and, if so, to what?

Then need to carry out a full oral examination with tongue spatula and a good torch.

Looking at mucous membranes, looking at and feeling the tongue—use gloved finger to feel the posterior third of tongue.

Look at the oropharynx—tonsils/fauces.

Then need to examine the chest and axillae.

Then need to examine the abdomen—spleen/other nodes.

Answer 2.4:
- FBC
- Bioprofile including liver function tests

- Chest X-ray
- Sputum for micro- and culture and for AFB
- Mantoux test.

Answer 2.5:
- Ask for an ENT opinion—they would carry out a video endoscopy of oropharynx and larynx.
- You can ask them to endoscope the esophagus at the same procedure.

Answer 2.6: We need a tissue diagnosis from the lump.

Answer 2.7:
- FNAC
- Open biopsy.

Answer 2.8: Open excisional biopsy of one of the nodes is performed. The histology shows the diagnosis is a reticulosis of the non-Hodgkin variety.

Answer 2.9:
- Chest X-ray
- CT of chest, abdomen and head and neck. Bone marrow.

TUTORIAL 7: Nipple Discharge, Breast Lumps and Breast Pain

Answer 1: The protocol listed here is that used at Penang Medical College and has been used in Module 1.

Examine with patient sitting on edge of examination couch first:

Remember:
- Look, Feel, Move
- Breast, Areola, Nipple.

Look: Right and left disparity in size/lumps/skin tethering abnormal skin changes, distended veins, then areola changes, then nipple changes or differences.
Raise arms—look for tethering/mass.

Feel:
- By quadrants, systematically:
- Describe lump by set criteria (site, size, shape, surface, etc.)
- Do not forget move (i.e. fixity to skin and pectoralis muscle), then examine areola and nipple.
- Examine normal breast first and then the other.
- Feel axillae correct way: ant/post/medial walls and apex.
- Feel supraclavicular areas.

Then lie paient down on 1 pillow, hand behind head and repeat whole sequence.

Check for ascites and liver enlargement.

CASE SCENARIOS

Answer 2.1:
- When did you first notice the discharge?
- How did you notice it?
- How often does it occur and how much blood is there?
- Is the discharge from one or both breasts?
- Is it always the same color?
- Why does she think it is blood?
- Does it happen without you poking or pushing on the breast?
- Do you still have periods and is the discharge related to these?
- Any other breast symptoms—pain/lumps/skin changes?
- Any recent history of trauma to breast?

Answer 2.2:
- Carry out a full breast examination.
- Test the discharge with a dipstick test for presence of blood or look at under microscope for red blood cells.
- Obtain mammograms.

Answer 2.3: Most likely diagnosis is mammary duct ectasia if discharge is from one nipple only, fibrocystic disease, if from both nipples (less likely intraduct papilloma).

Answer 3.1:
- Intraduct papilloma/carcinoma
- Carcinoma breast (rare)
- Paget's disease of nipple
- Duct ectasia
- Injury.

Answer 3.2:
- Full breast examination.
- See, if blood comes from single duct opening—more likely duct papilloma/carcinoma.
- If there are no other signs suggestive of cancer of breast (including mammograms), the management would be duct exploration (microdochotomy).

Answer 4.1:
- Hot   (Calor)
- Painful   (Dolor)
- Red   (Rugor)
- Swollen   (Tumor)

Answer 4.2: Principles of treating breast infection are:
1. Give appropriate antibiotics to reduce the formation of abscess (i.e. if cellulitis only).
2. If an abscess is suspected confirm by aspirating pus before considering drainage.
3. Exclude cancer in a solid, non-settling lesion (with mammograms and cytology).

In this case, we are dealing with lactating infection. The options are:
- Incision and drainage (I + D) or
- Repeated aspiration, preferably under ultrasound guidance with covering antibiotics. (organisms = *Staph. aureus*, *Staph. epididimis* or *Streptococcus*)
- Antibiotic of choice: flucloxacillin.
- Encourage the patient to continue to breastfeed—helps duct to secrete milk and not block, i.e. helps drainage).

Answer 5.1a:
- *Two types:* Pericanalicular which are small and hard, found in younger women with signs of a 'breast mouse.'
- Intracanalicular which are 'cauliflower like' on cut section, softer on palpation, bigger and can occur in the younger patient or an older patient at time of menopause.

Answer 5.1b:
- Triple assessment
- Clinical examination
- FNAC
- Mammograms/US.

Answer 5.1c: Yes, if fibroadenoma diameter is less than 3 cm (if larger should be removed to exclude cystosarcoma phylloides).

Remember a fibroadenoma should be regarded as an aberrance of normal breast tissue and about 30% either disappear or become smaller within 2 years.

Answer 6.1: Refer her to a general surgeon with an interest in breast diseases.

Answer 6.2: After full breast examination the surgeon decides that this is most probably a cyst with a history and signs of fibrocystic disease.

He will aspirate the cyst—see what comes out and palpate to make sure, it has disappeared.

Answer 6.3:
- Mammograms.
- Cytology of the cyst fluid is not necessary but can be sent if you wish.
- Follow-up in 2 weeks' time to check the results and make sure the cyst has not refilled.

Answer 6.4: This is the normal mammogram of a young lady. As you see the breast tissue is very dense and it would be difficult to see the changes of a carcinoma—hence an US may help.

Answer 6.5: This is a normal mammogram in a fatty breast.

Answer 6.6: This is a mammogram showing fibrocystic disease.

Answer 6.7: Cancer of the right breast. The mammographic changes of breast cancer are not always as straightforward as this case.

Answer 6.8:
- Review of all patients sent for investigation and treatment in the breast clinic.
- Surgeons/radiologists/pathologists/oncologist/nurses: All present to discuss each case and decide on the management and follow-up.

Answer 7.1: Redness around a retracted right nipple. Elevated lesion with central defect at 2 o'clock.

Answer 7.2: Mammary duct ectasia with mammary duct fistula.

Answer 7.3: With age the subareolar ducts dilate and shorten, called duct ectasia. Debris builds up in the ducts and can lead to a cheesy white discharge. Also the nipple retracts (becomes slit-like). Can become infected giving an abscess or fistula.

Importance is to distinguish from carcinoma or Paget's disease. Surgery may be required, if symptoms are troublesome.

Answer 8.1:
- Paget's disease of the nipple (until excluded).
- Eczema.

Answer 8.2: Tell her this may be something serious but treatable and send her to breast clinic.

Answer 9.1: You should tell her that this is a screening program (explain this) to try and pick-up breast cancer at an earlier stage (and therefore more likely curable). The incidence of breast cancer increases with age and it would be sensible for her to have this check. The test involves a special X-ray which, apart from a little discomfort, will not upset her.

She will get the results very quickly.

Answer 9.2: The principles of a disease suitable for a screening program are:
1. The disease is common or a known high-risk group is identified.
2. The natural history of the disease is known and shows that the screened for 'abnormality' will lead to improved prognosis, if identified and treated.
3. Sensitivity and specificity for the screened abnormality should be acceptable.
4. The 'test' should be cheap, easy to carryout and patient compliant.
5. Effective treatment is available for the early disease.
6. Test noninvasive as possible.
7. Cost effective.

The UK breast screening program is typical.
- Its purpose is to detect breast cancer at an early stage, mammography is the screening tool.
- Women over the age of 50 years are offered free mammography screening on a 3 year rolling basis.
- It is thought that there is a 35% reduction in mortality from breast cancer among screened women aged 50–69 years. This means that for 1 in 500 screened, 1 life will be saved.
- There is a risk of harm from overdiagnosis but it is thought that between 2 and 2.5 lives are saved for every over-diagnosed case.
- These figures are quoted from NHS Breast Cancer Screening Programme: *http://www.cancerscreening.nhs.uk/save-lives.html*
- Note that there are some groups who are critical of mammographic sceening on both socioeconomic grounds and over-diagnosis and treatment.

Answer 9.3: This is the 'hook wire' method of localizing a nonpalpable breast lesion found on mammography. The technique is to enable the surgeon to carry out an accurate biopsy of the suspect area.

TUTORIAL 8: Difficulty in Passing Urine (Prostate)

CASE SCENARIOS

Answer 1.1:
- How long is it since you passed urine?
- Have you had this problem before?
- Over the last few months have you been having difficulty passing urine?
- If he does not volunteer the information—ask directly:
  - Pain on passing urine/passing urine more often in the daytime/night-time with ratio/passing blood in the urine?
  - Do you have difficulty starting the stream? Is the flow good? Does it stop? Do you leak any urine?

Answer 1.2: See Table 8.1.

Table 8.1 Classification of urinary symptoms

Obstructive (voiding) symptoms	Irritative/storage symptoms
Hesitancy	Frequency
Difficulty in starting	Dysuria (painful micturition)
Poor/intermittent stream	Urgency
Terminal dribbling	Urge incontinence
Incomplete emptying	Nocturia

Answer 1.3: Acute urinary retention probably subsequent to benign prostatic hypertrophy.

Answer 1.4: Inability to pass urine, usually of sudden onset and accompanied by lower abdominal pain.

Answer 1.5: Persistent passage of small amounts of urine, despite a full bladder—usually pain free.

Answer 1.6: Look at him generally: Is he in pain? Is he drowsy? Any signs of anemia, jaundice, dehydration or weight loss?
- Examine his abdomen
  I: Any visible mass?
  P: Is the bladder palpable?
  Percussion: Can the bladder be percussed?

Answer 1.7: Have a routine:
- Explain to the patient what you are going to do. Always best to have a chaperone or nurse present.
- Make sure he is covered appropriately and the screens are closed (privacy).
- Bring the patient's buttocks to the edge of the bed in the L lateral position with his knees half drawn up
- Wear gloves that fit; lubricate index finger.
- Inspect the anal area.
- Gently press backwards at 6 o'clock on the anal verge—relaxes the sphincters.
- Examine each quadrant of the rectum in turn, noting any abnormality.
- If abnormality detected re-examine that area.
- Warn the patient and then press upwards once to reach about 10–12 cm feeling for any intrarectal swelling
- Then assess the prostate—use the S's—size shape surface + 'C' consistency. Define each lobe in this way and the median groove.

Answer 1.8: The prostate may be difficult to assess because the patient is in discomfort and also because the full bladder pushes the prostate down and makes it feel larger than it may be.

If prostate is assessable—you would expect it to be smooth with bilobar enlargement, median groove palpable and of rubbery consistency (changes of benign prostatic hypertrophy).

Answer 1.9: See Figure 8.1.

Answer 1.10:
- BPH = transition zone
- Prostatic cancer = peripheral zone

Answer 1.11: Acute retention of urine due to presumed benign prostatic hypertrophy.

Answer 1.12:
1. Ring-up your senior. Tell him the patient's history and your findings. Tell him you propose to catheterize the patient and seek his permission to proceed with this.

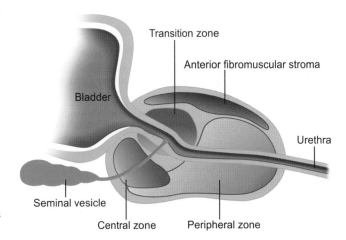

Fig. 8.1 Anatomy of prostate (schematic)

2. Explain to the patient what you think is wrong with him and explain what you are going to do to him.

Answer 1.13: I am Dr Beans, the House Officer who will be helping to look after you. We think you have got an enlarged prostate gland which is stopping you passing urine. You need to have a small tube, called a catheter, passed into your bladder to empty the bladder.
- I am going to do this for you, if you agree. Do not worry, it may be a little uncomfortable but will not hurt you. First of all, I will clean the area around your penis with some antiseptic. Then I will put some local anesthetic into the penis to stop the procedure hurting you. Once the tube is in place, we will fix it in the bladder by blowing up a balloon in the catheter end and then join it to a bag to collect the urine.
- To start with we will empty the bladder of the urine slowly.
- Do you have any questions? If not, I will get on with it.

Answer 1.14:
- Single lumen, double lumen, and triple lumen.
- French gauge (Fr): 8–24.
- Soft rubber Foley; simplastic; and hard rubber.

Answer 1.15: Soft rubber Foley catheter—try size 16/18 to start with.

Answer 1.16: Call your senior before you do any damage to the urethra.

Answer 1.17: By intermittently clamping the catheter for 5 minutes after, say, each 300 mL urine has drained (use a 'gate clamp').

If the bladder is quickly decompressed, then it is more likely to bleed.

Answer 1.18:

1. Routine charts: P/BP/temp/RR. Input/Output.
2. Catheter care: Daily washing of meatus and glans with soapy water.
   Check to make sure catheter is draining properly.
   Check for temperature and 'cloudy urine'.
   Empty urine bag as necessary.

Answer 1.19:

1. FBC—Hb for anemia. WCC for evidence of infection.
2. U and E and creatinine clearance as baseline renal function studies.
3. MSU/CSU to identify infection.
4. Ultrasound scan of ureters and kidneys to detect back pressure effects.

Note: In this case, the patient is catheterized.

You should be familiar with other basic urological investigations which may be carried out, if indicated:

a. PSA, if prostate feels abnormal on DRE—note the PSA will likely be raised in a patient who has been catheterized or had anorectal US because of the manipulation.
b. US scan of the bladder to exclude bladder stone and measure the size of prostate transvesically.
c. Transrectal US and biopsy, if malignancy is suspected.
d. Urine flow measurements—to quantify the reduction in urinary stream (flowmetry).
e. Cystoscopy to assess bladder neck and bladder particularly, if bladder cancer is suspected.

Answer 1.20: See Figure 8.2.

Answer 1.21:

> *Emergency acute retention:* Catheterization
> *Conservative:* No Rx—watch and wait
> *Medical:* • Alpha blockers
> • 5-alpha reductase inhibitors
> *Surgery:* • TURP
> • Open prostatectomy.

Answer 1.22: TURP (transurethral resection of prostate), unless the gland was very big.

Answer 2.1: Nodular enlargement, hard, irregular, loss of median sulcus.

Answer 2.2: Metastatic spread.

Answer 2.3:

1. FBC
2. U+E
3. LFTs, serum calcium
4. PSA
5. MSU

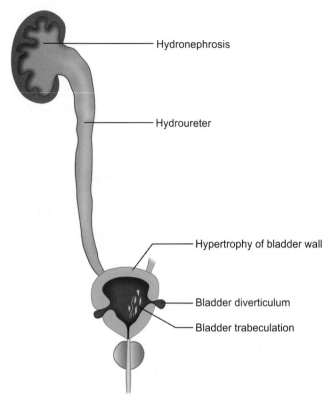

Fig. 8.2 Anatomical structural consequences of prostatic obstruction

6. Chest X-ray
7. Lumbar spine and pelvis X-rays
8. Transrectal US and biopsy
9. May need bone scan.

Answer 2.4a: Suggests an Fe-deficiency anemia: low Hb, low MCV, low MCH, low MCHC.

WCC at upper limit may suggest some infection—possibly in the urine, so you will arrange for an MSU.

Answer 2.4b: Either dehydrated or has a degree of renal failure.

Answer 2.4c: They are normal.

Answer 2.4d: A small number of red blood cells are commonly found on microscopy of urine. Microscopic hematuria is abnormal when the number seen on microscopy is greater than 3–5 per high powered field. Microscopic hematuria is often present in patients with prostatic cancer but is not, of course, diagnostic of it.

A PSA of 56 ng/mL is significantly elevated and suggests he has prostatic carcinoma. If the PSA is >10 ng/mL there is a 70% chance, the patient will have prostatic cancer. PSA levels in the hundreds suggest presence of bony metastases.

Answer 2.4e: Normal.

Answer 2.4f: Multiple sclerotic deposits in pelvic bones.

Answer 2.5:
- Usually, done as an outpatient procedure and takes about 10 minutes.
- The patient lies in the left lateral position.
- An ultrasound probe is covered with a condom and lubricated and inserted into the anus.
- Ultrasound scan is carried out and viewed on monitor. Guided biopsies are usually taken.

Answer 2.6:
- Nearly, all are adenocarcinomas (Fig. 8.6).
- Most are in the peripheral part of the gland.
- Most are multifocal.
- Gleason score is used to 'quantitate' degree of malignancy.

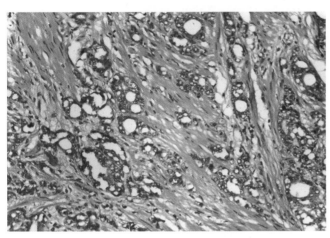

Fig. 8.6 H + E stain; histology of carcinoma prostate
(*Courtesy:* CDC, Atlanta, USA)

Answer 2.7: Bone scan showing areas of increased radioactive uptake in the spine and pelvis suggestive of multiple bony metastases.

Answer 2.8: This is an intravenous pyelogram (IVP or IVU).
Consent the patient with explanation of procedure.
Patient is asked to neither eat nor drink for 8 hours before the procedure; also asked to take a mild laxative. Patient lies flat on X-ray table. A plain X-ray is taken first (called a KUB—kidneys, urethra, bladder). Then an iodine-based contrast medium is given IV and serial X-rays taken at specified intervals, e.g. 5 minutes, then 15 minutes and so on.

Some films are taken with abdominal compression. The procedure takes about one hour but may take up to 4 hours, if excretion is slow.

Answer 2.9: Have they had a similar X-ray before and did they have any problems with it? Are they allergic to iodine or shell fish and is there any chance of being pregnant?

Answer 2.10:
- Either a KUB or plain abdomen X-ray.
- Shows radiodense opacities on L side.
- Positions of opacity in relation to vertebrae would suggest these are kidney stones.

TUTORIAL 9: Scrotal Swellings

CASE SCENARIOS

Answer 1.1:
- When did the pain start?
- What were you doing, when it came on?
- Has it got better or worse? How bad is the pain?
- Are you able to walk about?
- Where exactly is the pain?
- Has it gone anywhere else, e.g. into your tummy?
- Have you been sick?
- Do you have a fever?
- Can you pass your water OK, have a pee?
- Have you had this pain before?
- Have you fallen and injured your testicles?
- Have you been playing any sports which might have caused the injury?

Answer 1.2:
- Torsion of testis
- Epididymitis
- Orchitis
- Appendicitis
- Strangulated hernia.

Answer 1.3:
- General examination
- Full abdominal examination with inspection and palpation of hernial orifices and scrotum.

Answer 1.4:
General and Abdomen:
Is he in pain?
Is he flushed and hot?
Tachycardia.
Any signs of localized or general peritonitis?
Any evidence of a hernia?
Scrotum
Is there any difference between the right and left sides?
Where does he say the pain is?
Is the right testis tender? Is it swollen? What is its lie? Is it elevated?
Is there any edema of the scrotal skin?
Is there any reddening of the scrotum?
Is there relief of pain on elevating the scrotum? [Prehn's sign—Prehn's sign positive, i.e. relief of pain on elevating testis means diagnosis more likely epididymitis; no relief of pain (Prehn negative) more likely torsion]
Is other testis normal? What is its lie?
Any penile abnormality?

Answer 1.5: Torsion of the testis—until proven otherwise.

Answer 1.6: Page the on-call surgical resident/medical officer (or urologist) and ask him to see the patient urgently.

Answer 1.7: FBC and bioprofile. Ultrasound is the investigation of choice for diagnosis but in the presence of a high index of suspicion surgery should not be delayed to wait for an ultrasound.

Answer 1.8: Book an emergency theater and explore the right scrotum through a scrotal incision under GA.

Answer 1.9: Testicular torsion with testis probably still viable.

Answer 1.10:
- Untwist the torsion and observe the testis for signs of viability (*see* Fig. 9.2B).
- Fix testis in scrotum.
- Fix testis on other side.

Answer 1.11: Orchidectomy (removal of the testis) because the testis is nonviable.

Answer 1.12: 100% salvage rate, if untwisted within 6 hours of pain starting
- 20% viability, if left >12 hours.
- 0%, if left >24 hours.

Answer 1.13a: The Americans say 30–70% success rate.

Answer 1.13b: See Figure 9.4.

Answer 1.13c: Figure 9.5A to C.

Answer 2.1:
- Hydrocele
- Hernia
- Tumor—much less likely.

Answer 2.2:

Protocol:

Examination of male genitalia:
- Patient supine to start with.
- Examiner preferably wearing gloves (nonsterile).

Inspection:
1. Inspect the penis—including the glands and meatus-dorsal and ventral surface look for size, shape, skin color, discharge, any discrete abnormality, e.g. ulcer/lump—use appropriate protocol to describe (e.g. size, shape, surface, etc. or for an ulcer: Base Edge Depth Discharge). Retract prepuce, if indicated.
2. Inspect—the scrotum from front and then lift up and look underneath; looking for any difference in size or shape (Left versus Right), any skin abnormality, any lumps, ulcer.

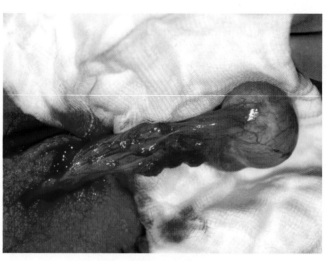
Fig. 9.2B Testis untwisted and viable

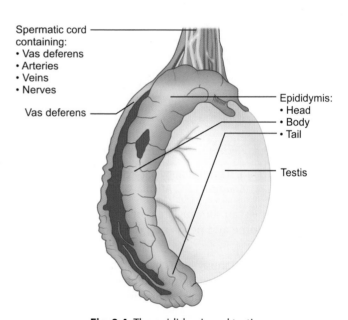
Fig. 9.4 The epididymis and testis

Palpation:
3. Palpate—palpate the contents of the scrotum starting with the normal side first. Compare right to left side.
   Identify and palpate:
   - Testis
   - Epididymis
   - Cord (feel vas deferens and vessels)
4. *If swelling is felt:* Determine four facts:
   a. Is the swelling confined to the scrotum? (i.e. can you get above it?)

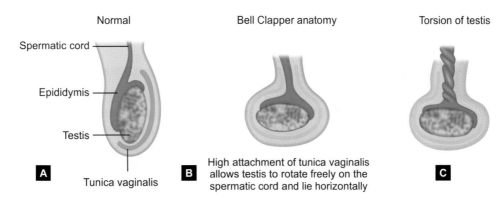

Normal · Bell Clapper anatomy · Torsion of testis

Spermatic cord

Epididymis

Testis

A

Tunica vaginalis

B High attachment of tunica vaginalis allows testis to rotate freely on the spermatic cord and lie horizontally

C

Figs 9.5A to C Anatomy predisposing to torsion of testis. (A) Normal; (B) Bell Clapper anatomy; (C) Torsion of testis

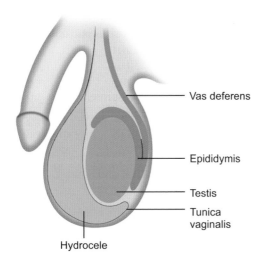

Vas deferens

Epididymis

Testis

Tunica vaginalis

Hydrocele

Fig. 9.7 Anatomy of hydrocele

b. Can the testis and epididymis be defined?
c. Is the swelling transilluminable?
d. Is the swelling tender?
5. Define the characteristics of any swelling using the standard protocol (SSS, etc.).
6. • Finally, stand the patient up:
   • Is the swelling still palpable or is a new one present? (e.g. varicocele)
   • Can you get above it? (i.e. Is it inguino-scrotal or scrotal?)

Answer 2.3: Hydrocele.

Answer 2.4: See Figure 9.7.
• A hydrocele is a collection of fluid in the tunica vaginalis.
• The causes will be discussed later.
• Because of the anatomical relationship of the tunica, the testis lies at the 'back' of the hydrocele. The pathognomic sign of a hydrocele is that it transilluminates.

Answer 2.5: Yes, in babies and young children, often associated with hernias.

Answer 2.6: See Figure 9.8. Noncommunicating hydrocele—when hydrocele is squeezed—the swelling does not go away.

Communicating hydrocele—when sac is squeezed the swelling gradually goes away and then comes back again. The 'open' processus vaginalis is an indirect inguinal hernia.

Management:
• If the infant presents with the signs of a hernia and a hydrocele, then a herniotomy is carried out.
• If a hydrocele is present with an obliterated tunica or if it is still communicating most of these disappear in the first year, if left alone. If persists then ligation of the persistant processus vaginalis (PPV) is carried out.

Answer 2.7:
• *Idiopathic*
• *Infection:* Epididymo-orchitis
• *Infection:* Filariasis
• *Trauma:* + hematocele
• Tumor
• Torsion.

Answer 2.8: Idiopathic hydrocele—because it is common and the history is suggestive-gradual onset, no pain, no trauma, no history of infection.

Answer 2.9: Ultrasound.

Answer 2.10: Fluid-filled sac surrounding a normal testis, consistent with a diagnosis of hydrocele.

Answer 2.11: The patient is usually offered surgery.

Answer 2.12: Jaboulay operation which involves turning the sac inside out and suturing it loosely behind the chord (Fig. 9.10).

Answer 2.13: Yes—aspiration, but the sac often refills.

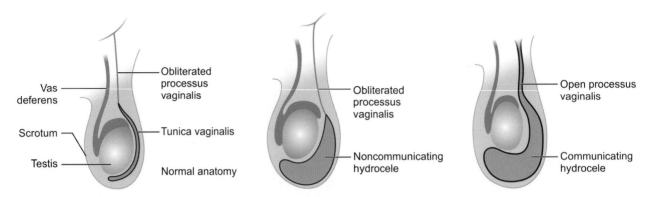

Fig. 9.8 Hydrocele in infants

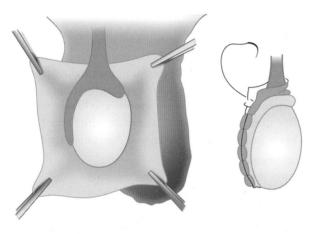

Tunica opened and fluid drained

Sac is partially excised and then reversed behind the epididymis with running suture for hemostasis

Fig. 9.10 Jaboulay procedure for hydrocele

Answer 2.14: Send it for micro, C+S, AFBs and cell cytology. FEEL the testis after you have aspirated to make sure, it is normal.

Answer 2.15:
Yes: MSU.
Feel his prostate and send venous blood for a PSA level.

Answer 3.1:
- General practitioners have for a long time offered Well Women Screening usually involving a breast examination and cervical smear—as well as a general medical history and BP check.
- This was really introduced to identify breast and cervical cancer in asymptomatic women.
  Now, many practitioners offer a Well Man Screening service as well as a general medical check-up. It will include testis examination in the younger man (to identify testicular tumors) and prostate examination in the older man (tumor and BPH).

Answer 3.2: Ultrasound scan of the testes.

Answer 3.3:
- FBC
- U and E
- Chest X-ray
- Tumor markers—alpha-fetoproteins. Beta-hCG and LDH
- CT of abdomen and thorax.

Answer 3.4:
Via lymph nodes—to para-aortic glands and into chest.
Via the bloodstream to liver and lungs.

Answer 3.5:
Stage 1   Limited to testis.
Stage 2   Abdominal lymphadenopathy.
Stage 3   Nodal involvement above the diaphragm.
Stage 4   Liver/lung metastases.

Answer 3.6:
- 90% of primary testicular tumors are derived from germ cells
- These are either:
  - Seminoma—50% most in young 30–40 years
    or
  - Nonseminomatous (mainly teratoma)—30%—20–30 years
  - Non-germ cell tumors are:
    Rarer = Gonadal stromal tumors – Sertoli and Leydig
    Lymphomas – older men.

Answer 3.7:
- Three serum tumor markers have a role in testicular cancer:
  1. Beta-hCG (human chorionic gonadotropin)
  2. Alpha-fetoproteins (AFP)
  3. Lactate dehydrogenase (LDH).
  AFP and/or β-hCG are elevated in 80–85% of non-seminomatous germ cell tumors.

- Beta-hCG is elevated in <25% of seminomas and AFP is not elevated in pure seminomas.
- LDH is a less specific marker. Its level correlates with the volume of tumor. It is elevated in 80% of advanced testicular cancer.
- Note that these markers are helpful in diagnosis and prognosis but their main use is in follow-up after primary treatment.

TUTORIAL 10: Burns

CASE SCENARIOS

Answer 1.1:
- Cool the burn down—best by running cold water over it for 20 minutes if possible.
- Reassure the patient as you do this.
- Wrap the arm loosely in a clean dry towel or cover with cling film.
- Take the patient to hospital.
- Cling film is very good as when applied loosely keeps the area clean and reduces pain.

Answer 1.2:
- How was the burn caused?
- What immediate treatment was carried out?
- What symptoms does she have now?
- What is Mrs M's general health like—any serious illness?
- Is she taking medications or drugs?

Answer 1.3:
- First you need to know the type of burn being treated—in this case, we know it is a thermal injury.
- Next need to assess the extent of the burn, its depth and any special problems likely to be associated with the burn, e.g. because of its site.

Remember:
- Cause
- Extent
- Depth
- Problems.

Answer 1.4:
Rule of 'Nines' (*see* Fig. 10.3)
Surface area covered by the patient's hand with fingers open is 1%.

Answer 1.5: <5% of body area.

Answer 1.6: This is a very confusing topic because different people use different terms and often mix them up.

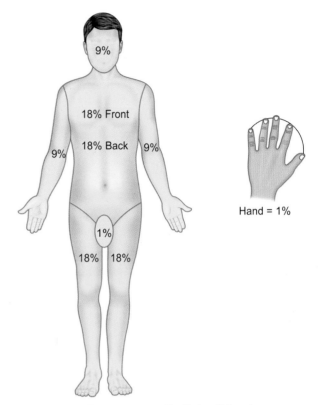

Fig. 10.3 Burns: The 'Rule of Nines'

Table 10.1 Terminology of burn depth	
Newer terminology	*Old terminology*
Superficial (epidermis)	1st degree
Partial thickness: Superficial dermal	2nd degree superficial
Partial thickness: Deep dermal	2nd degree deep
Full thickness	3rd degree

The schemes are summarized here in Table 10.1. It should be noted that the terms 1st degree, 2nd degree and 3rd degree are now rarely used. You are advised to use:
- Superficial (epidermal)
- Partial thickness:
  - Superficial dermal
  - Deep dermal
- Full thickness.

Answer 1.7: Partial thickness—superficial dermal .

Answer 1.8: Figure 10.4.

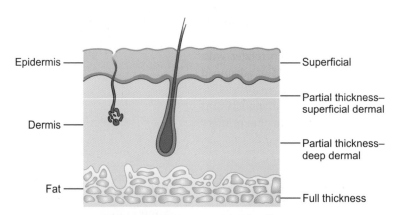

Fig. 10.4 Assessment of depth of burn

Table 10.2 Assessment and treatment of burns (*Courtesy:* Miss Lim Lay Hooi, Head, Plastic Surgery, Penang General Hospital)

Name	Depth	Appearance	Characteristic	Treatment
Superficial	Superficial, involves epidermis only	Reddish like a sunburn	Painful; heals without scarring; may have hyperpigmentation	Soothing ointment
Partial thickness superficial and deep dermal	Varying thickness of epidermis and dermis	Superficial dermal pink and blistered *Deep dermal:* Blotchy red and white	Painful; some heal without scarring; deeper areas heal with contractures, if not operated	Sterile dressing for superficial. Deeper dermal may need operation to prevent contractures and deformity
Full thickness	Epidermis and dermis through into fat	Whitish, grayish, leather-like	No sensation; will not heal	Excision and grafting required

Answer 1.9: Table 10.2.

Remember this excellent table, most of what you need to know is contained in it.

Answer 1.10:

As a guide to: (a) Treatment
 (b) Prognosis
 (c) Likely complications

Answer 1.11:

- The doctor will explain that the burn is not too serious (superficial dermal) and should heal quickly in about 14 days.
- The burn should be cleaned using a solution containing a mild antiseptic and saline as soon as possible. The wound will then be covered with a sterile dressing using either paraffin gauze or an evaporative dressing. It is then covered by sterile cotton gauze squares, cotton wool and a crepe bandage. The dressing should be reviewed at the OP department or clinic daily and left in place, unless it soaks through, for about 8–10 days. It will be painful at first which will be helped by taking paracetamol 4–6 hourly. Mrs M should be warned that if she develops a fever,

increasing pain in the burn area or swelling of the arm, she must immediately inform the doctors at the clinic. A bacteriology swab should be taken at initial treatment of the burn and at each subsequent dressing change.

- Note that in the UK now, nearly all burns over 3% (and all child burns) are treated in a regional burns unit.
- Any burn of the genitalia, hands and sole of the feet are better managed by a specialist burns doctor.

In children, NAI (nonaccidental injury) must be considered.

Answer 2.1: Initial assessment is as for a trauma case on the ABC principle:

(AIRWAY/BREATHING/CIRCULATION).

Although he is breathing, he has physical evidence of inadequate lung oxygenation with indicators of a significant inhalation injury. He will already have a high flow oxygen mask on but he will require endotracheal intubation—so ask the nurses to call the anesthetist on call. While you are waiting—insert a wide bore IV line and start it running with Hartmann's solution taking the bloods off as you do this: FBC, bioprofile, X-match, blood gases, and carboxyhemoglobin level.

Insert a urinary catheter and connect him to a 'dinamap', if he is not already on one (continuous monitoring of pulse/BP/ECG/CVP/oxygen saturation). A CVP line will probably be needed, but this is not urgent and the anesthetist can help with this. Do not examine the airway yourself with a scope as this may cause larynygospasm.

Now estimate the extent of his injury.

Remember: Cause/Extent/Depth/Problems as your guideline

Answer 2.2: About 45% – head + face = 9 + ½ back = 9 + R-arm = 9 + R-leg = 18, Total = 45%

Answer 2.3: Partial thickness (will probably be mixed superficial and deep dermal).

Answer 2.4: Mixed partial and full thickness (if a patient is conscious, you can test for sensation with pinprick).

Answer 2.5: >15% is regarded as a major burn (10% for children) and is best managed by a burns center or specialist.

Answer 2.6: Cover with sterile towels.

Answer 2.7: Use a formula such as the Parkland Formula (you do not need to remember the exact details—these should be available in the ICU/HDU—only remember principles).

Weight in kg × % area burn × 4 = Volume in mL to be replaced in 24 hours (this is using Hartmann's solution).

Give one half of total over first 8 hours and rest over next 16 hours.

Note: Whatever formula you use always monitor urine output to assess effectiveness. Aim for 1 mL per kg/hour.

Answer 2.8:
- Many different regimes—just remember one 'simple' guide, e.g.:
- *Partial thickness, superficial:* Clean with antiseptic, cover with tulle gras (jelonet).
- *Partial thickness deep dermal:* Clean with antiseptic, remove large blisters and dead tissue and put on flamazine cream (contains sulphadiazine)—redo daily.
- May need grafting.
- 3rd degree will need excision and grafting usually at 3–5th day.

Answer 2.9:
1. Lung problems because of the inhalation—respiratory failure with atelectasis and pneumonia or, if severe, RDS (hence ventilation/ICU care).
2. Infection from the burns themselves or from urinary catheter/lines (hence IV antibiotics, if indicated).

3. Severe hypovolemia from inadequate fluid replacement added to the consequences of SIRS (close watch on clinical hydration status, urine output/CVP).

(SIRS = Systemic Inflammatory Response Syndrome-revise this, if you cannot remember the details)
4. GI: Stress ulcers (prophylactic H_2-antagonists/proton pump inhibitors).
5. Local problems of the burns to his face; circumferential burn of his leg and arm.

Answer 3.1: Partial thickness, mixed superficial and deep dermal—because pale pink of superficial dermal, and blotchy red and white of deep dermal.

Check this on your table (Answer 1.9, Table 10.2).

Answer 3.2:
- Clean with antiseptic. Remove any large blisters and dead tissue.
- Cover with flamazine and sterile dressing.
- If the burn is to be reviewed by the burn surgeon apply temporary dressing with jelonet, gauze, BeBand and crepe as the flamazine will prevent assessment of burn depth.
- Deeper areas may need operation to prevent contractures.
- Partial thickness burns can be cleaned with the patient sedated using IV morphine or oromorph.

Answer 4.1:
- Electric.
- Full thickness.

Note in electrical burns you must examine for entry and exit wounds. Any arc can have caused muscle damage so a CK reading, urine for myoglobin and an ECG should be performed. The patient should be observed for 24 hours.

Answer 5.1:
- Sunburn—1st degree, superficial.
- Treat with soothing ointment.

Answer 5.2: See Table 10.3.

Table 10.3 First-aid treatment of burns

- In flame/fire, extinguish any flames on the clothes or drag person away from source
- In electric burn, either switch off current source or move person away using wooden pole (do not touch him)
- Assess ABC—start CPR, if necessary
- Remove the patient's clothing, if necessary, to assess the burned area
- If thermal/chemical burn wash with running water (large amounts—small amounts can make some chemical burns worse)
- Remove any jewellery metal objects (retain heat/cause constriction)
- Cover burns and patient with clean blanket/cloth
- Ask someone to send for ambulance and/or fire brigade

TUTORIAL 11: Fluid and Electrolyte Balance

Answer 1: Summary of most important conclusions from **British Consensus Document:**

Fluid and Electrolyte Management

Types of Fluids

1. When crystalloid resuscitation or replacement is indicated Hartmann's solution (Ringer's lactate acetate) should replace routinely used 0.9% Normal Saline except when the patient has hypochloremic acidosis from either vomiting or gastric aspiration.

2. Excessive use of dextrose 4%/0.18% saline and 5% dextrose should be used with caution to prevent hyponatremia—especially in the elderly or in children.

   They should not be used for resuscitation or replacement but only for maintenance.

Distinguish between maintenance and replacement requirements:

3. *Maintenance (per day):*
   - *Sodium:* 50–100 mmol/L
   - *Potassium:* 40–80 mmol/L
   - *Fluid:* 1.5 – 2.5 L (Hartmann's solution)

4. *Replacement:*
   - *Crystalloid solution with appropriate potassium supplement:*
     – Used in excessive losses from gastric aspiration/vomiting
     – 0.9% normal saline—in hypochloremia
   - *Hartmann's solution (balanced electrolyte solution):*
     – Used in saline depletion (e.g. excessive diuretic exposure)
     – Used in volume losses from diarrhea, ileostomy, small bowel fistula, ileus, obstruction.

Preoperative fluid management:

5. Unless the patient is obstructed or diabetic, they do not need to be starved for 6–8 hours preoperatively—may give free fluids up to 2 hours preoperative.

6. Administration of carbohydrate rich drinks 2–3 hours preoperatively enhances recovery because of better insulin mobilization.

Bowel Preparation:

7. Preoperative mechanical bowel preparation should be avoided.
   - May complicate intra- and postoperative management of fluid and electrolyte balance.
   - Where mechanical bowel preparation is used, fluid and electrolyte derangements should be corrected with IV therapy using Hartmann's solution.

Note: This is still disputed by some especially, if low anterior resection of the bowel is contemplated.

Hypovolemia:

8. *Assessment of hypovolemia:*
   - *Flow-based measurements—recommended:*
     – Transesophageal Doppler or pulse contour analysis for measurement of stroke volume and cardiac output, reflects vascular filling and hence fluid requirement.
     – If not available must rely on:
   - *Clinical assessment:*
     – Measurements of end organ function are particularly important-urine output but remember, this can be altered by the metabolic response to surgery and by cardiovascular disease.
     – Other valuable parameters include pulse rate, respiratory rate, arterial pressure, capillary refill time and presence of peripheral cyanosis.

9. *Types of fluid management:*
   - Hemorrhagic hypovolemia should be treated with either a balanced crystalloid solution or a suitable colloid until packed red cells are available.
   - Hypovolemia due to severe inflammation (e.g. infection, peritonitis, pancreatitis, or burns) should be treated with colloid or a balanced crystalloid.
   - Monitor for fluid overload especially in severely ill patient with impaired renal function.

10. *Test fluid bolus:*
    - If hypovolemia is in doubt and central venous pressure is not raised, the response to a bolus infusion of 250 mL of suitable colloid or crystalloid should be tested.
    - Clinical re-assessment 15 minutes later.

Postoperative fluid management:

11. Details of fluid administered must be recorded and easily accessible.

12. Assess the preoperative and perioperative fluid given and fluid lost when the patient leaves the recovery room and arrives on the ward, HDU or ICU, and tailor the patient's postoperative fluid regime accordingly.

13. Return to oral fluid administration and discontinuing of IV fluids should be achieved as early as possible to prevent fluid overload and electrolyte imbalances, i.e. fast-track recovery programs.

14. In patients requiring continued IV fluids (because unable to take orally), the fluids used should be sodium poor and low volume until the metabolic effects of surgery have returned to normal. After this, the IV fluid and electrolytes given should be maintenance volume + replacement as necessary.

Answer 2a:

Urea:	(2.5–6.7 mmol/L) = BUN
Na	(135–145 mmol/L)
K	(3.5–5 mmol/L)
Cl	(98–106 mmol/L)
HCO_3	(21–28 mmol/L)
Creatinine	(70–150 umol/L)

Answer 2b:

- Chemical bioprofile—as used in UK
- Will include:
- Urea and Electrolytes (as above)
- Liver Function Tests
    Total bilirubin: 3–17 umol/L
    Direct bilirubin: 1–5.1 umol/L

ALP	: 30–130 IU/L (alkaline phosphatase)
AST	: 7–40 IU/L (aspartate aminotransferase or SGOT)
ALT	: 0–42 IU/L (alanine aminotransferase or SGPT)
GGT	: 7–58 IU/L (gamma-glutamyl transpepsidase)
LDH	: 70–250 IU/L (lactate dehydrogenase)

Note: Alkaline phosphate and Gamma-GT are indicators of cholestasis, AST and ALT are indicators of hepatocellular disease.

Total protein and albumin/globulin ratio 60–80 g/L
alb = 35–50 g/L glob = 20–40 g/L
A/G: 1–1.8
Calcium: Ionized: 1–1.25 mmol/L Total = 2.12–2.65 mmol/L
Phosphate: 0.8–1.55 mmol/L
Glucose: < 6 mmol/L (fasting)   Random 3.6–11.1
Magnesium 0.75–1.05 mmol/L

Answer 2c:

ABG = Arterial blood gases	pH	7.35–7.45
	PaO_2	10.6 kPa
	$PaCO_2$	4.7–6.0 kPa
	HCO_3	21–28 mmol/L
	B Xs	+/– 2 mmol/L

O_2 sat   95–100%

Answer 3a:

Water	1 liter
Ca	2 mmol
K	5 mmol
HCO_3	29 mmol
Cl	111mmol
Na	131 mmol

Answer 3b:

Water	1 liter
Na	153 mmol/L
Cl	153 mmol/L

Answer 3c:

Water	1 liter
Dextrose	50 g

Answer 3d:

Water	1 liter
Polygeline	35 g
Ca	6.25 mmol
Cl	145 mmol
Na	145 mmol
K	5.1 mmol

Answer 3e:

Protein (95% albumin)	50 g/L
Na	145 mmol/L
K	0.25 mmol/L
Cl	145 mmol/L
Ca	—

Note: You do not need to remember the electrolyte content of Haemaccel/PPF/gelufusin. You are asked to record them, so that you know they contain electrolytes.

Answer 4a:
Orally:
Use as liquid or effervescent form, e.g. Sando K: effervescent potassium bicarbonate and chloride equivalent to 12 mmol K^+ and 8 mmol Cl (1–2 tablets per day). Kay-Cee-L syrup: 1 mmol/mL each of K and Cl (10–50 mL/day in divided doses).
    Slow release tablets have caused GI tract ulceration and are best avoided.
IV: Vials of 20 mmol potassium chloride (*Note:* Dangerous—use slow infusion) usually in 1 liter Hartmann's/0.9 N saline or 1 liter dextrose 5%.

Remember: Each 0.3 mmol/L reduction in the serum potassium represents 100 mmol/L deficit in body stores. For example, a patient with a serum potassium of 2.6 mmol/L will require at least 300 mmol of K to correct this.

Answer 4b:
Orally: Either dietary or by supplements.
Dietary: Bananas, fruit and vegetables.
Supplements:
Calcium Sandoz syrup: Calcium glubionate and calcium lactobionate
    2.27 mmol/5 mL (5–10 mL)
Calci-chew tabs–calcium carbonate (1–2 tabs)
IV: In hypocalcemic tetany use 10% calcium gluconate solution.

Slow 10 mL = 2.25 mmol Ca (use ECG monitor to be safe) followed by slow continuous infusion of 40 mL (9 mmol) over 24 hours (monitor plasma Ca).

Answer 4c:

Poorly absorbed from GI tract.

In hypomagnesemia associated with excess loss of gastro-intestinal fluid replace with:

Magnesium sulfate: 10–20 mmol mg/day given IV

Often given as part of TPN.

Answer 4d:

IV: Usually needed in severe metabolic acidosis (pH < 7.1). Mild metabolic acidosis usually responds to volume replacement with appropriate fluid.

IV by slow infusion (strong solution up to 8.4% or weaker solution 1.26%).

Answer 5:

Fluid:

Insensible skin loss: 600 mL

(*Note:* Can go up with fever and will depend on surrounding humidity and temperature.)

Insensible from respiration: 400 mL

                                                    (can go up with tachypnea)

Kidneys (urine):   1500 mL

Feces: 100 mL

Total = 2600 mL/day (Replace as water)

Electrolytes:

Lose   1 mmol Na per kg

                1 mmol K per kg

Simple to remember MAINTENANCE = 2 1 1
- 2 L fluid
- 1 mmol/kg Na
- 1 mmol/kg K

Remember the following:

Daily intake and output of water in adults (70 kg man)

Input (mL)	total:	2600
• Fluids		1300
• Solids		1000
• Metabolism		300

Output (mL)	total:	2600
• Urine		1500
• Lungs		400 ⎤ insensible loss
• Skin		600 ⎦
• Feces		100

Maintainance requirements: 2:1:1

Water	2000 mL
Na	1 mmol per kg
K	1 mmol per kg

Daily intake altered by:

Fever	: Add 10%* for each degree above 38°C
Sweating	: Add 10–15%*
Tachypnea	: Add 25–50% (50%, if RR doubled)*
Hypermetabolic	: Add 25–50%*

Replace as water except for sweating when added sodium is necessary.

*percentage of total insensible loss

Chart 11.2 Daily intravenous fluid-order chart						
Name	MANN					
First Name	REGINALD					
Reg. No.						
Ward	GEN SURGERY					
Bag/Bottle Order	State infusion fluid/blood, volume to be given period of infusion and drip site, if applicable			State drug and dosage to be added	Doctor's initials	Blood bottle/bag no. infusion batch no. to be confirmed by nurse
1	HARTMANN's	500 mL	6 hours		ℓ	
2	DEXTROSE 5%	500 mL	6 hours		ℓ	
3	DEXTROSE 5%	500 mL	6 hours		ℓ	
4	DEXTROSE 5%	500 mL	6 hours		ℓ	
5						
6						
7						
8						

Chart 11.4 Daily intravenous fluid-order chart				
Name	MANN			
First Name	REGINALD			
Reg. No.				
Ward	GEN SURGERY			
Bag/Bottle Order	State infusion fluid/blood, volume to be given period of infusion and drip site if applicable	State drug and dosage to be added	Doctor's initials	Blood bottle/bag no. infusion batch no. to be confirmed by nurse
1	DEXTROSE 5% 500 mL 6 hours		✓	
2	HARTMANN's 500 mL 6 hours		✓	
3	DEXTROSE 5% 500 mL 6 hours		✓	
4	HARTMANN's 5% 500 mL 6 hours		✓	
5				
6				
7				
8				

Answer 6: Minimum volume to excrete the solute load is 500 mL/day. Should aim for 50 mL/hour or at least 1200 mL/day.

Answer 7: For diarrhea: Hartmann's solution: volume for volume. For vomiting of gastric contents: 0.9 N saline and added K.

Answer 8: Yes—patient loses chloride and hydrogen ions so replace with 0.9 N saline.

Answer 9: Usually, use Hartmann's + K supplement when indicated.

CASE SCENARIOS

Answer 10.1: Clinically assess his hydration status:
1. Pulse/BP/skin turgor/dry tongue/temperature/peripheries.
2. Check his urine output/CVP.
3. Look at the anesthetic chart from theater—see what fluids, he has been given, what his urine output has been and whether his fluid losses would appear to have been replaced. Also check to see, if there has been any excessive intraoperative blood loss, and if so has there been any intraoperative transfusion.
4. Look at the surgeon's operation note, which should be summarized in the notes together with the postoperative instructions—have there been any problems, e.g. excess blood loss, long operating time/tissue damage (3rd space loss)?

Answer 10.2:
Dinamap giving continuous monitoring of pulse/BP/ECG/O_2 sat
Recorded 1 hourly P/BP/temperature/RR
Recorded 1 hourly CVP
Input/output chart with 1 hourly urine output
The IV fluid chart for you to fill out.

Answer 10.3:
Ice orally, hourly
Routine readings as above.

Intravenous Fluids:
Hartmann's solution 500 mL over 6 hours.
Dextrose 5% 1.5 liter over 18 hours (500 mL over 6 hours × 3) (because he would appear to be in reasonable fluid balance both clinically and from urine output and his theater losses in terms of blood have not been high and have been replaced), 2 liters of fluid (as per Consensus guidelines). No electrolytes (see metabolic response to surgery)
(*see* Chart 11.2, page 188).

Answer 10.4: The patient is in a +ve input balance of 690 mL.

His urine output has been reasonable with 50 mL the last 2 hours.

The U and Es from the night before would indicate he was dehydrated at this time.

This would appear to have been corrected by the overnight IV fluid input.

(Note his urea was raised at 14-strictly speaking this could be due to a prerenal or renal cause—if in doubt, this could be clarified by performing urine osmolality. If raised the patient is dehydrated and needs fluid, replaced as ECF—Hartmann's).

So, • You just need to provide his 'normal' fluid loss for the next 24 hours (i.e. maintenance)
   • Usually this would be 1.5–2 liters water (better to know weight—this patient is 70 kg)
      – 1 mmol/kg Na
      – 1 mmol/kg K

But: In the immediate postoperative period, the body tends to retain sodium (and hence water) as well, as part of the metabolic response to injury. There is increased excretion of potassium in the urine in exchange for sodium. However, because of cell lysis following surgery, there is an increase of serum potassium in spite of increased excretion. For these reasons in the first 48 hours postoperative—it is usual to give only 2 liters of fluid and no added electrolytes other than those in the balanced electrolyte solution (Unless, there are abnormalities in input/output/electrolytes which dictate otherwise).

The 'homeostatic' mechanism returns to normal in 48–72 hours.

So, the suggested regime is as shown in Chart 11.4, page 189:
   500 mL 5% dextrose over 6 hours
   500 mL Hartmann's over 6 hours
   500 mL 5% dextrose over 6 hours
   500 mL Hartmann's over 6 hours

Note: Although the electrolyte requirements are low in the immediate postoperative period if 5% dextrose only were used, the patient would almost certainly be water overloaded.

Answer 10.5: There was 400 mL blood loss in theater and no blood given. His immediate postoperative Hb was 9 g/dL—at that time he was probably a little dehydrated.

Provided there has been no further significant blood loss (e.g. from his drain), then there is no indication to transfuse him at this stage. Note that there has been a move away from blood transfusion both in theater and postoperatively as there is a suggestion that it may influence the patient's cancer outcome. This is in addition to the other side effects of blood transfusion.

Clearly, the above decision will be reviewed in the patient's routine twice daily assessment.

Answer 10.6:
1. The patient has started to vomit.
2. Since he started to vomit his oral input has quite correctly been stopped.

3. His clinical condition would suggest dehydration. His urine output is gradually diminishing and his CVP has fallen which would fit with volume depletion.

The most likely cause is that he has developed a postoperative ileus with sequestration of fluid into his gut (considered as a third space loss). Postoperative gastric stasis may also have occurred and he may be becoming septic.

Answer 10.7:
1. Ask the nurses to pass a nasogastric tube and show you what he has vomited (this is slightly greenish, contains mucus and is odorless—suggestive of gastric contents rather than small bowel).
2. Talk to the Registrar or the Consultant and ask their advice.

Answer 11.1:
• Due to lack of oral intake and the vomiting, he has become depleted in body water, sodium and potassium. His fluid replacement should be with great care because of his age. He will benefit from a central line for CVP monitoring and a bladder catheter to measure urinary output.
• The volume replacement in this case will probably be best provided by using 0.9N saline with added potassium.

Answer 12.1:
• He is overloaded; has developed hyponatremia due to excess IV fluids of water only (remember 5% dextrose in fluid terms is water)
• *Restrict his fluid intake*
   IV: Use 0.9 N saline in his IV line and give him say 1500 mL over next 24 hours. Check his K—this may correct as the hyponatremia is corrected.

TUTORIAL 12: Patient 1 Varicose Veins
Patient 2 Ulcer on Leg

CASE SCENARIOS

Answer 1.1:
• When did she first notice she had varicose veins?
• Did they affect one leg or both to start with?
• Have the veins become gradually worse?
• Why do they bother her?
• Is it correct that the swelling and aching have only occurred in the last year?
• Is the swelling and aching present in the morning?
• What does she do to help these symptoms?
• Did she take the contraceptive pill or has she at any time had a deep venous thrombosis or clot in the leg?
• How many children has she had?
• Any swelling of her legs during or after pregnancy?

- Any recent increase in her weight?
- Has she had any serious illnesses or operations recently?
- Is she on any medications or drugs?

Answer 1.2: To answer this, you need a knowledge of the basic anatomy and venous physiology of the normal lower limb.

The venous drainage of the lower limb consists of the superficial system (long saphenous and short saphenous veins) and the deep veins of the calf and thigh. These two systems are connected by communicating veins.

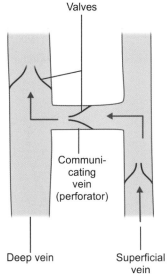

Fig. 12.1 *Venous blood flow:* Valves direct blood flow from superficial to deep

The normal venous return is driven by left ventricular contraction which is assisted in the lower limbs by the negative intrathoracic pressure of inspiration and the pumping action of the calf muscles.

In the normal situation, the venous blood flow is directed from superficial to deep by the presence of valves in the superficial, deep and communicating veins (Fig. 12.1).
From the clinical point of view the important valves are at:

- The saphenofemoral junction in the groin
- The short saphenous to popliteal vein in the popliteal fossa
- Communicators (perforators) along the medial side of the leg below the knee and at mid thigh level above the knee.

Varicose veins occur when the valves are damaged in either the superficial or communicator systems and the direction of flow then becomes from deep to superficial.

If the deep valves are damaged the pressure in the deep system is raised and blood refluxes into the superficial system.

Varicose veins can be either primary or secondary. In primary disease it is thought there is a structural deficit in the vein wall—this may be inherited and is made worse by

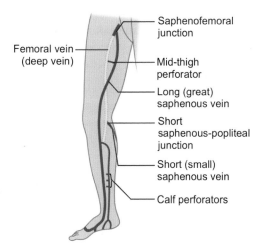

Fig. 12.2 Normal venous return of leg

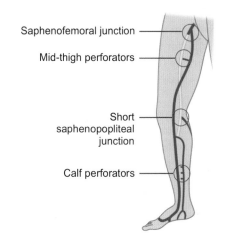

Fig. 12.3 Major sites of venous incompetence

obesity and the hormonal changes of pregnancy. This leads to venous dilation and secondary incompetence of the valves.

In secondary disease, the valves are damaged by superficial or deep venous thrombosis, proximal obstruction from injury or tumor or by the increased pressure of an arteriovenous fistula.

Answer 1.3: Figure 12.2.

Answer 1.4: Figure 12.3.

Answer 1.5: He will look for the extent and severity of the varicose veins with the patient standing, i.e. the distribution of the varicose veins. Flexing the hip and knee will enhance filling.

He will look to see, if the long saphenous system or the short saphenous system is involved or both.

He will examine the leg for evidence of varicose eczema, lipodermatosclerosis and ulceration.

Answer 1.6: Dr S explains to Mrs P that her varicose veins are quite advanced. He says that she can help herself by losing some weight, wearing compression stockings and trying to avoid standing for long periods.   (Communication skills)

Answer 1.7: The long saphenous vein starts on the dorsum of the foot, passes medially and upwards, anterior to the medial malleolus across the calf to the knee crease and then upwards and laterally across the thigh to enter the femoral vein at the saphenofemoral junction immediately medial to the femoral artery.

The short saphenous vein passes from the lateral venous arch on the dorsum of the foot upwards over the posterior surface of the calf in the midline and enters the popliteal vein slightly above the knee crease.

If long saphenous varicosities are present (90% of cases) first examine to see, if there is saphenofemoral incompetence using the classical Trendelenberg test. If this is negative, you then have to perform the Tourniquet test (Fig. 12.4).

Then examine for below knee perforators by feeling for the defects in the deep fascia.
(*Note:* These tests have largely been replaced by the use of the hand-held Doppler.)

Signs of venous hypertension will be lipodermatosclerosis, leg swelling and ulceration.

Examine her abdomen to make sure, there is no pelvic mass or malignant groin glands (causing obstruction and secondary VVs).

Answer 1.8: A saphena varix is a dilatation of the long saphenous vein immediately before it enters the femoral vein. It presents as a soft swelling in the groin on standing which goes away when the patient lies flat.

Answer 1.9:
1. Femoral hernia
2. Saphena varix
3. Femoral aneurysm
4. Enlarged lymph node
5. Lipoma
6. Sebaceous cyst.

Answer 1.10: Bilateral saphenofemoral ligation. Strip from groin to knee and avulsion of below-knee perforators.

The indications for surgery are ulceration, impending ulceration (pigmentation) and severity of symptoms, but remember cosmesis is often involved (Figs 12.5A to C).

Answer 2.1: She almost certainly developed a DVT at the time of her child birth.

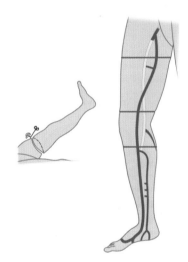

Fig. 12.4 The 'tourniquet test'

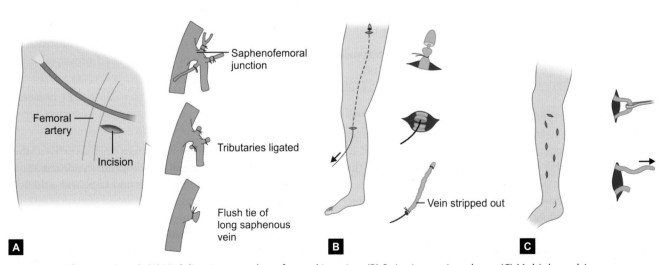

Figs 12.5A to C (A) High ligation at saphenofemoral junction; (B) Stripping groin to knee; (C) Multiple avulsions

Answer 2.2:

- There is an ulcer on the 'gaiter' area of the L leg lying above the medial malleolus — Site
- It is approximately 3.5 × 2.5 cm in size — Size
- It is almost ovoid in shape — Shape
- Its base contains reddish green granulation tissue — B
- Its edge appears sloping — E

Depth—shallow—1-2 mm — D

Discharge—non seen — D

Surroundings—pigmentation and thickening of skin — S

Answer 2.3:

Look: Site/Size/Shape/+ 'BEDDS'

Feel : Temperature/pulses/tenderness/induratation/ sensation

Move: Look at small muscles for wasting/fixation

Now check back, and see if you have covered all the points in your description of the ulcer.

Answer 2.4: The most common causes are:

Venous—Superficial insufficiency. Deep insufficiency.

Arterial—Large vessel disease. Small vessel disease.

Neuropatic (Diabetic).

Common things occur commonly, but remember there are other causes of chronic ulcers:

- Infection—including TB and Syphilis
- Trauma—single or repeated (including pressure)
- Ischemia
- Edema
- Denervation
- Malignancy.

Remember the other causes of a neuropathic ulcer:

- *Peripheral nerve lesions:* Diabetes, nerve injuries, leprosy.
- *Spinal cord lesions:* Spina bifida, tabes dorsalis, syringomyelia.

Answer 2.5:

Arterial: M>F >60 years old.
Risks: smoking, diabetes, hypertension, hyperlipidemia.
History of PVD/coronary/cerebrovascular disease.

Symptoms: Usually painful (unless diabetic).

Site: Pressure areas.

Signs: Punched out, indolent.
Dark green or black slough. Sometimes tendon or bone may be visible. No granulation tissue.
Thin leg because of muscle wasting.

Venous: F>M 40–60 years old.
Risk factors: DVT/VV's.
History of DVT in 20%.

Symptoms: One-third have pain but not severe.

Site: Most in gaiter area—usually above medial malleolus.

Signs: Edge irregular, depth shallow, base shows granulations. Surrounding lipodermatosclerosis and skin thickening.

Diabetic: Just think of the diabetic foot.
Combination of ischemia, neuropathy and immunocompromisation.
Gives Sepsis/Ulceration/Gangrene.
So you get:
- Painless ulceration at sites of trauma and pressure areas (sensory)
- Long and short flexors and extensors of calf and sole affected gives toe dorsi flexion (*motor*)
- Dry, scaly, fissured skin (autonomic).
Ulcers may be painless, infected and in abnormal positions.
Foot may be warm with pulses present.
Accompanying gangrene of toes/foot.

Answer 2.6:

- Dry, scaly and fissured skin (may be shiny) thickened toe nails.
- Cool temperature.
- Absent pulses.
- Wasted small muscles.

Answer 2.7: Varicose ulcer.

Answer 2.8: Lipodermatosclerosis refers to the skin changes of the lower limbs that often occur in a patient with chronic venous insufficiency (consequent to venous hypertension) It is a type of inflammation of the subcutaneous fat with the following characteristics:

1. Hardening of the skin
2. Dark pigmentation
3. Small white scarred areas
4. Swelling and redness
5. Inverted 'champagne bottle' appearance
6. Ulceration.

The etiopathology is probably a mixture of tissue hypoxia, leakage of proteins into the interstitium and leukocyte activation caused by the venous hypertension. The skin pigmentation comes from breakdown of red blood cells.

Answer 2.9:

- FBC
- Bioprofile
- Doppler or duplex US
- If absent pulses or reduced APBI, do CT/MRI arteriogram

- If doubt about diagnosis:
  – Blood glucose
  – Lipid profile
  – Rheumatoid serology.

Answer 2.10:
1. Control (reduce) the venous hypertension as far as possible by graded bandaging of legs or bed rest.
2. Dress the ulcer daily with simple cleaning with saline or betadine + non-stick dressing. No antibiotics unless cellulitis.
3. Consider surgery for valve incompetence (e.g. high tie and avulsions), provided deep veins are patent. Sometimes a skin graft may be used. Best done when ulcer is healed, but if healing is very slow may be considered earlier.

Answer 2.11: These are the compression bandages used for controlling the venous hypertension—must be carefully applied by experienced nurse (often referred to as the Charing Cross type of application).

TUTORIAL 13: Loin Pain (Renal)

CASE SCENARIO

Answer 1.1:
- When did the pain start?
- Where was it when it started?
- Did it come on suddenly or gradually?
- Have you had it before?
- How bad is it?
- Does it come and go or is it constant?
- Do you have any time, when there is no pain?
- Is it getting worse?
- Has it moved anywhere?
- What makes it better or worse?
- Have you noticed any blood in the urine?
- Have you had any problems passing urine?
- Have you had a fever?
- Have you vomited?
- Have you had any recent illness?

Answer 1.2:

Renal causes:
- Ureteric calculi
  Much less commonly:
  - Tumor (clot colic)
  - Pyelonephritis
  - Stricture
  - Retroperitoneal fibrosis
  - Papillary necrosis.

Non-renal causes: Acute appendicitis.

Answer 1.3:
- Is he alert, conscious and orientated?
- Is he in any obvious distress?
- Is he fevered?
- Is he well nourished?
- Is he clinically dehydrated?
- Is he clinically anemic or jaundiced?
- Any signs in lips or mouth?
- Any signs in hands/arms?
- Pulse/BP/RR/temperature/peripheries?

Abdomen:		
	• Inspection:	Moving with respiration
		Distension
		Skin changes/scars
		Visible mass/veins/pulsations
		Umbilcal abnormalities
	• Palpation:	Tenderness/guarding/rebound
		Organomegaly
	• Percussion:	Dullness/ascites
	• Auscultation:	Bowel sounds
	• Groins/external genitalia:	Hernia/nodes/swelling/ulceration
	• PR:	Mass/blood/tenderness
	• Legs:	Look /feel/move – query any abnormality

Answer 1.4: Most likely ureteric colic.

Answer 1.5:
- FBC
- Urea/electrolytes and creatinine
- Urine dipstick
- MSU
- KUB
- CT (urological).

Answer 1.6:
- Hb in N limits (13.5–18 g/dL)
- WCC upper limit N ($4–11 \times 10^9$/L)—may indicate infection
- Platelets = N ($150–40 \times 10^9$/L).

Answer 1.7:
- 4 hourly P/BP/RR/temperature
- Input/output chart.

Answer 1.8:
Yes, ask nurse to:
- Dipstick test urine.
- Sieve the urine looking for stones.

Answer 1.9:
- Write him up for an analgesic and antiemetic–pethidine 50-100 mg IM 4-6 hourly p.r.n., Stemetil 25 mg IM 4-6 hourly p.r.n..
- Put up IV drip.

Answer 1.10: Normal.

Answer 1.11:

pH
- Normal is 4.5 to 8
- This test is not usually contributory to most common clinical scenarios, but may sometimes be helpful in investigating patients with stone disease and urinary tract infections. For example, alkaline urine indicates infection with a urea splitting organism (e.g. *Proteus*). Urinary pH is usually acidic in patients with uric acid and cystine stones and alkalinization of urine is part of treatment (use potassium citrate).

Specific gravity:
- Normal is 1.001 to 1.035.
- Shows the concentration of urine and reflects hydration status and may be helpful when assessing renal/ endocrine/water balance disorders.
- High SG found in dehydration, diabetes, inappropriate ADH secretion.
- Low value in diabetes insipidus, overhydration, renal failure.

Glucose:
- Normal patient has no glucose in the urine
- Extremely important test. Glucose in the urine usually implies diabetes mellitus
- Diabetes mellitus will be confirmed if:
  Random plasma glucose is >11.1 mmol/L*
  Fasting plasma glucose is >7.0 mmol/L*

*WHO criteria

(Glucose tolerance testing and HbA1c may also be used depending on the clinical context)

Remember that a small proportion of patients who have glycosuria will have a low renal threshold for glucose (i.e. do not have diabetes mellitus). This is most common in pregnancy and children. Other metabolic causes of glycosuria are rare, e.g. Fanconi syndrome, Cushing's syndrome.

Ketonuria:
- Ketones will appear in the urine when there is reduced food intake and fat is being metabolised instead of carbohydrate. They appear in very large quantities in uncontrolled type 1 diabetics (Diabetic ketoacidosis).

Nitrites and leukocyte esterase:
- Normal urine is negative.
- Very useful test in routine work.
- Identifies UTI—bacteria breakdown nitrates to nitrites, leukocyte esterase is produced by neutrophils and indicates infection.
- A negative result for nitrites and leukocyte esterase usually excludes UTI

Protein:
- Negative in normal patient, present in renal disease and cardiac disease.
- Low readings suggest cardiac disease and sometimes inflammation and smoking.

Note: Bence-Jones protein does not show on dipstick.

Bilirubin/urobilinogen:
- Normal urine is negative
- In obstructive jaundice, the urine contains bilirubin but no urobilinogen. In early hepatocellular, jaundice, there is urobilinogen but no bilirubin. In late hepatocellular jaundice, the findings become like those of obstructive jaundice (cholestasis). See also Module 2 Tutorial 2.

Blood:
- Usually negative in normal patient. Positive in renal causes glomerulonephritis, IgA nephropathy, interstitial nephritis, polycystic kidney and neoplasia and in extrarenal causes: UTI, stones, hypertension, sickle cell disease.

Note: It has been established in Well Person Clinics that a small number of healthy people will exhibit dipstick hematuria without detectable pathology.

Urine from catheterized patients will usually test positive for blood, protein and leukocytes (and this does not necessarily imply infection).

(If you want to read more, look at the excellent article in Student BMJ 2009:17:b 260 by Subramonian, MacDonald, Vijapurapu and Yadav, on which the above is based.)

Answer 1.12:
- 3 x plus of glucose—may be diabetic and will need fasting blood glucose.
- Nitrites indicate UTI.
- Blood may indicate renal pathology.
- Bilirubin and urobilinogen may indicate hepatocellular dysfunction—do LFTs.

Answer 1.13: Indicates urinary tract infection (UTI).

Answer 1.14: KUB stands for Kidneys/Ureters/Bladder. For the X-ray to cover the area of these organs, the film must be from above T12 down to and including the whole bony pelvis. A plain abdominal X-ray usually shows a more limited area.

Answer 1.15: The presence of a radiopaque calculus.

Answer 1.16: Radiopaque, calcified opacity in pelvis suggestive of a right ureteric calculus.

Answer 1.17: The stone is less than 4 mm in diameter so conservative treatment would be initial management with:
- Nonsteroidal analgesia (e.g. ibuprofen/volterol).
- Antispasmodic (e.g. buscopan).
- High fluid intake.
  Failure to pass stone within 48 hours—intervention will be necessary.
- Extracorporeal Shock Wave Lithotripsy (ESWL) followed by analgesia, high fluid intake.

Answer 1.18: The kidneys lie at T12 to L1/2.

The ureter passes downwards in the line of the tips of the lumbar transverse processes until, it reaches the pelvis where it passes over the sacroiliac joint passing downwards, outwards and then inwards to enter the bladder at the level of the sacrococcygeal junction.

Answer 1.19:
- Calcium oxalate (40%)
- Calcium phosphate (15%)
- Mixed oxalate/phosphate (20%)
- Struvite (15%)
- Uric acid (10%)

Answer 1.20:
1. Increased urinary concentration of constituents, e.g. calcium/dehydration.
2. Presence of promoter substances, e.g. infection.
3. Reduction in concentration of inhibitors.

Note:
- 90% are idiopathic
  - 10% are due to: Hyperparathyroidism
    Vitamin D excess
    Primary hyperoxaluria.

Answer 1.21:
- There is an irregular radiodense opacity lying on the right side of the film which because of its relationship to the vertebrae and ribs would appear to be in the position of the right kidney.
- The density has the shape of the calyces of the kidney.

Answer 1.22: Staghorn calculus of right kidney.

Answer 1.23: Calcium magnesium ammonium phosphate.

Answer 1.24: Intravenous pyelogram (IVP) showing a large stone in the left ureter with hydronephrosis.

Answer 1.25: A double J stent passing from left kidney down the left ureter into the bladder.

Answer 1.26: Large bladder calculus.

Management and House Officer Tasks

TUTORIAL 1: Neck Swellings

INSTRUCTIONS

a. Make sure you have reread the chapters in your standard surgical textbook on thyroid problems and neck swellings.
b. Revise your answers from the Case Scenarios in **Module 2 Tutorial 6**—Neck Swellings.
c. Try and answer the Module 3 tutorial without the books or your notes, then look up any points you are not sure about, then redo the tutorial and check your answers.

A lot of work but worth it, if you get the patient in the finals!!

Question 1: Case scenario

A bit of revision to make sure you have carried out the instructions:

> A 30-year-old lady presents with a solitary swelling in the right lobe of her thyroid gland. No lymph nodes are palpable and she is clinically euthyroid.

Question 1.1: What is your differential diagnosis?

Question 1.2: You see her in the OP clinic with your consultant. He agrees with your assessment and asks you to arrange the appropriate investigations.

Make a list of these investigations.

Question 2: Case scenario

> A 55-year-old lady presents at the OP clinic with a swelling in the neck. She has had it for many years. She has noticed that it involves both sides of her neck and over the last year has grown bigger. Recently, she has become a little breathless at rest—she particularly notices this at night in bed. She has no symptoms of thyrotoxicosis or myxedema and is otherwise fit and well. The rest of her 'protocoled history' is noncontributory.

A picture of the patient's neck is shown in Figure 1.1.

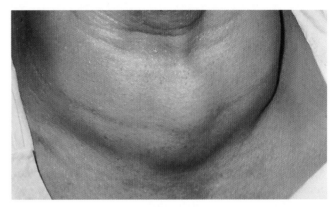

Fig. 1.1

On examination, inspection shows a large irregular swelling involving the right and left anterior triangles and the midline. There are no obvious scars; the overlying skin is normal. There are no obvious arterial or venous pulsations. The swelling moves up and down when she swallows and does not move when she puts out her tongue. On palpation from behind, the swelling measures about 14 cm × 10 cm, it moves on swallowing and appears to involve both the left and right lobes of the thyroid gland and the isthmus. It is irregular. There are several separate nodules which vary in size between 2 cm and 4 cm diameter. The swellings are firm in consistency, smooth-surfaced and have well-demarcated edges. The swelling is non-tender, does not pulsate and none of the nodules transilluminate. The carotid pulses are palpable, the skin moves freely over the swelling but it appears to be 'fixed' deeply. There are no palpable neck nodes. The trachea is not palpable, auscultation is negative but Pemberton's sign appears to be positive—in that she is a little plethoric and breathless when asked to elevate her arms.

Question 2.1: What is your differential diagnosis? Make a list.

Question 2.2: What complications of her disease is she likely exhibiting?

Her thyroid function tests are normal as are her thyroid antibodies. The ultrasound scan of the R lobe of her thyroid is shown here.

Question 2.3: What does it show (Fig. 1.2)?

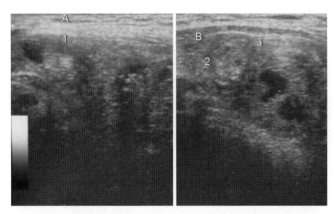

Fig. 1.2 Ultrasound scan of thyroid gland

Fine-needle aspiration cytology (FNAC) of the dominant nodule is reported as showing no malignant cells.

A diagnosis of multinodular goiter with tracheal compression is made and the patient is advised to have surgery.

Question 2.4: Would a preoperative CT scan be indicated and, if so, why?

Question 2.5: What investigation is this and what does it show (Fig. 1.3)?

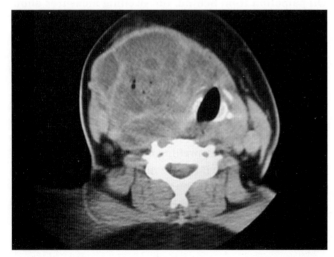

Fig. 1.3

Question 2.6: What operation do you think the patient in Question 2: Case scenario would be advised to undergo?

She is admitted to the ward for the operation; you are the house officer/intern looking after her.

Question 2.7: What investigations will you arrange before her surgery—make a list and give reasons for ordering them.

Question 2.8: What do you see on this X-ray (Fig. 1.4)?

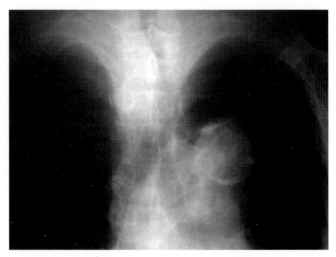

Fig. 1.4 Plain X-ray of chest/neck

Question 2.9: Write down here how you would consent this patient for the operation (in bullet point form, i.e. exactly what you would say to the patient so she understands it).

The lady undergoes an uncomplicated near total thyroidectomy. 12 hours postoperatively, the nurse on the ward bleeps you and says she is very breathless and blue. When you examine her she is dypsneic, tachycardic, and has stridor. The neck is bruised and the suction drains have not drained any blood.

Question 2.10: What is the likely cause of her problems?

Question 2.11: What would you do?

Question 3: Case scenario

On the morning ward, round the man in bed 3 who is 2 days after a total thyroidectomy for a carcinoma says he has noticed some tingling in his fingers.

Question 3.1: What would you be worried about? What would you do?

Question 3.2: Write down the drug order for the oral calcium.

Question 3.3: If the tetany is severe and your consultant advises IV calcium—what concentration would you give—would it be diluted and how much would you give?

What special precautions will you take while giving it?

Question 4: Case scenario

A 65-year-old lady presents at the OP clinic with a swelling on her neck. This is shown in the Figure 1.5.

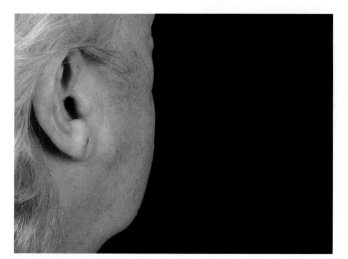

Fig. 1.5 Reproduced from Surgery (Oxford) 27, 12, Thevasagayam MS, Parker A. Diagnosis and management of neck lumps, p 523-9, 2009, with permission Elsevier

Question 4.1: What questions will you ask her for the presenting history?

The patient says that she thinks she has had a small swelling there for a long time. She thinks for about 5 or 6 years. It did not bother her until recently, when it has become bigger. It does not hurt but people have started to comment on it. She has no other symptoms and is fit and well.

Question 4.2: What do you think this swelling is?

On examination, the swelling is at the angle of the mandible, it is deep to the skin which moves feely over it. It is 2.5 cm in diameter, ovoid in shape, has a well-defined edge and is firm in consistency. It is non-painful. Does not transilluminate or pulsate. It appears to be deeply fixed. There are no lymph nodes to palpate.

Question 4.3: With this information, there are two specific elements of examination you should now carry out. What are they?

Question 4.4: What are you looking in the mouth for?

Question 4.5: How do you test the facial nerve function?

Question 4.6: Name the three *common* types of parotid tumor—are there any suggestive signs clinically which help identify which type of tumor it is?

Clinically, this would appear to be a mixed parotid tumor (pleomorphic adenoma).

Question 4.7: What investigations will you do?

Question 4.8: What treatment would you advise in this case?

Finally 2 short cases:

Question 5: What do you see in this picture (Fig. 1.6)?

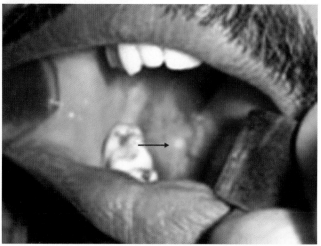

Fig. 1.6 Courtesy of SRB's Manual of Surgery

Question 5.1: How might this patient present?

Question 5.2: What would you recommend as treatment in this case?

Question 6: What do you think is the cause of this swelling shown in Figure 1.7?

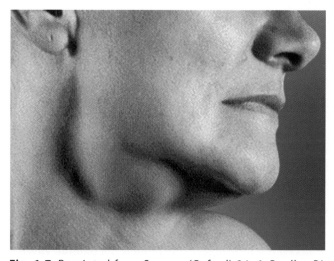

Fig. 1.7 Reprinted from Surgery (Oxford) 24, 6, Bradley PJ. Pathology and treatment of salivary gland conditions, p 304-11, 2006, with permission Elsevier

Question 6.1: What is the name of this X-ray and what does it show (Fig. 1.8)?

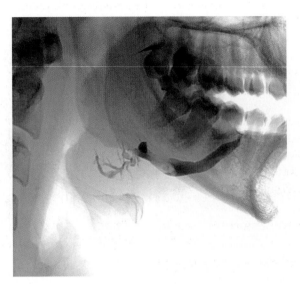

Fig. 1.8 With permission Professor Dr Prepageran AL Narayanan UMMC, KL, Malaysia

TUTORIAL 2: Breast Diseases

INSTRUCTIONS

a. Read the chapter on breast diseases in your standard surgical textbook.
b. Revise the content of the tutorials on breast diseases in Module 1 and Module 2.
c. Try and answer as much of the tutorial for Module 3 without your notes. Make a list of what you do not know or are not sure about. Read it up.
d. Then go through the cases in Module 3 again.

Question 1: Case scenario

A 45-year-old lady presents with a lump in her right breast. She noticed this while showering.

Question 1.1: What questions will you ask her about the lump?

Question 1.2: What questions will you ask her to cover the risk factors for breast cancer?

She says that she first noticed the lump while showering about 1 month ago. She has had painful lumpy breasts especially at her period times and thought it would go away after her period finished. However, it has not done so—she thinks it is a little bigger. The lump is not painful. There is no nipple discharge, and she has not noticed any change in the overlying skin. She does not usually check her own breasts but since she noticed the lump she has checked the other side and cannot feel any swellings.

She is married with 3 children—all girls, who are 23, 18 and 16 years old. She breastfed all the children. Her periods started when she was 13 years old and she is still having them regularly. She took the oral contraceptive pill for 12 years but not for the last 5 years.

She is not on any other medications. Her mother developed breast cancer when she was 80 years of age but she does not think she died of it. She has 3 sisters one of whom she thinks has had a breast operation but she is not in contact with her.

She is otherwise fit and well. Her appetite is good and she has not lost weight. She has no bony pains. The rest of her protocoled history is negative.

Question 1.3: When you examine this lady, list the signs that will make you think that the lump is malignant.

On examination, she looks well, she is not clinically anemic or jaundiced. She is well nourished. On examination of her breasts, the left side is normal.
These are the findings on the right side:

Inspection: There is no obvious swelling in the breast even when her arms are elevated. There is no asymmetry with the left side. There are no visible skin changes or scars to see. There are no distended veins. The nipple and areola appear normal and the same as the left side.

On palpation: There is a 2 cm diameter swelling in the right upper outer quadrant at the 10 o'clock position, 3 cm out from the areolar. It is firm in consistency, round in shape with a slightly irregular edge. It is not attached to the skin or to the deep structures. The nipple and areola are normal.

On palpation of the axilla, there is a firm 1 cm node palpable on the medial wall, it is mobile. There are no nodes in the L-axilla or the supraclavicular areas and on examination of the abdomen, there is no ascites and the liver is not palpable.

Question 1.4: Draw how you would record the breast findings in the patient's notes, if you were the house officer taking the history:

Question 1.5: What investigations would the surgeon arrange for this lady?

Question 1.6: What do you think he should say to the patient at this stage?

The mammograms are reported as showing a 2 cm lesion in the upper outer quadrant of the right breast with the characteristics of a carcinoma.

The FNAC carried out at the clinic shows malignant cells (C5)

C1 = Insufficient for diagnosis
C2 = Cells present, all benign, no suspicious features
C3 = Cells suspicious, probably benign
C4 = Cells suspicious, probably malignant
C5 = Definitely malignant
Chest X-ray is negative.

Note: Patients with small breast cancers (<4 cm) have a low incidence of detectable metastatic disease and in many breast units do not routinely have bone scan or CT done unless they have suggestive symptoms.

Question 1.7: On the TNM staging protocol, how would you stage this lady at present? (see Module 1, Tutorial 11)

In summary, therefore, we have a premenopausal 45-year-old lady with a 2 cm right upper outer quadrant breast carcinoma which clinically is staged T2, N1, M0.

Question 1.8: What operation would she be advised to have to remove the lump?

Question 1.9: Is there any alternative to this?

Question 1.10: Breast conserving surgery is planned. How would you stage her axilla?

She is advised to have a lumpectomy and axillary clearance.

Question 1.11: Write how you would consent her for the operation.

The histology is reported as an intraduct carcinoma with 1.5 cm clearance. Three of 13 lymph nodes are shown to be involved in the axillary clearance fat. Immune staining shows she is estrogen receptor positive.

Question 1.12: Does she require radiotherapy? Yes/No

Question 1.13: Where to?

Question 1.14: Why does she not need DXR to the axilla?

Question 1.15: What hormonal therapy would you advise for this lady and why?

Question 1.16: Who would be present at the multidisciplinary meeting to discuss this lady's management preoperatively?

Question 1.17: What is the importance of such meetings?

Question 2: Case scenario

You will recognize this lady from Module 1 Tutorial 11:

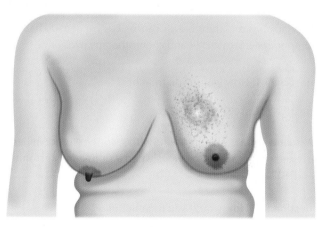

Fig. 2.2

As you can see in Figure 2.2, there is an obvious swelling.

Question 2.1: Do you see other physical signs on the picture which may influence the patient's management?

This situation is termed locally advanced breast cancer (LABC).

You will also hear breast surgeons talking about:

Operable breast tumors (those < 5 cm in diameter, no skin or deep fixation and with mobile axillary nodes) or advanced or metastatic cancer—where there is fixation or fixed nodes or distal metastases.

Question 2.2: What is a simple mastectomy?

Question 2.3: Why may a simple mastectomy be difficult in patients with locally advanced disease?

Question 2.4: What therapy might you recommend before you operate on this lady?

Question 2.5: What do you understand by immediate reconstruction after a mastectomy?

Question 2.6: How is this done?

If you do not know what a TRAM flap is—look it up yourself in either a surgical textbook or on the net. If you do this, you will be more likely to remember it.

Question 2.7: What does the terminal care of a breast cancer patient involve?

Question 3: Case scenario

The patient shown in Figure 2.3 has very advanced breast cancer:

Question 3.1: What treatment is this lady likely to be offered (Fig. 2.3)?

Question 4: Case scenario

This lady has recurrent breast cancer, having already had a lumpectomy, breast DXR and chemotherapy (Fig. 2.4).

Question 4.1: How would you treat her?

Question 5: Case scenario

At follow-up, a patient presents with recurrent tumor in her mastectomy scar. She previously had a simple mastectomy and axillary clearance.

Question 5.1: How would you treat her now?

Question 6: Case scenario

Question 6.1: What complication is shown in Figure 2.5

Question 6.2: Why has it developed?

Question 6.3: What can you do about it?

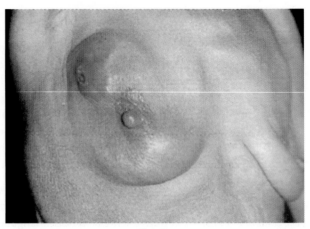

Fig. 2.3

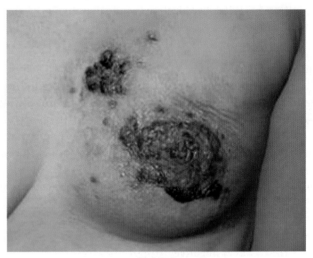

Fig. 2.4

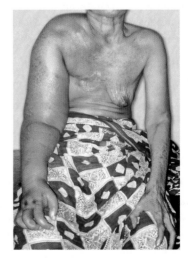

Fig. 2.5

TUTORIAL 3: Upper Gastrointestinal Cases

Please revise the relevant upper gastrointestinal tutorials you have already completed (Module 1 Tutorials 5 and 6, and Module 2 Tutorial 1).

We are going to 'revisit' some of the patients for 'revision purposes', and where appropriate, expand on their management.

Question 1: Case scenario

> Mr T is a 72-year-old laborer who presents with an 8-week history of difficulty in swallowing. He can only eat liquid food. He has a long history of heartburn, has been a heavy smoker for 50 years and drinks 3 bottles of beer a day.

Figure 3.1 is one of the films from the X-rays arranged by his GP.

Question 1.1: What type of X-ray is it?

Question 1.2: What does it show?

Figure 3.2 is a picture of the upper gastrointestinal endoscopy carried out on Mr T.

Question 1.3: What does it show?

A biopsy was taken at the endoscopy and the histology is confirmatory of malignancy.

Question 1.4: What type of carcinoma is it likely to be?

Question 1.5: What investigation is shown in Figure 3.3, and what is the purpose of performing this investigation in a patient with esophageal cancer?

Question 1.6: What factors decide if a patient with cancer of the esophagus should be advised to have surgery?

The type of operation depends on the site of the tumor in the esophagus, especially its relationship to the bifurcation of the trachea.

Question 1.7: List the type of operation used for:
a. A cancer at the gastroesophageal junction or in the lower third of esophagus.
b. In the lower third or mid third but below the carina.
c. At the carina or in the upper third.

You do not need to know anymore than this as an undergraduate, but it will help if you just draw the operations in simple outline, so that if you have to help manage such operations as a House Surgeon/Intern, you are familiar with their format.

Question 1.8: Make outline drawings of:
a. Total gastrectomy and Roux-en-Y.
b. Thoracoabdominal gastroesophagectomy.
c. A 3-stage esophagectomy with colonic interposition.

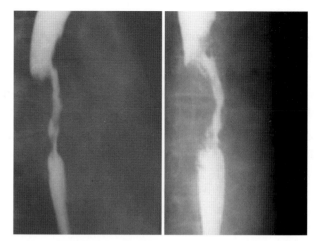

Fig. 3.1 With permission Dr Sumer Sethi

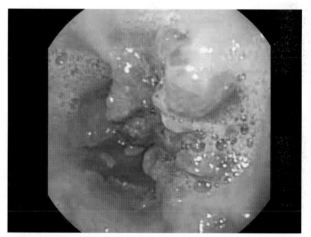

Fig. 3.2 Reprinted from Surgery (Oxford) 29, 11, Griffin MS and Wahed S, Oesophageal cancer. p 557-562, 2011, with permission Elsevier.

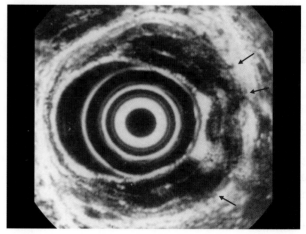

Fig. 3.3 Reproduced from Surgery (Oxford) 26, 11, Griffin MS and Dunn l. p 458-62, 2008, with permission Elsevier

As a house officer you may well have to look after a patient who has undergone an esophagectomy and has developed problems.

Question 1.9: List, in outline only, the complications which may occur with this operation.

Question 1.10: What would you think might be the problem if, in his original history, Mr T had complained of hoarseness in addition to his dysphagia.

Question 1.11: What might be the problem, if he said in his history that he had started to cough up very dirty sputum at night?

We will now consider INOPERABLE cancer of esophagus.

Question 1.12: List the methods which are available for palliation of esophageal cancer.

Question 2: Case scenario

You will remember Mr F, he is the 46-year-old man who had a 2-year history of indigestion and was discussed in Tutorial 6 of Module 1. He was diagnosed as having a duodenal ulcer on endoscopy, see Figure 3.7.

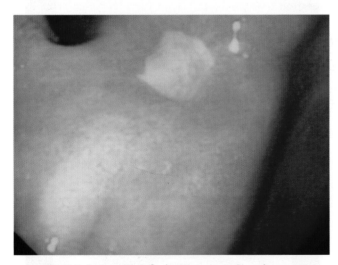

Fig. 3.7 Patient Mr F: findings at upper GI endoscopy

Question 2.1: You are the house officer, how would you consent Mr F for his endoscopy?

Not only must be in a language that he can understand but must also show that you know how the procedure is carried out and have given some thought as to what concerns the patient might have about the procedure.

All endoscopy units now have very good patient information leaflets and these are often sent to the patient with his appointment. If this is done, ask him if he has

read the leaflet, if he understands it and if he has any questions.

If he has not had any previous information you must make sure he is provided with the patient information either before or after you have explained it to him. Very often the patient information forms part of the patient consent form.

When you have answered this question (and only then) go onto the web and download an actual hospital patient information leaflet for upper gastrointestinal endoscopy, see how it compares with your own answer (excellent patient information given on: *www.patient.co.uk/health/ gastroscopy-endoscopy*).

Question 2.2: If the patient has an ulcer or gastritis, what test is routinely carried out with the endoscopy?

Question 2.3: How is the urease test done?

Mr F is HP positive.

Question 2.4: In outline only using bullet points summarize current concepts of the etiology of a duodenal ulcer.

Question 2.5: Write below what you understand by the term triple therapy for treatment of HP.

Question 2.6: You are Mr F's GP: write out a prescription for his triple therapy exactly, as if you were giving it to him in the surgery. The prescription pad is:

Dr PM Boggs MB CHB MRCGP
Riverside Surgery
Riverside Rd
HUMBER
Rx:

Question 2.7: What treatment should he have when he has completed the course?

As you know from Module 1 Mr F is admitted 18 months later with an acute abdomen.

We are going to consider this admission in more detail now.

You are the house officer/intern on duty when Mr F is admitted to the surgical ward. He was diagnosed about two years ago as having a DU and received antibiotics. He says his symptoms cleared up for a year but he has been having indigestion again for 6 months, usually before eating, and waking him in the middle of the night. He has been taking Rennies and bought some Zantac over the counter. This morning, two hours ago, he developed upper abdominal pain which has become very severe and has spread over his whole abdomen. He has been vomiting.

On examination, he looks ill and in pain. He is pale, has sunken eyes and a dry tongue. His pulse is 100/min and BP 100/60. His peripheries are cold. His abdomen

does not move with respiration and shows diffuse board-like rigidity and guarding. There are no bowel sounds present.

You make a clinical diagnosis of a perforated duodenal ulcer with peritonitis.

Question 2.8: Describe exactly how you would manage him in practical terms, i.e. what would you do as the house officer, in bullet form, but including ALL practical details—including fluids, drugs, instructions and investigations. This should be in chronological order. Think about it, then rough out a list of what you would do and then enter it here.

Do this carefully, it is not the knowledge you can easily copy from a textbook, but it is what you will be doing as a house officer.

Question 2.9: These are the results of his investigations. Comment on each one and any action you will take.

FBC: Hb   16 g/dL
      MCV   80 fl
      PCV   40%
      WCC $14.000 \times 10^9/L$
      Neutrophils $9 \times 10^9/L$
      Lymphocytes $2 \times 10^9/L$
      Platelets $200 \times 10^9/L$

Before doing so write in the normal values for each parameter.

Question 2.10:

Urea and electrolytes:

Na   140 mmol/L
K   3 mmol/L
Cl   126 mmol/L
Urea   12 mmol/L
Creatinine   0.14 mmol/L

Write in the normal values and comment on the results.

The patient's serum amylase is 200 u/L

Question 2.11: Comment on this result.

His Erect chest X-ray is shown in Figure 3.9.

Question 2.12: What does this show?

Question 2.13: What do you understand by the term *lateral decubitus* X-ray and when is it indicated?

He is tachycardic and hypotensive with cold peripheries with the abdominal signs of peritonitis. When you catheterize him only 200 mL of urine come out and it is very concentrated.

Question 2.14: What does this mean to you about his clinical condition?

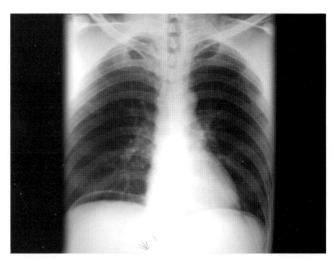

Fig. 3.9 Erect chest X-ray

Question 2.15: What action would now be indicated in his fluid balance?

At this stage, as the house officer or intern you should be seeking more senior help.

In addition to the above the Registrar asks you to start him on antibiotics.

Question 2.16: List the antibiotics you would use—type, dose, mode of administration and frequency of administration.

With the extra fluid his pulse rate comes down to 90/min and BP to 120/80. His peripheries warm up and his urine output rises to 60 mL per minute. The Specialist Registrar says to put 20 mmol KCl in his next liter of Hartmann's and run it in over 2 hours. The Consultant says to get him ready for theater.

Question 2.17: Write a check list of things you, as the House Officer, should have done before he goes to theater.

Question 2.18: What operation is the patient likely to undergo? What will be carried out by the Surgeon?

Question 2.19: Describe how you would consent the patient for operation. To do this you must know what operation the specialist is likely to carry and be able to put it into a language that the patient understands.

Question 2.20: What procedure has been carried out on the patient in Figure 3.10?

In this case (Fig. 3.10), the catheter is placed into the SVC via the subclavian vein; sometimes it is placed via the internal jugular (a route favored by anesthetists—Fig. 3.11) Figure 3.12 shows a CVP insertion kit—a sterile, pre-prepared set containing the necessary equipment for inserting the line.

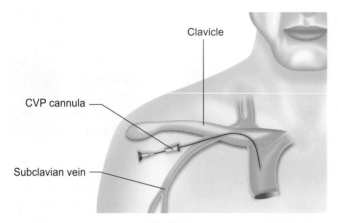

Clavicle

CVP cannula

Subclavian vein

Fig. 3.10

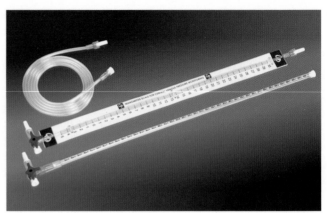

Fig. 3.13

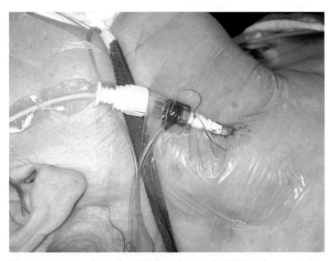

Fig. 3.11 Internal jugular CVP line Copyright RCSI with permission

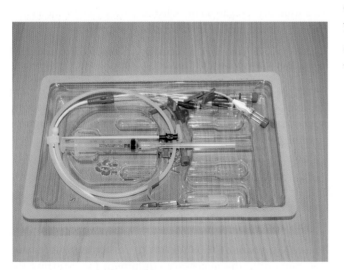

Fig. 3.12 CVP insertion kit

Question 2.21: How is the procedure carried out?

You should have seen the procedure in the Skills Laboratory and should attempt to see an insertion in the hospital.

Question 2.22: What investigation must always be done after insertion and why?

Question 2.23: What is a CVP line used for?

Question 2.24: What are the complications of a CVP line?

Question 2.25: What is shown in Figure 3.13. Explain how you set up and calibrate the instrument.

A CVP line is inserted in our patient who has peritonitis.

Question 2.26: If the CVP reading is low (<3 cm H_2O); what will you do?

Question 2.27: If the CVP reading is 5–10 cm H_2O; what will you do?

Question 2.28: If the CVP reading is high, say, 14 cm H_2O; what does this suggest to you?

TUTORIAL 4: Hepatobiliary

Question 1: Case scenario

Please look back and re-read Patient 1 in the Jaundice Tutorial of Module 2, Tutorial 2.

You will recall that this was a 35-year-old lady who was admitted with obstructive jaundice. She had an ERCP carried out and the gallstones removed from her common bile duct.

She was discharged from hospital and the jaundice settled over the course of the next week. When seen at the OP clinic 3 weeks later, she was fit and well with a normal liver function tests and white cell count.

The surgeon decided to admit her next week for surgery.

Question 1.1: Why would he admit her? What are the options for the patient?

Question 1.2: Describe briefly how these 2 operations are performed. Please note that the detail required is that sufficient for you to obtain informed consent for the operation from the patient (as you will be doing as a house officer).

Question 1.3: What are the advantages of laparoscopic cholecystectomy?

You are the house officer/intern who admits this lady for her operation. You take her history and examine her, she has had no further problems since discharge and there are no physical signs in her abdomen.

You do not identify any other problems in her problem-orientated history.

Question 1.4: What preoperative management will this lady require? Include the doses and method of administration of any drugs you prescribe.

Question 2: Case scenario

A 60-year-old patient, known to have gallstones, is admitted as an emergency to the surgical ward with fever, chills and rigors, jaundice and abdominal pain. She is diabetic for which she takes oral hypoglycemics.

On examination, she is a little confused, has scleral icterus and is clinically dehydrated. She has a temperature of 40°C, She has a tachycardia. Her BP is 100/60. Her peripheries are cold. Her abdomen is jaundiced and she is tender in the RUQ and epigastrium. Bowel sounds are present.

Question 2.1: What is the name given to the symptom/sign complex this lady is showing?

Question 2.2: What do you think it is due to in this case?

Question 2.3: If you had performed a problem-based history and examination on this lady, what are the likely list of *problems*?

You are the house officer/intern called to see her: You elicit the history as above—helped by her husband. She has been unwell for 48 hours now.

Question 2.4: Using bullet points list the exact management you would institute for this patient—including details of investigation and surgical therapeutics—alongside each bullet point explain why you are doing this.

Question 2.5: What organisms are likely to be causing the ascending cholangitis? What antibiotics are you likely to give—including dose and method of administration? What analgesic are you going to use—dose and route?

Question 2.6: What intervention is this patient likely to need?

Question 2.7: Do you think the patient will require vitamin K, if so why and how will you give it?

Question 2.8: How do you think this patient's diabetes is going to be managed?

TUTORIAL 5: Jaundice and Weight Loss (Pancreas)

To start with please look back to Question 2: Case scenario in *Module 1 Tutorial 7* and Question 2: Case scenario in *Module 2 Tutorial 2*. Redo as many of the questions about these cases as you can without looking at your answers. Then re-read the chapter in your book about neoplasia of the pancreas.

Just to make sure you have done this, here are a few questions:

Question 1: Describe the classical 'core' history and examination findings in a patient with carcinoma of the head of the pancreas.

Question 2: What is the anatomical distribution and histology of neoplasms of the pancreas?

Question 3: What do you understand by a periampullary carcinoma?

Question 4: What information and investigations will help you in making a diagnosis of cancer of the pancreas?

Now we come back to Patient 2 from Module 1 Tutorial 7.

Question 5: Case scenario 1

This is a 73-year-old lady who has been feeling unwell for many weeks. She has a poor appetite and has lost 6 kg in weight. About a month ago, she became jaundiced and this has gradually become worse. She has had no abdominal pain until about 3 weeks ago—she now has a dull abdominal ache. She has dark urine and itchy skin. On examination of her abdomen apart from evidence of weight loss and jaundice, there are no physical signs.

Question 5.1: These are her investigations—please comment on them:

Question 5.1a:

Hb is 10 g/dL

U and Es = normal

Question 5.1b: LFTs Bilirubin is 40

alkaline phosphate is elevated

enzymes are normal

serum albumin is at lower limit of normal

Question 5.1c: CA 19-9 is elevated.

Other investigations:

Clotting screen is normal

CXR—normal

The ultrasound scan of her abdomen shows a dilated common bile duct but no gallstones.

See Figure 5.1.

Question 5.2: What investigation will you order next?

The CT scan is shown below in Figure 5.2.

Question 5.3: What does it show?

Using the arterial and venous phases of the CT the portal vein is not involved, the fat plane between the superior mesenteric artery and vein is preserved and there are no enlarged peri-pancreatic lymph nodes. The liver is clear of metastases.

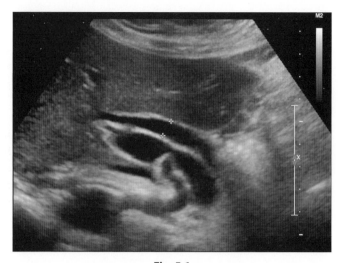

Fig. 5.1

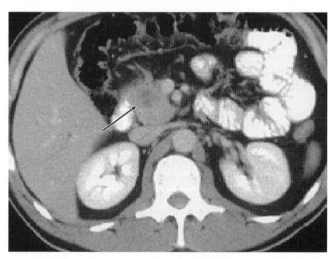

Fig. 5.2 Courtesy of Professor N Karanja and Dr Tony Lopez, Guildford, UK

At the multidisciplinary meeting, the surgeon reviews the X-rays with the radiologists and it is agreed that this is a carcinoma of the pancreas and that it may be resectable.

Question 5.4: What operation would the surgeon have in mind?

Question 5.5: Draw the operation in outline (all you need to know is an outline of the procedure—so that if you are the house officer looking after a patient who has undergone a Whipple's operation, you will know what has been done).

Further information:

Treatment options for CA pancreas:

1. Resection, if possible.

    Note that about 80% are non-resectable because of the presence of peritoneal or liver metastases, spread to lymph nodes or extensive involvement of portal vein and/ or superior mesenteric artery and vein.

2. Palliation: with stenting, if bile duct obstruction alone

with triple bypass if bile duct and duodenal obstruction

with radiation + chemotherapy in some cases.

Question 6: Case scenario

Chronic Abdominal Pain (Pancreas)

A 63-year-old man is seen at the clinic with a 3-year history of abdominal pain. The pain is in the epigastrium and radiates through to the back. To start with, he had it every 2 or 3 months and it was worse when he had been drinking alcohol. He describes it as a 'dull boring' pain. Recently, he has been getting it much more often—for 2 or 3 days each week and it would not go away until he takes pain killers. He has been admitted to hospital twice but discharged himself after he had been given pain killers.

He has lost 14 lbs in weight in the last year and recently has started to vomit when the pain is bad. His bowel habit has changed—more frequent and he has difficulty in flushing the toilet.

On examination, he looks unwell and has clearly lost weight. He is not clinically anemic or jaundiced. His abdomen has some red marks over the area around his umbilicus. There is tenderness in the epigastrium. There is no organomegaly and normal bowel sounds. PR is negative.

Question 6.1: What is your differential diagnosis?

Question 6.2: What investigations will you order initially?

These are the results:

Hb = 11 g/dL, WCC = normal

U and Es normal

LFTs normal bilirubin; raised enzymes and alkaline phosphate

Serum albumin lower limit of normal

Amylase normal

Urine dipstick shows 3+ glucose

CA 19-9 = normal

Chest X-ray = normal

Question 6.3: His abdominal X-ray is shown in Figure 5.4. What does it show?

Question 6.4: What do you think is the diagnosis now?

Question 6.5: What other investigations will the consultant now order?

The results come back:

GTT shows fasting BS = 7.2 mmol; at 2 hrs = 12.7 mmol

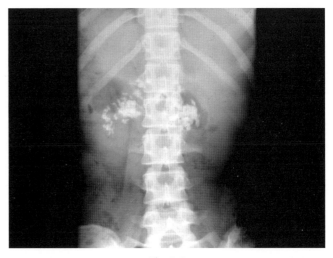

Fig. 5.4

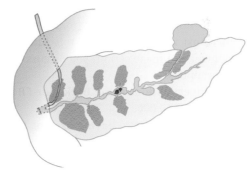

Fig. 5.5

Question 6.6: What does this indicate?

Stool fat = 15 g/24 hours (normal = 5–7 g/24 hours)

Question 6.7: What does this indicate?

A simulated drawing of the changes seen on the patient's ERCP scan is shown (Fig. 5.5).

Similar changes would be seen on an MRICP (which is used more often nowadays).

Question 6.8: What abnormalities do you see?

Question 6.9: How will you manage this patient medically?

Question 6.10: Can surgery help?

Question 7: Case scenario 3

Severe Abdominal Pain (Pancreas)

Before starting, revise Question 1: Case scenario, Module 1 Tutorial 8:

A 40-year-old lady presents with sudden onset of severe generalized abdominal pain. She has been vomiting and feels very unwell. She has never had the pain before but in the past, has been investigated for gallstones.

On examination, she looks unwell and is in obvious pain. She is pale but not jaundiced. She is clinically dehydrated.

Her pulse is 100/min, BP 100/60, RR 20.

Temperature = 38°C and her peripheries are cold.

Her abdomen is diffusely tender with rebound tenderness and guarding.

No bowel sounds are present.

You are the house surgeon/intern who sees her first on the surgical ward.

Question 7.1: What is the diagnosis in *one word* (without a specific cause).

Question 7.2: *List in bullet points* exactly what you will do (i.e. how you will manage her).

This should be written down in the order you will do the specific tasks/investigations.

Remember, this is exactly what you will be doing as a house officer—not easily extracted from a textbook but probably the most important part of this tutorial. Do it carefully yourself, and make certain you discuss with your tutor any uncertainties.

The blood investigations come back: her FBC shows her to have a WCC of 15,000.

Her U and Es show her to have a urea of 14, others within normal limits. Her LFTs are normal.

Her serum amylase is 1200 IU

Imaging: Chest X-ray = N

Abdominal films: No free air

Multiple small bowel fluid levels

Gas in colon

Question 7.3: What is your diagnosis?

Question 7.4: How may acute pancreatic be classified CLINICALLY?

Question 7.5: In this lady how will you, as the intern, decide if she has got mild or severe acute pancreatitis?

Question 7.6: In addition to the investigation already performed, now you know she has acute pancreatitis, what other investigations will you order?

Note: You do *not* need to remember the absolute criteria of *Ranson's Score* or the *Glasgow Prognostic Score*—these should be on a protocoled form available in the Emergency Ward.

However, for completeness they are shown here:

Glasgow prognostic score (Modified Imrie's criteria)

Age > 55

BUN > 16 mmol/L

Albumin < 32 g/L

S. calcium < 2 mmol/L

Glucose > 10 in nondiabetic

LDH > 600 units/L

AST/ALT > 200

PaO_2 < 8 kPa (60 mm Hg)

WCC > 15×10^9

What you should know is that if 3 or more of the criteria are positive the patient has a severe disease.

Glasgow prognostic score can be remembered by the mnemonic: PANCREAAS: ie 2 'A's'

PO_2 < 8 kPA

Age > 55

Neutrophils > 15

Calcium < 2

Urea > 16

AST > 200 (LDH > 600)

Albumin < 32

S. glucose > 10

Question 7.7: What difference will a high Imrie score make to the patient's management?

Question 7.8: What complications are they likely to develop, if they have a severe disease?

Question 7.9: Make a list of the principles of management of a patient with severe acute pancreatitis.

TUTORIAL 6: Lower Gastrointestinal Tract

1. Please revise Module 1, Tutorial 9 (Rectal Bleeding) and make sure you know all of this.
2. Then revise Module 2, Tutorial 3 (Rectal Bleeding—investigations).

Only when you have done this should you proceed.

Try and answer this Tutorial without books or notes. Then look up the answers you do not know or are not sure about. Then repeat the tutorial as a top copy for revision.

All of this will take about 3 hours, but if you carry it out in this way you are more likely to retain the knowledge.

Here are a few questions to make sure you have looked at the relevant Module 1 and 2 sections:

Question 1.1a: What color is the blood in the bowel motions of a patient with a cancer of the descending colon most likely to be?

Question 1.1b: What color is the blood with a rectal cancer?

Question 1.1c: What is the difference between 'incomplete evacuation' and tenesmus? Who do they occur in?

Question 1.2: What imaging is required to clinically stage?
a. Colon cancer.
b. Rectal cancer.

Question 1.3: What are the names of the staging regimes used in colorectal cancer?

Question 1.4: What do you understand by the terms:
a. Neo-adjuvant therapy?
b. Adjuvant therapy?
c. Write below when these would be used in large bowel cancer (bullet form only).

Question 2: Case scenario

(The same patient from Module 1, Tutorial 9)

> He is a 65-year-old man with an adenocarcinoma at 18 cm from the anal verge.
> He is admitted to the ward for his surgery and you are the house officer/intern who admits him.
> He has already had the following investigations performed:
> FBC = N
> U + Es = N
> LFTs = N
> Chest X-ray = N
> CT = N (liver)

Question 2.1: What further blood investigations are required?

Question 2.2: What bowel preparation is required and what instruction will you give to the nurses?

Question 2.3: What preoperative prophylaxis will the patient require?

Question 2.4: For both DVT and antibiotic prophylaxis write out the drugs involved, their dosage and when they will be given.

Your Consultant says the patient requires an anterior resection.

Question 2.5: Draw this operation in outline.

The Consultant says it is unlikely that he will require a covering loop ileostomy but asks you to explain to the patient that there is a small possibility that this may need to be done and asks you to mark the site (the stoma nurse is away).

Question 2.6: Draw a simple diagram of a loop ileostomy.

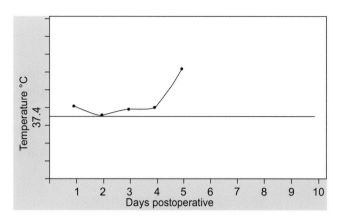

Fig. 6.4

Question 2.7: On a simple diagram of the abdomen mark in the site of the loop ileostomy and then write its anatomical location and explain how you would mark this on the patient.

The operation goes well. He has a high anterior resection performed with no ileostomy necessary.

On day 5 postoperative you (the house officer) are doing the morning ward round with the specialist and the patient complains of lower abdominal pain which started during the night and has gradually become worse. He is on free fluids and his IV line was taken down yesterday.

On examination: He looks unwell

> **pulse 100/min   BP 100/60**
> **RR = increased**
> **His peripheries are cold and clammy**

Abdomen examination   Marked lower abdominal tenderness, rebound and guarding incision not inflamed
> **Drain = out**
> **Urinary catheter out**
> **No bowel sounds on auscultation**

His temperature chart is shown in Figure 6.4.

Question 2.8: What do you think has happened?

Question 2.9: Make a list of the instructions the Consultant is likely to tell you to carry out, i.e. how will you manage this 'event'?

The patient begins a short period of resuscitation, during this he is taken to the CT room and a small quantity of gastrograffin is run into his rectum and a CT performed. This confirms an anastomotic leak.

Question 2.10: What action will the surgeon take?

Question 2.11: What will be the procedure most likely performed?

Now a few short Case scenarios.

Question 3: Case scenario

A 39-year-old man presents to his GP with severe cutting pain on defecation together with a streak of bright red blood on the toilet paper. He has had symptoms for 8 weeks' duration.

The Figure 6.5 shows the findings on inspection of his anus:

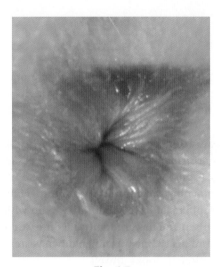

Fig. 6.5

Question 3.1: What is your diagnosis?

Question 3.2: What treatment will the GP advise?

The patient comes back 2 weeks later and is no better. The GP refers him to the Surgical Outpatient Clinic where he is still found to have a fissure.

Question 3.3: What options does the surgeon have in his treatment?

Question 4: Case scenario

A 35-year-old man complains to his GP of intermittent bright red bleeding on defecation. He has had this on and off for 2 years. He has no anal or abdominal pain and his bowel habit is regular.

Question 4.1: What is the likely diagnosis?

Question 4.2: How do you classify hemorrhoids? Make a table of the classification on one side and the treatment on the other.

Question 4.3: What procudure is depicted in Figure 6.6.

Question 4.4: What operation is shown in Figures 6.7A and B?

Question 4.5: You are the intern looking after a patient who has had a hemorrhoidectomy—what specific complications will you be watching for in the postoperative period?

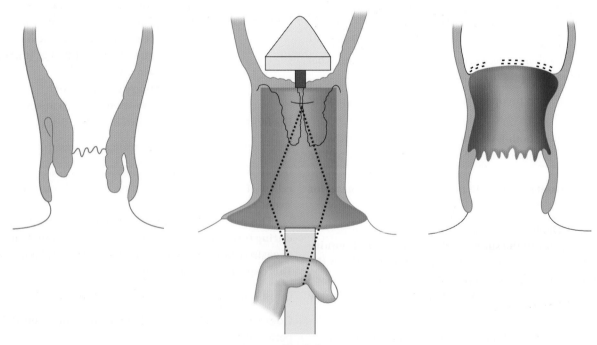

Fig. 6.6

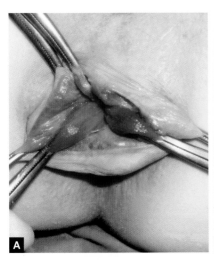
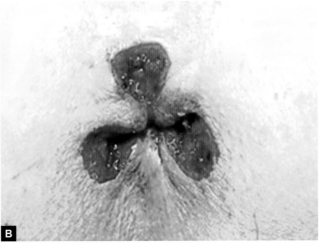

Figs 6.7A and B (A) Preoperative image; (B) postoperative image reproduced from
Surgery (Oxford) 21, 7, Acheson AG and Scholefield JH, Haemorrrhoids p165-167, 2003 with permission Elsevier

Question 5: Case scenario

An 18-year-old young man presents to A and E with severe perianal pain of 24 hours' duration. Figure 6.8 is a picture of his anal region.

Question 5.1: What is your diagnosis and what is the treatment?

Question 6: Case scenario

A 50-year-old man presents to his GP with a very sore and itchy bottom end. He says he has had this for 3 months—it is getting worse. He has noticed a smelly discharge and his underwear is always stained. His bowel habit is normal and he is otherwise fit and well.

Figure 6.9 is a picture of his anal area:.

Question 6.1: What is the diagnosis?

Question 6.2: What is the management? Outline in a few words only:

Now we return to Question 2: Case scenario, where we ended with Question 2.11, and continue.

Question 7: Draw in outline the types of intestinal stoma you will come across on the surgical ward.

Write how you will recognize the different stomas when you examine the patients abdomen.

Question 8: List the complications of a stoma.

We are now going to consider some stomal and anorectal conditions which you may encounter on the wards or in the clinic.

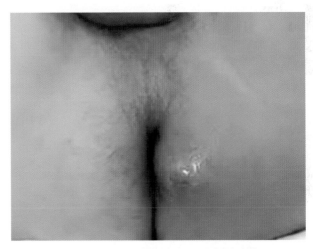

Fig. 6.8 With permission Surgicalexam

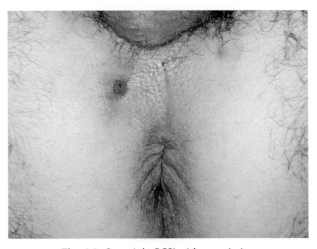

Fig. 6.9 Copyright RCSI with permission

Question 9: Look at the following pictures and write your diagnosis (or what you think it is) for each and, where appropriate, the treatment.

Question 9a: What type of stoma is this (Fig. 6.14)?

Question 9b: What anorectal condition is shown here (Fig. 6.15) and what would be the treatment?

Question 9c: What type of stoma is shown (Fig. 6.16).

Question 9d: What is the diagnosis and treatment of the anorectal condition illustrated in Figure 6.17.

Question 9e: The illustration shown in Figure 6.18 shows the natal cleft of an adult, male patient. What condition does he have and what is the treatment?

Question 9f: This patient presents with perianal itching. What is the diagnosis and treatment (Fig. 6.19)?

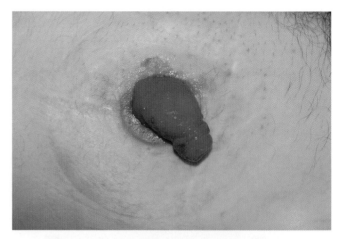

Fig. 6.16 With permission Welland Medical Ltd

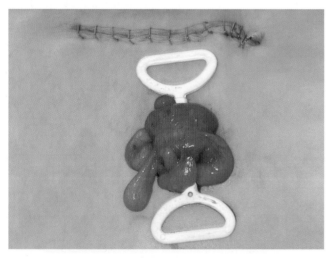

Fig. 6.14 Copyright RCSI with permission

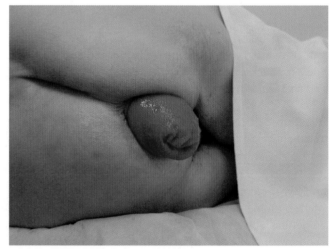

Fig. 6.17

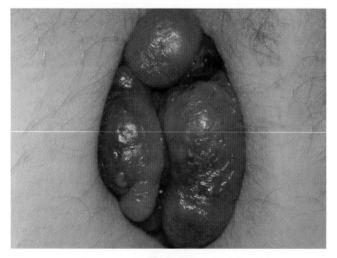

Fig. 6.15

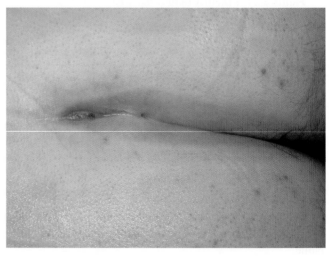

Fig. 6.18 Copyright RCSI with permission

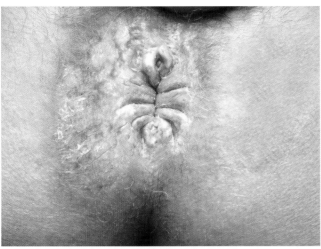

Fig. 6.19

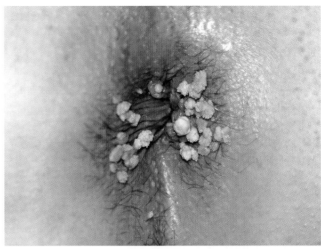
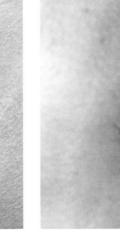

Fig. 6.21

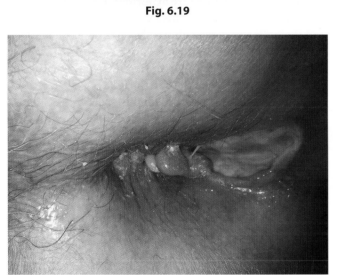

Fig. 6.20

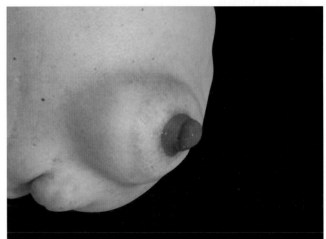

Fig. 6.22 Courtesy of Welland Medical Ltd

Question 9g: What malignant anal condition is shown in Figure 6.20 and what is the treatment?

Question 9h: What is the diagnosis and treatment of this perianal disease (Fig. 6.21)?

Question 9i: What condition has this patient developed and what is the management (Fig. 6.22)?

Question 9j: What stomal complication is shown in Figure 6.23?

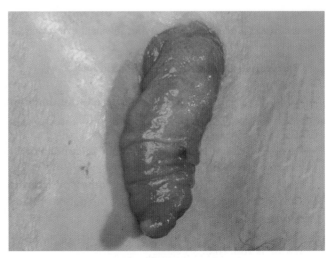

Fig. 6.23

TUTORIAL 7: Vascular Disease (Arterial)

INSTRUCTIONS

- Look back at your answers for *Module 1, Tutorial 3*: Symptoms and Signs of Vascular Diseases
- Look at your answers to *Module 1, Tutorials 14 and 15* (Vascular Disease)
- Look at your answers to *Module 2, Tutorials 5 and 12* (Vascular Disease)
- Revise any lecture notes you have on Vascular Disease or read the relevant sections in your surgical textbook.

Now

- Without notes and books try and answer the following case scenarios.
- When you have finished look-up the sections, you do not know, or need to check and redo the Tutorial.

Question 1: Case scenario

A 65-year-old obese man presents to the A and E Department because of severe right-sided cramping calf pain. It came on when he was hurrying to catch an airline flight.

On direct questioning, he says the pain went away in a few minutes when he stood and rested.

When he thinks about it, for some months now he has noticed some pain in his leg when he has been out walking.

He does not recall any trauma to his leg recently.

He has just flown on a long haul flight for 8 hours.

He has a past history of chronic back pain.

He is a smoker and drinks 3 units of alcohol per day.

Question 1.1: List what you think may be the differential diagnosis.

Question 1.2: With this history, what physical examinations you will perform.

The findings on examination are as follows:
On general examination:
He is alert, conscious and orientated and does not appear in any distress.
He is markedly overweight.
He does not appear clinically anemic or jaundiced.
He is well hydrated.
He has *arcus senilis* of both eyes and some xanthelasma.
Hands: No fingernail abnormalities/no palmar pallor/erythema.
His pulse is 80 per minute, regular and of good volume.
His BP is 160/100.

His RR and temperature are normal.
His peripheries are well perfused.
Examination of his cardiovascular system shows the following:
- **Radial pulses N and equal.**
- **Both carotid pulses are present with no bruits.**
- **JVP not raised.**
- **HS present and normal; RS normal expansion, no added sounds.**

Abdominal examination: **Normal with no obvious arterial pulsation or mass to palpate. No bruits heard.**

Examination of his limbs:

Inspection: **The limbs are of normal color. There is some loss of hair over the toes of his right foot and the skin is dry and the nails thickened. There are no discolored areas or ulcers but he has some obvious varicose veins.**

On palpation: **Feeling with the back of the hand, the right limb is slightly cooler than the left.**

Capillary filling is reduced on the right.

Examination of the peripheral pulses is shown in Figure 7.1.

On elevation of the right lower limb, the leg becomes pale at 45°.

There is some blushing when the leg is then made dependent.

Left leg: **No limb paleness on elevation or blushing on dependency.**

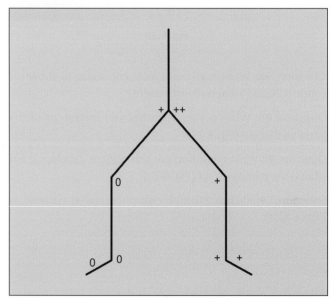

Fig. 7.1 Schematic recording of patient's peripheral pulses

Sensation: There are no sensory changes detectable in his lower limbs.

Movement: Full leg movements are present with normal tone and power of all muscle groups.

Straight leg raising is negative.

Others: No muscle wasting.

No calf tenderness.

No tenderness over lumbar spine.

Diameters at mid-calf level are equal.

Question 1.3: What is your diagnosis?

You tell the patient that you think he has intermittent claudication.

He asks you to explain this to him. Please note his occupation was a science and biology teacher at A-Level standard!

Question 1.4: What will you say to him?

He wants to know in detail how atherosclerosis develops.

Question 1.5: What will you say to him?

He wants to know the natural history of peripheral vascular disease (PVD).

Question 1.6: What will you say to him?

He wants to know how he will be managed.

You tell him that he needs to see a vascular surgeon for full assessment but he insists you tell him about likely management.

First of all, he wants to know what tests he will have to undergo.

Question 1.7: Make a list of the tests you think are indicated.

He wants to know the risk factors for PVD.

Question 1.8: What will you tell him?

After this, he wants to know how he is likely to be treated. You tell him that it will depend on the extent of the PVD in his right leg—either medically or surgically. He says, if his is not bad enough for surgery, how will he be treated? He has been reading about cholesterol levels and wants to know about this?

Question 1.9: Using your list of risk factors—make a table of best medical management.

You have told him that he will probably not need surgery unless there is a threat of him losing his limb. He wants to know what he should look out for.

Question 1.10: What will you tell him?

The patient obtains an urgent referral to the vascular surgeon.

The surgeon agrees with your diagnosis and confirms your assessment on clinical examination.

He arranges for:

1.	FBC	= N
2.	U and E	= N
3.	Cholesterol	= 7 mmol/L
4.	Lipids	= High triglycerides
5.	Blood glucose	= N
6.	ECG	= N
7.	Serial BP readings	BP is between 90/100 diastolic all the time, systolic 160/180 mm Hg
8.	Chest X-ray	= N
9.	Ankle brachial ratio	= 0.7
10.	An MR arteriogram	= Shows disease affecting the external iliac and superficial femoral artery in the region of the adductor canal. (See Fig. 7.2)

He is treated by 'best medical management', but one year later comes back to see the vascular surgeon because he can now only walk about 75 yards without pain. He is also getting some pain in his right foot at night.

On examination, he now has a weak femoral pulse on the right side and slight discoloration of his 4th and 5th R toes.

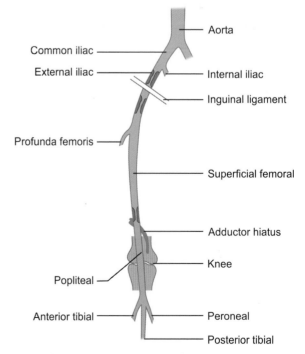

Fig. 7.2 Schematic image of MR arteriogram

Question 1.11: What new symptom is he describing?

Question 1.12: What does this and the leg changes indicate, and what needs to be done?

A further MR arteriogram is performed and shows extensive atherosclerosis in the superficial femoral artery, collaterals and some narrowing of the common and external iliac arteries (See Fig. 7.3).

Question 1.13: What options does the surgeon have?

Question 1.14: The patient is advised to have a percutaneous angioplasty of his right aortoiliac region.

Write here how you would explain this to the patient.

Question 1.15: Following this, the patient is advised to have a right-sided femoropopliteal bypass graft.

Draw a simple diagram of this procedure so that you can explain it to the patient.

Question 1.16: What is an extra anatomic bypass and give an example.

The patient's surgery is initially successful but one year later, he comes back with severe rest pain and an occluded graft. Attempts at salvage are unsuccessful and it is decided he needs an amputation.

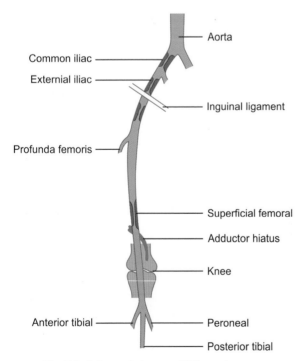

Fig. 7.3 Schematic image of MR arteriogram

Question 1.17: What are the indications for limb amputation? List them.

Question 1.18: Draw a lower limb and put in the common lower limb amputation sites and name the operations.

Question 2: Case scenario

A patient is transferred urgently from an outlying hospital with an acutely ischemic limb.

You are the surgical officer on duty and are called to see the patient on the ward.

The patient, who gives a long history of PVD, says his leg became acutely painful 12 hours ago and has become worse. He cannot move it now and it has become discolored.

On examination, he is very unwell. He is pale, in great pain and breathing rapidly. His pulse is 100 per minute and irregular and his BP is 100/60.

His foot is shown in Figure 7.7.

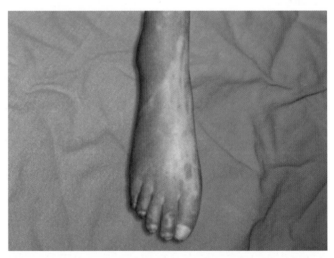

Fig. 7.7 Reproduced from Puppula S, Patel J Fig 7 in Acute limb ischaemia: Imaging, 2009;21:109-21 with kind permission of The British Institute of Radiology

Question 2.1: Do you think his limb is salvageable?

Question 2.2: List the clinical features which suggest limb salvage is too late.

Question 3: Case scenario

Next week you are on-call and another patient is admitted under the vascular service with an acutely ischemic limb. You are called to see him.

A 68-year-old man was quite well until 2 hours ago when his left leg suddenly became very painful. The pain has become worse and he says he cannot move his leg now. He has noticed it is much paler than the other side. He has never had anything like this before. He is fit and well and walks 3 miles a day. He is taking some tablets from his doctor for an irregular heart beat.

On Examination:

He looks unwell and in obvious pain.

Pulse 100 per min, poor volume, irregular.

BP 100/80.

Examination of his left leg shows it to be pale, cold and with no pulses below the femoral pulse. He says he cannot move his toes and when you squeeze his calf it causes him pain. He has loss of light touch on the dorsum of the foot.

The right limb is normal in color, has full peripheral pulses, full movement and sensation.

Question 3.1: What is your diagnosis?

Question 3.2: Why do you not think it is acute on chronic ischemia due to thrombosis of a leg with PVD? List your reasons:

You are the 2nd year surgical trainee called to help the House Officer.

Question 3.3: List how you would manage this gentleman in order of priority.

The vascular surgeon comes to see him urgently and agrees with your diagnosis. He seems pleased with your initial management.

Question 3.4: What will he arrange to do?

TUTORIAL 8: The Acute Abdomen

In Module 1, Tutorial 20 you were asked to make a table (Table 20.1/20.2) with the *core history and examination of the common acute abdominal conditions*. Please revise these: the model table is also available (Table 8.1) to facilitate this.

The next part of this tutorial will consist of a series of short histories, relevant physical findings and, if appropriate, results of indicated examinations. These are similar to the content of a Modified Essay Questions (MEQ) now commonly used in your assessment examinations.

Work through the cases—make your diagnosis and, where asked, list the management in bullet form. Do this without textbooks or notes and then go back, read up the relevant facts and check your answers. We will be covering several common acute surgical conditions.

Question 1: Case scenario

A 40-year-old female is admitted with a 2-day history of abdominal pain. On direct questioning, the pain is in the RUQ and is severe and continuous. It came on suddenly, has remained there ever since and has become gradually worse. She has never had it before but has a long history of abdominal discomfort. She does not particularly associate this with fatty foods. She feels unwell and thinks she has a fever. On examination, she is febrile, tachycardic and has marked right upper quadrant tenderness and guarding. Bowel sounds are normal.

Question 1.1: What is the likely diagnosis?

Her WCC is $12,000 \times 10^9$/L. Her urine dipstick shows the presence of bilirubin. Her LFTs are normal. Amylase = 140 units.

Question 1.2: What imaging will you request?

The ultrasound shows a thickened gallbladder containing multiple stones.

Question 1.3: How will you manage this lady? If medications of any sort are advised you must give name, dose, method of administration and for how long.

Question 1.4: What is the place of ERCP in a symptomatic patient with known gallstones?

Question 2: Case scenario

A 59-year-old English lady is admitted to hospital from a hotel where she is staying on holiday.

Two days ago, she first noticed a lower abdominal ache which has become worse and is now present over the whole of her lower abdomen. She feels unwell and fevered. She is not hungry. Her bowels have not worked for 2 days. She says that she has had a lot of trouble with her bowels over the last 3 years—sometimes they are loose and sometimes constipated. She has not noticed any blood. She has had colicky lower abdominal pain on and off for the last 3 years but nothing as bad as this.

Table 8.1 Acute abdominal pain—core knowledge

Diagnostic features of abdominal pain							
Disorder	Localization	Character	Aggravating factors	Relieving factors	Visceral symptoms	Major physical signs	Diagnostic test
Acute pancreatitis	Epigastric and left hypochondrium radiating to back	Severe, constant pain		May improve when sitting forward	Nausea, vomiting	Tachycardia, shock, tender upper abdomen with guarding. Bruising in flanks	Raised serum and urinary amylase
Acute cholecystitis/ biliary colic	Right hypochondrium/ epigastric radiating to right scapula and shoulder	Initially colicky, becomes contiuous	Palpation over the gallbladder bed (below 10th rib in right upper quadrant)		Nausea, vomiting, may have fever and rigors	Tender right hypochondrium, positive Murphy's sign, may be jaundiced	Biliary tract ultrasound, ERCP
Renal colic (Ureteric stones)	Loin pain radiating to groin, and in males the scrotum	Severe colicky/ constant/ intermittent			Nausea, vomiting, frequency	Microscopic or obvious hematuria	Abdominal radiograph (90% stones visible) IVP or CT urogram
Intestinal obstruction	*Large bowel:* Lower abdomen *Small intestine:* Periumbilical	colicky	Food, drink		*Large bowel:* Constipation, vomitting occurs later *Small intestine:* Vomiting, constipation occurs later	Abdominal distension empty rectum	Radiograph of abdomen shows air-fluid levels in bowel or do CT scan abdo
Acute appendicitis	Initially, periumbilical pain, later localizes to right iliac fossa	Initially dull, later intense	Movement, hip extension	Lying still	Nausea, anorexia, vomiting	Fever, tenderness and guarding in the right iliac fossa	CT scan, laparoscopy
Perforated peptic ulcer	Sudden onset of epigastric pain. May radiate to the shoulder and extend to whole abdomen	Severe, persistent	Movement	Lying still	Nausea, vomiting	Fever, tachycardia, hypotension shock, rigid abdomen with rebound tenderness	Chest radiograph reveals air under the diaphragm, CT scan abdo
Ruptured ectopic pregnancy	Lower abdomen	Sudden onset, severe pain	Movement	Lying still		Tachycardia, hypotension, shock. Lower abdominal tenderness may become generalized. Guarding and rebound tenderness, tender cervix	Positive pregnancy test, anemia ultrasound
Ruptured aortic aneurysm	Pain radiating to the back	Moderately severe			Nausea, sweating	Pulsatile tender mass, hypotension, shock, oliguria/ anuria	Abdominal radiograph (calcification), ultrasound angiography

Abbreviations: abdo, abdominal; CT, computed tomography; ERCP, endoscopic retrograde cholangiopancreatography; IVP, intravenous pyelogram

On examination, she has temperature of 38°C. Pulse 90/min, BP normal. There is marked lower abdominal tenderness, maximum in the left lower quadrant with rebound. Bowel sounds are present. On rectal examination, she is tender in the left Pouch of Douglas.

Question 2.1: What is your differential diagnosis?

> **The initial investigations are as follows:**
> Hb = N   WCC = $13,000 \times 10^9$/L   LFTs = N,
> Amylase = N   CXR = N
> Abdo films: No free gas, no fluid levels.

Question 2.2: Do these investigations help and why?

> **The consultant comes on the ward round and asks you to do one further investigation.**

Question 2.3: What do you think it would be?

> **The radiologist reports the CT scan as showing severe left-sided diverticular disease with thickening and edema of the sigmoid colon with a possible small abscess adjacent to sigmoid colon. Some free fluid in the pelvis.**

Question 2.4: What is your diagnosis now?

Question 2.5: Using bullet points write below how this patient will be managed initially.

Question 2.6: You are the house officer/intern. What will you be looking out for in terms of complications?

Question 3: Case scenario

A 57-year-old man is admitted to the ward with abdominal pain. It came on suddenly while he was driving to work and has been present ever since. It is severe, colicky in nature and comes on every 10 minutes or so. Between the severe bouts, he has a dull ache in his abdomen. The pain is around the umbilicus and radiates across his whole abdomen. He has never had any pain like this since he had a burst ulcer at the age of 30. He has vomited 3 times since the pain started—greenish, acidy fluid. He had a normal bowel action yesterday—his bowels have not worked today but he passed wind when he got up this morning. He took some Gaviscon but it has not helped. He is diabetic on insulin and took his normal insulin this morning with his breakfast.

He is otherwise well. On direct questioning, he has had some indigestion over the years but he just takes Rennies for this. He remembers that he was told there were problems when he had the anesthetic for his ulcer operation but he does not know what they were.

Rest of his PMH, FH, SH, ROS are unremarkable.

Drugs = Sol. insulin 12 units night and morning. He tests his own blood sugars daily and attends the diabetic clinic at the hospital twice a year. His diabetes has always been well controlled.

He is allergic to penicillin—brings him out in a rash.

Question 3.1: With this history, what are you thinking may be the differential diagnosis?

On Examination:
General: He is alert and orientated. He is in pain. He is not clinically anemic or jaundiced. His eyes are sunken and his tongue dry. He is well nourished. No intraoral pathology, dental hygiene is good.

> Hands moist and warm. No other signs.
> P = 100, BP 120/80, RR = 20, Temp = 38°C, Peripheries well perfused.

Neck: Marked scoliosis, fat short neck.
Abdomen: Moving normally with respiration, not distended, midline upper abdominal scar—bulges on coughing, mild tenderness over whole abdomen. No guarding or rebound. No organomegally.
>   Bowels sounds = hyperactive in runs.
>   Easily reducible Left inguinal hernia (when this is pointed out he says, yes, he has noticed a swelling there at times for 2 years—never troubled him)
>   PR: Empty rectum.

Question 3.2: What is your differential diagnosis now?

Question 3.3: Now, this is a problem-orientated history, you are the house officer dealing with him—list the patient's problems and what you are going to do about them. (Think, Think, Think). Answer in bullet form, no details.

Question 3.4: You are the House Officer, list your management of this patient, i.e. exactly what you will do and in the order you will do it. You have taken the history, examined the patient, made a problem-orientated assessment. What will you do now?

Question 3.5: What will you start the IV with?

Question 3.6: What investigations will you order? List them:

> **These are the results:**
> Hb = N   WCC = $10,000 \times 10^9$/L
> Urea = 12 mmol/L   K = 3.2 mmol/L
> Amylase = N
> Blood glucose: = 4 mmol/L
> Dipstick urine = No glucose
> Chest X-ray shown in Figure 8.1

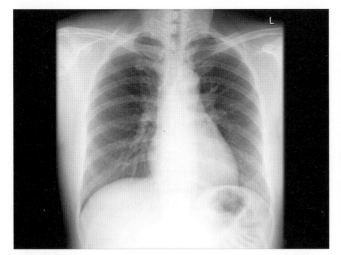

Fig. 8.1 Erect chest X-ray

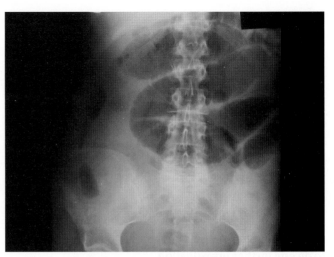

Fig. 8.3 Supine plain abdominal X-ray

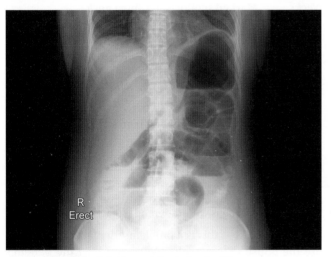

Fig 8.2 Erect plain abdominal X-ray

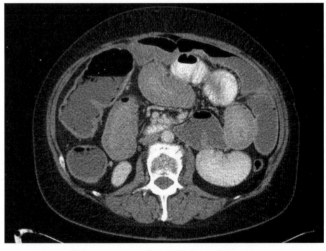

Fig. 8.4 Image from CT scan abdomen

Question 3.7: What do you see (Fig. 8.1)?

The plain abdominal X-rays are shown in Figures 8.2 and 8.3.

Question 3.8: What do you see in Figures 8.2 and 8.3? What is your diagnosis?

Question 3.9: What do you think is the likely cause of the obstruction in this case?

Question 3.10: List the common causes of small bowel obstruction in their order of frequency.

Question 3.11: What are the options for managing this patient? List in simple terms (one word each).

The patient is seen by the Registrar and Consultant and they decide on an initial course of conservative management.

The Consultant wants a nasogastric tube passed, the nurses are very busy and he asks you to do it.

Question 3.12: List in bullet form, how you would do it.

Question 3.13: What problems could develop during the period of *watch and wait*? What would you, the house officer, be checking? List them.

Question 3.14: What will you do about his diabetes?

Twelve hours later, the patient is complaining of continuing pain. When you examine him, he is more tender to the left of the umbilicus and his abdomen seems a little more distended.

His pulse rate on the hourly chart has gone up a little, BP = N and urine output is good (> 60 mL per hour), NG aspirate is not rising but you think it smells feculent.

You are worried about him and get the specialist to review him. He asks for an urgent CT scan and you go together to the X-ray department to discuss it with the radiologist.

The scan is shown in Figure 8.4.

Question 3.15: What do you see (Fig. 8.4)?

The Radiologist says the CT shows an obstruction at mid-small bowel level almost certainly due to adhesions. There is very little gas distal to the obstruction but no evidence of bowel ischemia.

The Consultant decides an operation is necessary and asks you to book the theater and speak to the anesthetist.

Question 3.16: Write in bullet form what you will tell the anesthetist about this patient—THINK!

The patient goes to theater. The surgeon opens the abdomen through a short incision below the umbilicus which he carefully extends upwards. There is a single band adhesion at mid-small bowel level with dilated, slightly congested bowel above and collapsed below. The small bowel is viable. The adhesions are released. He confirms the patient has an indirect inguinal hernia—uncomplicated and makes a note to speak to the patient about having it repaired in the future.

The Surgeon is able to close the incision in one layer repairing the small incisional hernia with no problems.

TUTORIAL 9: Patient 1: Varicose Veins
Patient 2: Leg Ulcer
Patient 3: A Swollen Leg

Please go back to *Module 2, Tutorial 12* (Varicose Veins) and go through your answers to the Question 1: Case scenario (Mrs P, who has varicose veins) (Mrs N, who has a varicose ulcer).

We are going to discuss their treatment in a little more detail, you will not be able to do this adequately if you do not look back at the previous cases.

Question 1: Case scenario

> *Mrs P:* Figure 9.1 is a picture of her legs. She has bilateral varicose veins with bilateral saphenofemoral incompetence and perforators above and below the knee.

The surgeon, Professor S, has decided she needs a bilateral saphenofemoral ligation, stripping from groin to knee and multiple avulsions.

Question 1.1: Please draw in simple outline form what this operation involves.

Professor S admits the patient for surgery and is called away to deal with a ruptured aortic aneurysm. He asks you to consent Mrs P for her operation.

Question 1.2: List in bullet form, what you will say to the patient (including an appropriate explanation of the common complications of the operation).

At the varicose veins clinic, you are asked to take the history and examine a lady who turns out to have minor varicose veins below the knee on her right leg only, with no saphenofemoral incompetence or perforators above the knee. She is getting married and wants her leg to look

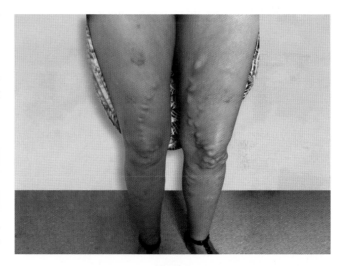

Fig. 9.1

nice! The surgeon says he thinks the varicose veins can be treated by injections.

Question 1.3: Write how the injection of varicose veins is performed including the after care.

This lady is on the oral contraceptive pill.

Question 1.4: Does this make any difference?

She also has some small spidery blue and red patches of superficial veins (See Figure 9.4).

Question 1.5: Can anything be done about these?

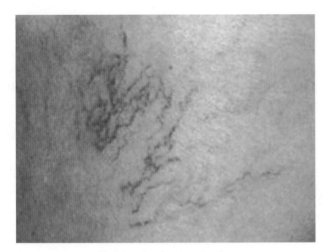

Fig. 9.4 'Spider veins' on leg

Question 2: Case scenario

Now we will look at Patient 2, similar to Mrs N, from Module 2.

Mrs S has a varicose ulcer, this is shown in Figure 9.5.

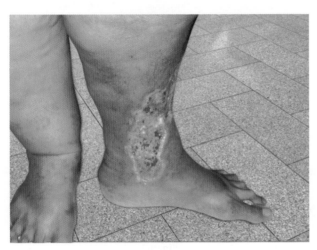

Fig. 9.5

She is admitted for treatment to the surgical ward.

Question 2.1: What investigations will you, as the HO, arrange for her?

Mrs N has normal peripheral pulses and her ABPI is 0.9.

Question 2.2: What does this indicate?

Her FBC, U and Es, lipid profile, TFTs, Rh serology and blood glucose are all normal.

Duplex scanning confirms perforators below the knee and saphenofemoral incompetence.

Bacteriology swab: mixed growth of gram +ve and –ve organisms.

Question 2.3: List why each of these tests is necessary in this patient.

Question 2.4: How will this lady's ulcer be treated? Your answer should be under 3 main headings and should include why each of the treatments is being carried out.

Question 3: Case scenario

Mrs L is a 60-year-old Indian lady who lived most of her life in Tamil Nadu (India). She thinks that both of her legs have been swollen for some years. The right leg is now getting bigger and causing her some difficulty in walking. She has had some trouble with her heart over the years and has been taking water tablets and blood pressure tablets for 4 years.

Two years ago, she had an operation at which her 'womb' was removed, she says. The doctor told her she has cancer—she has not been back for follow-up for 18 months because she says she is frightened. She did not have radiotherapy.

When asked about other illnesses she says she remembers years ago that she had some pain in her right leg and was in bed for a few weeks. She thinks the leg was swollen and had red marks on it.

Question 3.1: With the above history—make a list of the possible diagnoses you are considering and why?

Question 3.2: Just to make sure you are thinking along the correct lines, make a table here of the causes of swelling of the legs. Divide this into bilateral and unilateral.

Do it without looking at the books, then check your table and alter it as necessary.

This is a picture of Mrs L's legs (Fig. 9.6).

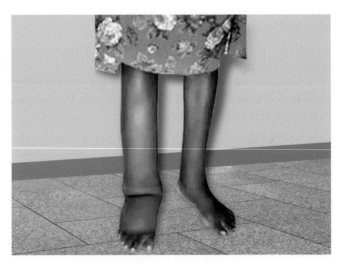

Fig. 9.6 Courtesy of CDC (Atlanta, USA)

On examination, there is swelling of the right leg up to the knee. The skin is discolored and is much thickened. There is no pitting edema. There are no varicose veins to see and no ulcers. She has difficulty in moving the leg and sensation is diminished over the whole of the lower leg. The peripheral pulses are not palpable except for the femoral pulse. There are multiple firm glands in the groin. No thrill is palpable and there is no bruit to be heard in the groin. The other leg is swollen to mid-calf level with pitting edema. No other skin changes. Normal sensation and movement. All the pulses are palpable. Examination of the abdomen shows a well-healed Pfannenstiel incision. No masses, no organomegally and no ascites. Rectal and vaginal examination are negative.

On examination of the cardiorespiratory systems, she has a slightly raised JVP and fine crepitations at both bases of the lungs.

Question 3.3: What do you think is the cause of the swollen right leg?

Question 3.4: What do you think is the cause of the swelling of the left leg?

You only need to know the very basics of lymphedema, so just answer the questions.

Question 3.5: What are the two classifications of lymphedema?

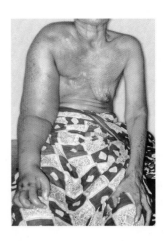

Fig. 9.10 Lymphedema of right arm

Question 3.6: What are the classical clinical features of lymphedema?

Question 3.7: How is the diagnosis made?

Question 3.8: What is the management?

Question 3.9: What is filariasis?

Question 3.10: What treatment is available for filariasis?

Question 3.11: How do you treat lymphedema of the arm due to radical breast surgery and radiotherapy (Fig. 9.10)?

TUTORIAL 10: Renal Problems

Reread the tutorials from *Module 1, Tutorials 2 and 13.*

Question 1: Case scenario

This patient is a 35-year-old man who has an 8-hour history of sudden onset of right loin pain. It is the worst pain he has ever had in his life. He has been rolling around the bed with pain. The pain radiates down the right side of his abdomen into his testicle. He has no problems passing urine and there is no blood in the urine. He is otherwise fit and well.

Question 1.1: This is a classical history of ureteric colic but list the other diseases which may present with flank or loin pain of sudden onset.

Question 1.2: List what you would specifically be looking for when you examine him, under the headings—general and specific.

On Examination:

The patient is lying still at present because he says the pain has gone away.

He does not look ill or fevered.

Temp = N, Pulse 80/min, BP 120/80

Inspection of his abdomen shows normal movement with respiration, no bruising, no abdominal or loin mass.

Palpation shows no tenderness or guarding.

External genitalia normal.

No bony tenderness over spine, full leg movements.

Rectal examination not done.

You make a provisional diagnosis of ureteric colic.

Question 1.3: What might you expect to find on urine dipstick testing?

Question 1.4: What would you be looking for on the KUB?

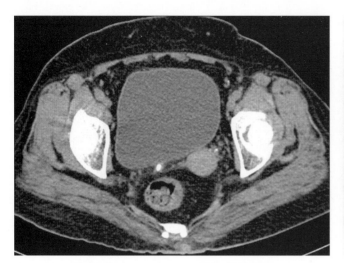

Fig. 10.2 Image from urological CT scan

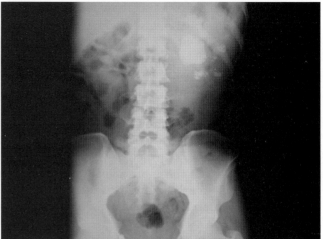

Fig. 10.3 KUB plain abdominal X-ray

Question 1.5: If you saw a radiopaque calcification suggestive of a ureteric stone what line of anatomical landmarks should it lie in?

This is the urological CT of the patient (Fig. 10.2).

The radiologist says the stone is 4 mm and is at the ureterovesical junction.

Question 1.6: What are your treatment options with ureteric calculi (in general, not this specific case).

In this case, it is appropriate for him to be treated conservatively.

Question 1.7: How will you manage this patient with a stone of 4 mm diameter—give generic name, dose and frequency of any medications used.

Question 1.8: List the complications of medical management.

The patient is still having severe intermittent pain after 24 hours and wants something done about it.

Question 1.9: What will the consultant advise?

Question 1.10: What are the advantages and disadvantages of extracorporeal shock wave lithotripsy (ESWL)?

Question 1.11: If the ESWL is not successful, what are the alternatives?

Question 2: Case scenario

Figure 10.3 shows the KUB of a patient with a left-sided calcifications. CT shows the stones to lie in the kidney.

Question 2.1: How does the management of this patient differ from the patient in Question 1

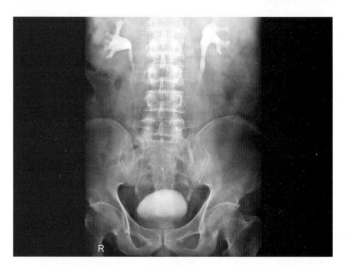

Fig. 10.4

Question 3: Case scenario

Figure 10.4 shows an investigation carried out on a patient with right flank pain.

Question 3.1: What type of X-ray is this (Fig. 10.4)?

Question 3.2: What questions will you ask the patient before carrying out the procedure?

Question 3.3: What would you do if the patient started to complain of feeling unwell as the dye was injected—becoming tachycardic and breathless?

Question 3.4: What abnormalities do you see in the IVP (Fig. 10.5)?

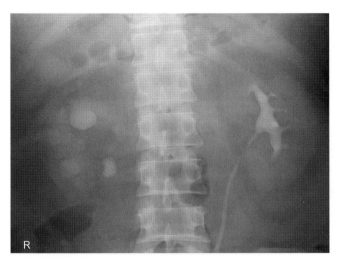

Fig. 10.5 Image from intravenous pyelogram (IVP)

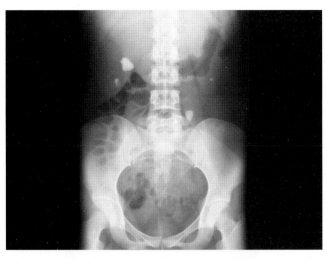

Fig. 10.6 KUB plain abdominal X-ray showing recurrent renal calculi

Question 3.5: Are there any problems associated with performing an IVP in a diabetic taking metformin?

Question 3.6: What would you do if you knew the patient was taking metformin and needed renal investigation?

Question 4: Case scenario

Figure 10.6 is the KUB of a patient with recurrent renal calculi.

Question 4.1: What are the causes of recurrent renal stones?

Question 4.2: What special investigations will the consultant order in this situation?

Question 4.3: What advice should the patient be given to try and prevent more stones from forming?

TUTORIAL 11: Testis/Scrotum/Penis

Remember the cases described are common clinical problems in many medical situations; for example, family medicine, surgery and general medicine. Before you answer this tutorial, revise your answers to *Module 2, Tutorial 9*.

Also revise undescended testis, phimosis and epi and hypospadias from your Pediatric module.

Question 1: Draw a simple diagram of the testis and epididymis.

Question 2: Case scenario

You are the surgical house officer on call and are asked to see a 65-year-old man in A and E who has a painful scrotum.

He first noticed the pain 24 hours ago; he has had it ever since and it is getting worse.

He has taken some paracetamol and this helps. The pain is in the right side of his scrotum and is worse when he walks about.

He gives a history of recent difficulty in passing urine but has had no frequency, nocturia or hematuria.

He is retired but used to be a sailor on cargo ships.

Question 2.1: What other questions will you ask him (from genitourinary point of view)?

He says he has had a fever. He has not noticed any discharge from his penis. He has never had this before. No history of trauma. He is married and has had no casual sexual contact recently. He says when he was a sailor it was different.

On examination, he has a temperature of 38°C. There are no signs in his abdomen.

His right scrotum is swollen and red and very tender. The testis feels enlarged and is tender and heavy.

It is not possible to feel his epididymis because it hurts him. The chord feels thickened in the scrotal neck. It is possible to get above the swelling and there is no evidence of hernia.

No penile discharge or abnormality of glans or shaft of penis are identified.

PR: enlarged prostate—both lobes enlarged uniformly and firm.

Figure 11.2 is a picture of his scrotum.

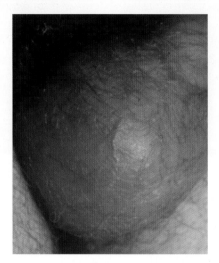

Fig. 11.2

Question 2.2: What is the likely diagnosis?

Question 2.3: How does this condition occur and in whom?

Question 2.4: What investigations will you arrange?

The urine examination comes back showing multiple white and red cells.

Culture awaited.

Question 2.5: Write how you will manage this man—in bullet point form.

Question 2.6: Write down below the presentation and treatment of mumps orchitis.

Question 3: Case scenario

A 78-year-old man presents at A and E with the appearance of his scrotum as shown in Figure 11.3.

Question 3.1: What is your diagnosis?

You are the surgical house officer/intern asked to see him.

Question 3.2: Are you worried about him and, if so, why?

Question 3.3: What is the etiopathology of this condition?

Question 3.4: How will he be managed?

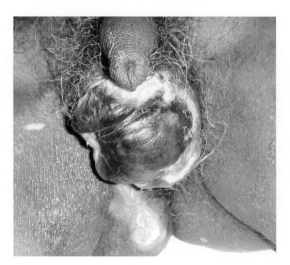

Fig. 11.3

Question 4: Case scenario

You will remember this young man from Module 2. He presented with a dull ache in his right testis of 3 months' duration and thinks the testis has become bigger and harder. He has seen a notice in his GP's surgery for 'well man screening' and wants to be checked.

On examination, his right testis is firm and enlarged compared to the other side. There appears to be a small hydrocele. The rest of the scrotal, abdominal and chest examination is normal.

Question 4.1: What will you say to him (You are the GP)?

Question 4.2: He says 'do you mean I have got cancer?' What will you say?

The GP refers him urgently to the hospital urologist.

Question 4.3: What investigations will the Urologist order?

These are the results:

FBC = N

U and Es = N

alpha fetoproteins, hCG and LDH not elevated

US: 4 × 4 cm mixed density mass in right testis suggestive of a tumor

L testis = N

Chest X-ray = N

CT abdomen and chest = N

Question 4.4: What procedure will the surgeon carry out now (With what precaution)?

The pathology report comes back indicating this is a seminoma.

Question 4.5a: Make a simple table outlining the pathology of testicular tumors.

Question 4.5b: How do you stage testicular tumors (simple table)?

Question 4.5c: How do you manage testicular cancer (simple table)?

Question 4.6: What stage is this young man? Will he need adjuvant therapy? What is his prognosis?

Question 4.7: Describe (in the words you would use to him) what you would say to the patient about his condition once you know the diagnosis and staging.

Now one or two shorter scenarios.

Question 5: Case scenario

A 22-year-old young man presents at the urology clinic. He says he has difficulty in having intercourse because his foreskin is too tight (Fig. 11.4).

Question 5.1: What questions will you ask?

Question 5.2: What is the likely diagnosis?

On examination, Figure 11.4 below shows the situation—the foreskin will not retract over the glands.

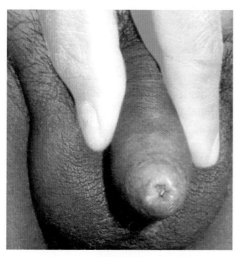

Fig. 11.4

Question 5.3: Why has he got this problem?

Question 5.4: What operation will the urologist advise?

Question 5.5: Describe in simple bullet points how the operation of circumcision is done.
You are the house officer/intern on the surgical ward.

Question 5.6: What complications can occur after a circumcision?

Question 6: Case scenario

A 30-year-old man comes to the GP clinic complaining of aching in his left scrotum. He has had it for 6 months. He has no other symptoms. When he is examined on the couch; the left and right scrotum, testes, epididymes, chords and inguinal regions are all normal except for a little fullness in the left scrotal neck.

Question 6.1: What simple instruction will the GP give the patient?

In the standing position, there is a soft compressible mass above the left testis.

Question 6.2: What is the diagnosis and what 'acronym' is used to describe the physical sign?

Question 6.3: What are the indications for treatment and what would you advise?

Question 7: Case scenario

A distraught young mother brings her 2-year-old son into the clinic because she cannot feel his right testis.

Question 7.1: Write down below a simple list of the causes for an 'apparently' absent right testis in a 2-year-old boy.

On further questioning, the mother thinks she has been able to feel the testis before but is not certain.
The child is otherwise healthy.

Question 7.2: What technique will you use to examine this boy's scrotum and groins?

When you examine him the testis is palpable at the neck of the scrotum and can be gently brought down into the scrotum.

Question 7.3: What is the diagnosis? Write how you will explain it to the mother, including the management. Will you arrange follow-up?

In a second child of similar age, the testis is identified in the inguinal canal but cannot be brought down.

Question 7.4: What is the diagnosis and what will you advise?

In a third child of similar age when you examine him you cannot identify any right testis, the left lies in the scrotum.

Question 7.5: What are the possibilities and what would you do?

TUTORIAL 12: Prostate and Bladder

Please first revise *Module 2, Tutorial 8* (Difficulty in Passing Urine)—much of the content will recur in this module. Try, then, to answer the following scenarios without reference to notes or books. Then look up what you do not know or are not sure about.

Question 1: Case scenario

Mr L is a 66-year-old laborer who comes to the clinic complaining of difficulty in passing urine for 4 months. By this he means that he has a poor stream.

Question 1.1: What is the likely cause of this symptom? NOT DISEASE but mechanism.

Question 1.2: What is the differential diagnosis you have in mind?

Question 1.3: What other questions will you ask him?

Question 1.4: What physical signs may indicate the urinary pathologies you have in mind when you come to examine him? List under GENERAL and SPECIFIC systems, i.e. what will you be specifically looking for?

In addition to his poor stream Mr L says he has been passing urine more frequently both day and night.

D/N ratio (before was = q 4 hours/0) and now: (D/N ratio = q 2 hours/2.)

Note: This is a good way of 'objectively' recording the facts.

D/N ratio is the number of times, he passes urine in Day -time compared to Night-time.

He has no dysuria or hematuria, no dribbling, no stress or urge incontinence. He has no abdominal or back pain, lower limb weakness or constipation. His appetite is good and he has no other problems.

O/E: He looks well, he is not anemic or jaundiced. He is well nourished and hydrated.

He has no physical signs in his hands, neck or abdomen.
Pulse = 70/min BP = 120/80
External genitalia = N
PR = smoothly enlarged prostate right lobe greater than left rubbery and firm
CVS/RS and neurological systems = N

Question 1.5: What is your diagnosis?

Question 1.6: What blood and urine investigations will you arrange?

Here are the results:
FBC = normal
U and Es = N
LFTs = N
PSA = N
Glucose = N
Urine dipstick = 3+ blood
MSU = red cells ++, no growth

Question 1.7: With these results available, what imaging will you arrange? Note he has hematuria, so other causes of this must be excluded.

The KUB and urological CT are negative.

Question 1.8: What procedure will you arrange now?

Question 1.9: How do you perform a cystoscopy? Answer here as though you were explaining it to the patient.

The cystoscopy shows no urethral stricture, an enlarged prostate and a normal bladder.

Question 1.10: What are your treatment options for a man with symptomatic BPH?

It is decided to treat him medically.

Question 1.11: List what medications can be used, their purpose and their common side effects.

Question 2: Case scenario

A 66-year-old gentleman presents with lower urinary tract symptoms. Investigations show him to have an elevated PSA. Transrectal ultrasound (TRUS) and biopsies confirm adenocarcinoma of the prostate.

Question 2.1: What imaging investigations will you order and why?

The investigations show the cancer is confined to his prostate. It is large and histology shows it to be well differentiated (Gleeson score < 6). No bony or other metastases.

Question 2.2: What are the treatment options for this patient?

Question 3: Case scenario

This patient presents with lower back pain and difficulty in passing urine. Investigations confirm a cancer of the prostate with bony metastases.

Question 3.1: How would you treat this patient?

Question 4: Case scenario

A 59-year-old man presents with a one-week history of painless hematuria—bright red and large in amounts. Abdominal examination is negative. Digital rectal examination shows a moderately enlarged benign feeling prostate.

Question 4.1: What examinations will you arrange?

His fexible cystoscopy shows the following finding in the bladder (see Fig. 12.1).

Question 4.2: Describe what you see.

Question 4.3: What environmental and occupational hazards may be relevant?

Question 4.4: How will this patient be managed?

Question 4.5: What is the operation of total cystectomy and ileal conduit? Make a simple drawing to show you know what it means.

Question 4.6: What is a TURP? How would you explain it to the patient?

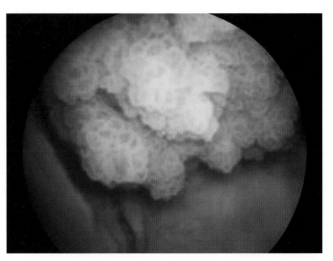

Fig. 12.1 Courtesy of Dr Ban Eng Lau

TUTORIAL 13: Fluid and Electrolyte Balance + Parenteral Nutrition

INSTRUCTIONS

Go back to *Module 2, Tutorial 11* (Fluid and Electrolytes) and work through it again. Reread the 4 articles which were recommended.

It is essential you have the information from that tutorial and understand it because we will be using it now.

REMEMBER in a few months' time you will be responsible for writing up the fluid balance charts so you better know what to do!!

REVISION

Question 1: List the normal values of the serum urea and electrolytes (you will be using them so often you should know them).

Question 2: List the normal values of arterial blood gases (ABG).

Question 3: List the fluid and electrolyte content of:
a. 1 liter Hartmann's solution (Ringer lactate)
b. 1 liter 0.9 N saline
c. 1 liter 5% dextrose

Question 4: In the perioperative period (i.e. preoperative/during the operation/postoperative) what are the guiding PRINCIPLES for management of the patient's fluids?

Give three short headings.

Question 5: List the normal insensible losses of a patient.

Question 6: How will this be affected by the patient's temperature and the ambient humidity and how would you correct for this?

Question 7: What do you understand by 3rd space sequestration?

Question 8: How do you allow for 'third spacing'?

Question 9a: What fluid will you use to replace gastric aspirate and why?

Question 9b: What fluid will you use to replace vomiting of small bowel content, diarrhea or small bowel fistula?

If in doubt with ongoing loss from fistula/ileostomy, use Hartmann's solution. Do not try to remember the table 'composition of some GI secretions'—look it up, if necessary—it is shown below for this reason!!! (Table 13.2)

An assessment of the patient's clinical status and the patient's fluid balance chart will enable you to work out what fluids and electrolytes the patient needs to keep them in balance.

The average fluid and electrolyte MAINTENANCE requirements of the postoperative patient (without any complicating losses) can be remembered by a simple formula which you can use to write up the fluid chart on a daily basis.

Table 13.2 Composition of some gastrointestinal secretions (From British Consensus Guidelines with permission)

Body secretion	Na^+ (mmol/L)	K^+ (mmol/L)	Cl^- (mmol/L)	HCO_3^- (mmol/L)	Volume (L/24 hr)
Saliva	2–85	0–20	16–23	14	0.5–1.5
Gastric juice	20–60	14	140	0–15	2–3
Pancreatic juice	125–138	8	56	85	0.7–2.5
Bile	145	5	105	30	0.6
Jejunal juice	140	5	135	8	—
Ileal juice	140	5	125	30	—
Ileostomy (adapted)	50	4	25	—	0.5
Colostomy	60	15	40	—	0.1–0.2
Diarrhea	30–140	30–70	—	20–80	Variable
Normal stool	20–40	30	—	—	0.1–0.25
Sweat (pilocarpine)	47–60	9	30–40	0–35	0.5 + variable
Visible sweat	58	10	45	—	0.5

Question 10: What is this formula?

In the first 2 or 3 days after surgery, the patient require less fluid, Na^+ and K^+.

Question 11: Why is this?

Question 12: What difference will it make to the fluids and electrolytes you write up?

Now, we are going to look at a patient who develops complications after her surgery.

Question 13: Case scenario

> Miss H is a 25-year-old lady who has Crohn's disease. This involves ileocecal disease and one more proximal segment of the small bowel, as shown in Figure 13.1.
>
> She fails to improve on medical therapy and it is decided that she needs surgery.
>
> The surgeon performs a limited right hemicolectomy to include the ileocecal disease and the distal ileal segment of Crohn's and a stricturoplasty on the more proximal segment.

Question 13.1: Make a simple drawing of what is performed in the operation so that you understand the situation when she comes back to the high dependency unit on the ward where you are the surgical house offices/intern.

When she comes back to the ward, she has an IV line, a CVP line, and a urinary catheter.

She is put on a monitor to measure her pulse, BP, ECG, CVP and O$_2$ sat.

She has a standard input and output chart and a urimeter.

She is conscious and talking.

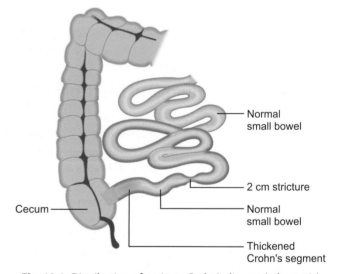

Fig. 13.1 Distribution of patients Crohn's disease (schematic)

Question 13.2: What is a urimeter and what do you use it for?

The anesthetist has not written up her postoperative fluids, so the high dependency nurse asks you to do it.

Question 13.3: What information will you look for:
a. In the anesthetist's operation record?
b. In the operation note?
c. In the recovery room records?
d. In the patient's readings?

The surgeon's operation note describes the operation as uneventful. There is less than 500 mL estimated blood loss.

She received 500 mL haemaccel and 2 liters of Hartmann's solution in theater and the recovery area.

In the recovery area, the pulse and BP were stable, CVP = +5, she had a urine output of 50 mL per hour.

On the ward, her pulse is 90/min, BP 120/80, CVP +5.

She is on ice cubes and sips of oral fluid as tolerated.

Urine output 50 mL per hour.

Suction drain in right abdomen: 200 mL serosanguinous fluid.

Question 13.4: Write her postoperative fluids on the chart below (Chart 13.1) for the next 16 hours (it is 6.00 pm). As was done in Module 2 either scan or download the 'charts' so you can fill them in.

You ask the nurse to send-off a postoperative FBC and U and Es and go-off duty (all staff now on 'shift work' because of the European Working Time Directives).

Next morning, you do the rounds with the Specialist Registrar.

The patient is well and sat up in bed talking. Pulse, BP, CVP all stable through the night. Temperature = 38°C.

Her fluid balance chart is shown on page 234 (Chart 13.3)- LOOK AT IT.

Question 13.5: What are your comments?

Question 13.6: Write up her IV fluids for the day on Chart 13.4 and explain why you have prescribed this fluid regime.

The Specialist Registrar checks the patient's clinical hydration status and reviews the fluid balance chart. He looks at the wound and the drain bag. He asks you to examine the patient's chest and legs.

Question 13.7: Why?

You look at her 6 pm blood results (immediately postoperative from previous evening).

Hb is 10 g/dL

U and Es = Normal.

Question 13.8: Would you do anything about her Hb?

Question 13.9: Can you give a guideline as to when transfusion is necessary in the postoperative patient (in the absence of overt bleeding).

The patient does well until postoperative day 6. She is on free fluids and a light diet and has all her lines and catheter out and her bowels have opened.

On the morning, ward round of day 6 postoperative she says she does not feel well. She has a fever (38°C), feels sick and has some pain in her RIF.

On examination: She has a tachycardia, normal BP. She is tender in the RIF but has normal bowel sounds.

The Specialist Registrar tells you to put her on nil-by-mouth and put her IV line back up. He arranges some plain abdominal films, plus FBC and U and Es.

These show her Hb is 9 g/dL, Urea is 10, Na is 133 and K normal. The plain X-rays show dilated small bowel with air-fluid levels but gas in the colon and rectum.

Question 13.10: What do you think is going on?

The Consultant comes to see her and agrees she may have leaked. He decides to manage her conservatively. He asks you to restart her antibiotics, put her back in the high dependency unit and get an urgent CT of abdomen.

The CT is reported as showing a fluid collection in the RIF with an accompanying ileus.

Question 13.11: What fluid will you write-up for her and why? Put in Chart 13.6.

Bag/Bottle Order	State infusion fluid/blood, volume to be given period of infusion and drip site, if applicable	State drug and dosage to be added	Doctor's initials	Blood bottle/bag no. infusion batch no. to be confirmed by nurse
Chart 13.1 Daily intravenous fluid-order chart				
Name				
First Name				
Reg. No.				
Ward				
1				
2				
3				
4				
5				
6				
7				
8				

Chart 13.3 Fluid chart, University Hospital

Day	Input						Output				
	Intravenous		Oral		Others		Urine	Feces	Vomit	n/g	Others Drain
Time	Type	Volume	Type	Volume	Type	Volume					
7.00 am											
8.00 am											
9.00 am											
10.00 am											
11.00 am											
12.00 pm											
1.00 pm											
2.00 pm											
AM											
2.00 pm											
3.00 pm											
4.00 pm											
5.00 pm	HARTMANN (8 hrs)										
6.00 pm		500	Ice	30 mL							
7.00 pm			Ice	30 mL			40				
8.00 pm			Ice	30 mL			30				200
9.00 pm			Ice	30 mL			30				
PM											
10.00 pm							40				
11.00 pm							60				
12.00 pm							50				
1.00 am							50				
2.00 am	DEXT 5% (8 hrs)						40				
3.00 am		500	Ice	30 mL			40				
4.00 am			Ice	30 mL			30				
5.00 am			Sips	30 mL			30				
6.00 am			Sips	60 mL			30				
7.00 am		(300)	Sips	40 mL			20				100
ON		800		310			490				300

Name:	Miss H	Total Intake:	1110
Consultant/Ward:	Mr. X Gen Surg	Total Output:	790
Unit No.:		Balance:	+320
		Date 04/05/2010 → 05/05/2010	

Chart 13.4 Daily intravenous fluid-order chart

Name				
First Name				
Reg. No.				
Ward				

Bag/Bottle Order	State infusion fluid/blood, volume to be given period of infusion and drip site, if applicable	State drug and dosage to be added	Doctor's initials	Blood bottle/bag no. infusion batch no. to be confirmed by nurse
1				
2				
3				
4				
5				
6				
7				
8				

Chart 13.6 Daily intravenous fluid-order chart

Name				
First Name				
Reg. No.				
Ward				

Bag/Bottle Order	State infusion fluid/blood, volume to be given period of infusion and drip site, if applicable	State drug and dosage to be added	Doctor's initials	Blood bottle/bag no. infusion batch no. to be confirmed by nurse
1				
2				
3				
4				
5				
6				
7				
8				

The consultant comes back to review her twice that day. She remains stable with no change in her abdominal signs.

It is decided to continue with conservative management under close observation.

Two days later, the lower end of her abdominal wound becomes red and painful. She is stable.

The Consultant says to remove two of the sutures. Pus comes out initially and 12 hours, later the wound starts to leak brownish fluid. However, she does not develop any signs of generalized peritonitis.

Question 13.12: What would be the signs of generalized peritonitis?

Following the discharge from the wound the patient says she feels better. The Consultant says she has definitely leaked but that he thinks it is 'contained'.

Question 13.13: What does he mean by this?

Her fluid balance chart the next day is shown in Chart 13.8 Her Hb is 8 g/dL Urea 6, Na 130, K 3.5 Cl 111 Bicarbonate: normal.

Chart 13.8 Fluid chart, University Hospital

Day	Input						Output				
	Intravenous		Oral		Others		Urine	Feces	Vomit	n/g	Others Fistula
Time	Type	Volume	Type	Volume	Type	Volume					
7.00 am	HARTMANN			30			200				100
8.00 am		500		30							
9.00 am				30							
10.00 am	↓			30			200				
11.00 am	DEXT 5%	500		30							100
12.00 pm		500		30							
1.00 pm				30							
2.00 pm				30							
AM			↑								100
2.00 pm	↓										
3.00 pm	HARTMANN						200				
4.00 pm		500									150
5.00 pm											
6.00 pm	↓										
7.00 pm	DEXT 5%	5%									
8.00 pm		500									250
9.00 pm							250				
PM				N							
10.00 pm	↓			B							
11.00 pm	DEXT	5%		M							150
12.00 pm		500									
1.00 am							300				
2.00 am	↓										
3.00 am	DEXT	5%									200
4.00 am		500									
5.00 am							250				
6.00 am											
7.00 am	↓			↓							100
ON	3000			240			1400				1150

Name:	Miss H		Total Intake:	3240
Consultant/Ward:	Mr X Gen Surg		Total Output:	2550
Unit No.:			Balance:	+690
			Date 12-13 May, 2010	

Chart 13.9	Daily intravenous fluid-order chart				
Name					
First Name					
Reg. No.					
Ward					
Bag/Bottle Order	State infusion fluid/blood, volume to be given period of infusion and drip site, if applicable	State drug and dosage to be added	Doctor's initials	Blood bottle/bag no. infusion batch no. to be confirmed by nurse
1				
2				
3				
4				
5				
6				
7				
8				

Question 13.14: Write up her IV fluids on the chart shown here (Chart 13.9) and explain why you have prescribed the fluid and electrolytes you have.

The Consultant says to get another CT and a fistulogram.

These show a collection in the RIF and a fistula from the R hemicolectomy anastomosis to the lower end of the wound.

As she is clinically well the consultant decides to continue conservative management.

He tells the specialist Registrar to get hold of the Nutrition Team and start her on TPN.

Question 13.15: What does he mean by this?

Question 13.16: How will it be given?

Question 13.17: What will be used?

When a patient is receiving TPN, they are usually looked after by the hospital or unit 'TPN' team—who are responsible for insertion of the line, its daily care and writing up the fluid regimes and additives. However, as the house officer you will be in contact with the patient much more—so you must know the potential problems of central lines and TPN administration and be on the 'look out' for them.

Question 13.18: What complications will you be watching for which may indicate a problem with the central line or the nutrition?

Question 13.19: What will you watch for clinically and what data and investigations will the 'TPN' team expect you to have available when they come to review the patient?

Over the course of the next 10 days, the fistula drainage decreases and turns to pus again. Two days later, it is dry. The patient remains well and says she is hungry.

The Consultant says to start her on enteral nutrition.

Question 13.20: What is enteral nutrition? In what circumstances is it used, how is it given and what complication may occur? Your answers should be short and simple—just the 'working' knowledge you need as a house officer.

The Consultant says to let her have free fluids, and if the fistula remains dry for 48 hours more to take the central line down. This is done. At day 21 postoperative she is taking a normal diet plus enteral supplements and goes home to be followed up at OP in two weeks. Mr X, the consultant, says to discharge her on E/C salazopyrine and 'Ensure'.

Question 13.21: As the House Officer/Intern you will be responsible for sending the GP a summary of the patient's in-patient care. This is very important and greatly appreciated by the GP, if carried out properly. Write a discharge summary for this patient.

TUTORIAL 14: Gastrointestinal Bleeding

Question 1: Case scenario

You are the House Officer/Intern on-call for A and E and are asked to see a 68-year-old man who has been vomiting blood.

Question 1.1: When you enter the cubicle in A and E, what will be your first actions?

Question 1.2: How would you ascertain that the patient has had a hematemesis?

Question 1.3: Describe how you will establish the IV line.
Note: When asked about the question of managing patients with an acute abdomen or GI bleeding students will start off with the 'stock' answer: Establish airway and then put in 2 large bore cannulae—this advice relates to the multiple trauma patients. Very few 'acute abdomens' or 'bleeders' have airway compromise (why should they?) and very few require two large bore cannulae!

Let us just say:

The patient has vomited a large amount of blood (at least two basins full of bright red blood on at least three occasions).

He is pale, sweating, and dypsneic, pulse 120, poor volume, BP systolic of 80 and peripheries are cold, i.e. his condition is critical.

Question 1.4: As the HO/SHO what would you do?

Question 1.5: What will the senior surgeon do?

However, in this case, on your initial quick assessment, the patient is alert and conscious, talking, does not look pale and says, he has vomited 2 cupfulls of bright red blood mixed with brownish fluid one hour ago.

He has a pulse of 80 per minute and a BP of 120/80. His peripheries are well perfused.

You put him on oxygen, put up his IV line and send off his bloods.

Question 1.6: What would you do then?

Question 1.7: What will be the importance of the rectal examination?

Question 1.8: What are the likely causes of hematemesis in this man?

Question 1.9: What is the Mallory-Weiss syndrome and how would you diagnose it?

Question 1.10: What is the incidence of the various causes of upper GI hemorrhage?

Question 1.11: What are the important features in a patient's history which will help you to make a diagnosis of the cause of his/her upper GI bleeding?

The patient gives a 4-day history of upper abdominal discomfort and belching for which he took some painkillers he got from his wife. He has had indigestion for years and takes a lot of Siamese Wind powder. No PH of note, no previous hospital admissions. He drinks one whisky a day and has done so for 30 years

Question 1.12: What do you think is the likely differential diagnosis in this case?

Question 1.13: Validate your differential diagnosis, i.e. say which of the patients symptoms fit with your diagnoses?

We have already outlined your initial management of this patient above.

Question 1.14: Repeat your initial management below in bullet point form without looking back.

The patient remains stable with no further hematemesis or melena in the first three hours of admission.

Question 1.15: What investigation will you arrange and with what urgency?

The endoscopy shows a 1.5 cm ulcer in the 1st part of the duodenum with adherent clot. No active bleeding. No varices.

Question 1.16: In this 68-year-old man with a DU and adherent clot, what will be the management?

Question 1.17: What management would the surgeon/gastroenterologist arrange after the endoscopy?

Question 1.18: What would the medical therapy be?

Question 1.19: What regime will you use for HP eradication? List including drugs, dose and length of time, they should be taken.

About 24 hours after the endoscopy, the patient has a further hematemesis of 500 mL bright red blood.

His pulse is up to 100/min, BP 80 systolic and he is shut down peripherally.

Question 1.20: You are the House Officer/Intern on call—what would you do?

The surgeon comes and examines the patient.

Question 1.21: What do you think are the surgeon's options in this 68-year-old man with one significant rebleed after injection and no significant comorbidity.

The Consultant advises that the resuscitation continue and that the patient should go to theater for surgery as soon as possible.

Question 1.22: Has the surgeon any EBM (evidence-based medicine) to back this up this decision?

You will have had an EBM module in your course and should be familiar with the principles and practice of EBM. The subject of management of the the acute bleeder with respect to the timing of surgery is an excellent topic to try out your EBM skills. So choose your appropriate search engines, select out those papers you consider most relevant, reference these, extract the information you want and formulate an opinion (be sure to annotate your search and results).

To obtain the answer to Question 1.22 a simple working summary for the practical evaluation and application of evidence-based medicine is included here—this is intended as a simplified *Aide de Memoire* which you might find useful. In no way, will it replace your formal EBM training.

Use the mnemonic **FIRE** as the guiding protocol:
> **F**ormulate a question
> **I**nformation search
> **R**eview of information
> **E**mploy results

STEP 1
For formulating the question, we will use the well-known mnemonic **PICO:**
> **P**atient 'group' (i.e. what group of patients are we talking about)
> **I**ntervention/diagnostic test/drug therapy
> **C**ontrol or standard
> **O**utcome; what 'effect' are you looking for.

Our example:
Patient group: Elderly male with rebleed after endoscopic injection of bleeding duodenal ulcer
Intervention : Endoscopic reinjection
Control: Surgery
Outcome: Is morbidity/mortality less with reinjection than with surgery

STEP 2: Information Research (**FIRE**)
Choose search engine, e.g.
1. Google
2. PubMed
3. Medical School Library e-journals
4. Cochrane Review Disc
   Decide on the keywords.
   Often just google e-medicine and the keywords.

Example: e-medicine management, rebleed, endoscopic injection, surgery
> Look for overview paper

Identify, if 'problem' is answered in overview.
Identify the best reference for the answer.
Download the 'abstract'.
See if this is appropriate, and if so download the full text (*Note:* Other useful 'quick' engines: TRIP EBM BMJ)

Now we come to the real problem area—the **R** of FIRE—review or appraisal of article. This is usually where the student starts to have difficulty. What is really needed for the average doctor is something, he can remember and apply to appraisal of all types of articles either at home, in the library or at the Journal Club (very important so you look good when asked!!!). It is all very well for the expert to have an appraisal format for each type of paper, e.g. systematic review or RCT or diagnostic test, if you really feel you need to do this download, the necessary guideline from AGREE for guidelines, CONSORT for RCTs/JAMA/How to read a paper?

However, for all situations and for the non-expert, it is suggested you use the sort of format suggested in the brilliant little book by Jorgen Nordemstrom, *Evidence Based Medicine in Sherlock Holmes Footsteps*: Blackwell, Oxford, 2007. This has been adapted to the mnemonic:

AMQERR
A: AIM has the aim of the study been clearly defined and is it justifiable, e.g. likely to be useful (i.e. new information).
M: METHODOLOGY: What sort of 'trial' is it (e.g. RCT, cohort study, etc). Has it been set-up properly with like groups, etc. Internal validity.
Q: QUALITY: Dropouts
> Bias
> Length of follow-up, etc.
E: EFFECT results.
R: RELIABILITY: Data EBM tools statistics clinical applicability.
R: RELEVENCE: What is the value to your patients—external validity?
This gives you the BASIC requisites.
VALIDITY and RELIABILTY and APPLICABILITY.

Question 1.23: However, the decision is made for the patient to have surgery. What will your actions be as the House Officer/Intern?

Question 1.24: This is a 68-year-old man with a long history of dyspepsia and one episode of hematemesis with a rebleed. What operation is he likely to undergo? Make a simple drawing of the operation (so that you will be able to explain it to the patient).

Question 1.25: What is a vagotomy?

Question 1.26: Would the patient we have been considering in this case scenario require a vagotomy, and if not why not?

Question 2: Case scenario

A 50-year-old hotel barman presents to A and E with a 500 mL vomit of fresh red blood. He is a known alcoholic with liver cirrhosis and has previously been shown to have esophageal varices at endoscopy.

Question 2.1: You are the Intern who is asked to see this patient. Write in bullet form his initial management.

The patient remains stable. Endoscopy shows the following at the lower end of the esophagus:

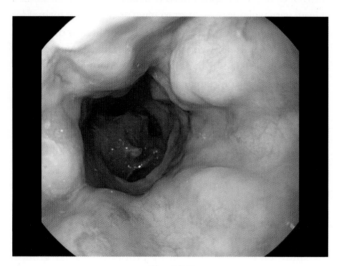

Fig. 14.5

Question 2.2: What do you see (in Fig. 14.5)?

Question 2.3: What are your treatment options?
The gastroenterologist elects to inject the varices.

Question 2.4: How is this done?
The patient returns to the ward and 24 hours later has a further significant hematemesis and melena.

Question 2.5: What would be the next step in management?
The patient continues to bleed and the Consultant tells the Specialist Registrar to put in a Sengstaken tube.

Question 2.6: What is a Sengstaken tube? How is it put in and how is it managed? Are there problems associated with its use?

Question 2.7: Are there any surgical options for this patient, if he continues to bleed?

Question 2.8: Are these operations used much nowadays?

Question 2.9: What is Transjugular Intrahepatic Porto Systemic Shunting (TIPSS)?

Question 2.10: Draw a simple flow chart to summarize the management of bleeding esophageal varices.

TUTORIAL 15: Irreducible Scrotal Swelling

We are starting to approach the end of the tutorials now and examinations are probably looming. This tutorial has been set-up in the form of a Modified Essay Question (MEQ). This type of assessment is often used in the final undergraduate examination. It tests not only factual knowledge, but also thinking and reasoning. You will see that the scenario is very typical of the situation you will soon be in as a House Officer.

As it is in MEQ format the 'answers' sometimes follow on the next section of the scenario. Do not pass onto the next section without answering the previous one (or 'cheat' by looking at the 'answer'), if you do, you are not helping anyone, especially yourself!!

(Note that in the examination situation you would not be given the next section until you have completed the current one).

Answer the questions as best you can without books or notes. Then check your answers.

Question 1: Case scenario

Mr R is 68-years-old and is admitted to the surgical ward as an emergency. He has had a swelling in his right groin for 5 years. He knows it is a hernia because his father had one.

Over the last few years, it has become bigger and more difficult to reduce. For the last 24 hours, the swelling has become painful and will not go away when he lies down. He has had some colicky lower abdominal pain and feels sick.

When asked about his PMH, he says he had a 'mild' heart attack 1 year ago. He smokes 20 cigarettes a day and has done so since he was a teenager. He always has a cough.
He is on atenolol.
You are the admitting House Officer/Intern.

Question 1.1: What will you ask about the 'mild heart attack'?

Question 1.2: What questions will you ask about his cough?

Mr R says he was admitted to the hospital with chest pain 1 year ago. He was in the CCU (coronary care unit) for 2 days. The doctor told him, he had a mild heart attack. He did not have any further investigations and has not had any trouble since. He does not get any chest pain and can walk 500 yards on the flat. He gets breathless when he runs and walking uphill in the winter. He has no palpitations and no ankle swelling.

He has had a cough for 10 years—worse in the winter. He brings up white phlegm—sometimes this becomes green and the doctor gives him antibiotics. He has not had any hemoptysis.

He takes atenolol for his BP—he got it from his GP. He takes it everyday and has his BP checked by the nurse at the surgery every 6 months—the nurse says it is well controlled.

Question 1.3: Write your summary of his history.

Question 1.4: When you come to examine him: what systems will you be focusing on and what signs will you be looking for? List these under 'General Examination' and Specific.

On examination: He is alert and orientated. He is not in any distress. He is not clinically anemic or jaundiced. He is well nourished and well hydrated. He has no cyanosis. He has no obvious intraoral pathology and his dentition is good.

There are no physical signs in his hands or arms.

His pulse is 80 per minute, regular and of good volume.

His BP is 140/85.

His RR is 20 per min, his temperature is 37.4°C.

CVS: JVP not elevated

Radial pulse as above. Both radials present and equal

Apex beat in 5th space

HS 1 and 2 normal with no added sounds

Carotid pulses present and no bruit

Leg pulses all present. No ankle edema.

RS: Equal AE (Right and left)

Scattered wheezes and crackles in both lung fields.

ABDO: Inspection: Abdomen moves normally with respiration

No distention. No visible peristalsis

No masses, no scars, no distended veins, pulsations

Umbilicus inverted and normal

Palpation: No tenderness or guarding. No mass. No organomegaly.

No ascites, hyperactive bowel sounds.

In his right scrotum, he has a large swelling extending up to the scrotal neck and into the groin.

It is not possible to get above it. It is tender. No skin changes and the testicle is palpable separately. The patient says he cannot reduce it and you do not try.

The left scrotum is normal and no hernia can be identified.

PR: Large benign feeling prostate.

Question 1.5: What is your primary diagnosis?

Question 1.6: Justify this diagnosis.

THIS IS A PROBLEM-BASED HISTORY.

Question 1.7: List this patient's problems which you, the HO/Intern have identified.

For each problem, write in bullet form exactly what you, the HO, are going to do about each of these problems.

You do the following:

1. *Irreducible RIH:* Put on NBM and insert IV cannula—as doing so take-off bloods for FBC, U and Es. Start on routine readings and input and output chart.

   Ask him if he needs any painkillers. Write up his fluid orders chart. Write up his medications including his DVT prophylaxis.

   Carry out an ECG and arrange for him to have a chest X-ray and because he is going for chest X-ray get him an erect and supine abdominal film as well.

2. *PH of MI:* Look at his ECG and chest X-ray. Make a note to tell the anesthetist of any changes.

3. *Cough:* Look at chest X-ray. Send off sputum for C and S. Arrange for the physiotherapist to come ASAP. Give a bedside spirometer.

4. Note that his BP is reasonable. Make sure his atenolol has been taken that day and is written up for it postoperatively.

5. Note that he has a large prostate. Will need to check he is passing urine pre and post-operatively (if he does not have a catheter in place post-operative).

6. Ring up Specialist Registrar, tell him you have a patient warded who has an irreducible inguinal hernia who you think will need surgery. Tell him, he has a PH of an MI and has probably got COPD, treated hypertension and a big prostate. Get him to look at the patient ASAP.

7. Speak to the patient.

The Specialist Registrar says to ring the anesthetist and book a theater.

Question 1.8: What will you say to the anesthetist?

Question 1.9: What will you say when you speak to the patient?

Knowing the Registrar and Consultant are coming, you chase up the investigations:

FBC: N.

U and Es: N.

Chest X-ray shows hyperinflated lung fields suggestive of COPD.

Abdominal X-rays: R scrotal mass. No fluid levels.

ECG: RBBB, changes of old MI.

The consultant comes to see the patient and agrees with your diagnosis; he asks you to book the emergency theater. You tell him it is arranged for 2 hours' time. He asks you to consent the patient.

Question 1.10: Write here EXACTLY what you will say to the patient (in words you would use to the patient).

The Registrar Anesthetist comes and thanks you for letting her know about the problem.

She notes the results which you have obtained for her. She rings her Consultant who says to do it under a spinal and he will come along and supervise. He says to make sure there is a bed in the high dependency unit.

The patient goes to the operating theater. The specialist asks you to scrub and gown up.

Question 1.11: In brief bullet form describe how do you do this? I am sure you will have been taught this in the skills laboratory and will have 'scrubbed up' in theater.

Question 1.12: What incision will the surgeon use?

Through a right groin incision, the Specialist confirms the findings of an irreducible right inguinal hernia (RIH) with omentum in the sac and into the scrotum.

Question 1.13: What operative steps will he carry out?

Question 1.14: What is a spinal anesthetic and what is an epidural anesthetic?

Question 1.15: What postoperative problems might a spinal or an epidural anesthetic cause for you, the HO/Intern?

TUTORIAL 16: Inflammatory Bowel Diseases: Ulcerative Colitis and Crohn's Disease

INTRODUCTION

These two case scenarios contain all the information you need to know (and more!) about inflammatory bowel disease (IBD). IBD is the collective term for two main diseases, namely ulcerative colitis (UC) and Crohn's disease. These are two very distinct conditions which do have a number of similarities; for this reason, you may find the two diseases somewhat confusing and difficult to separate in your memory. The table included after the two cases is very helpful in remembering the differences. IBD is not very common in the Far East but is much more common in the Western world. It is an important group of conditions as it often affects young people and may have a significant, but avoidable, impact on quality of life.

Question 1: Case scenario

> You are working as the surgical house officer. You are asked to see a 28-year-old Englishman who has just returned from back-packing around Malaysia and presented to casualty with diarrhea, rectal bleeding and abdominal pain.

Question 1.1: What questions do you want to ask him about his diarrhea?

He tells you that he has had loose stools for 3 months but thought it was just because he had picked up an infection whilst traveling. He reported opening his bowels up to 10 times per day and 2 times at night. Over the last month, there was blood mixed in with the diarrhea. Before his diarrhea started, he had always opened his bowels once per day and passed a firm stool with no bleeding. None of his friends had similar symptoms.

He then tells you his symptoms had got worse over the last few days and now he was opening his bowels up to 20 times per day. He was passing a lot more blood in the stool and now his tummy (abdomen) was painful and swollen. He mentioned he felt generally unwell and either felt very hot or very cold. He has not lost any weight recently but has had a reduced appetite for the last few weeks.

Question 1.2: What other aspects of the history (such as past, social or family history) should you ask him about?

He tells you he was previously fit and well until he went traveling 3 months ago and had no other medical problems. He had been traveling in Malaysia only and had stayed in back-packers hostels and hotels. He had not anything to eat that his friends had not eaten. He gave up smoking 6 months ago and drinks up to 30 units of alcohol per week. He has a girlfriend back in England and did not have any risk factors for blood-borne virus infection. No one in his family had any bowel problems. He does not take any medications regularly and does not have any allergies.

Question 1.3: You ask to examine him, what signs are you looking for?

On examination, you find his pulse is 110 per minute. BP 110/60, temperature 38.4°C, respiratory rate 20 per minute. He looks pale and uncomfortable.

His abdomen is slightly distended. It is generally tender though there is no guarding. Bowel sounds are diminished. On PR, there is a small amount of fresh blood on your finger.

Question 1.4: What is the differential diagnosis and why?

Question 1.5: What investigations do you request?

Question 1.6: You decide this is an acute presentation of ulcerative colitis. You are about to present to your Consultant. How do you assess the severity of the UC?

If you are not sure, look up Truelove and Witt criteria.

Your patient has a hemoglobin of 10.3 g/dL and ESR is 40 mm/hr. Based on these results and his clinical findings you decide this is a severe flare of UC.

He is transferred to the surgical ward. His abdominal X-rays have not shown any toxic dilatation but suggest the whole of the colon is affected. A very careful flexible sigmoidoscopy was performed by the surgical registrar which showed inflamed, ulcerated mucosa in the rectum. Biopsies taken carefully have shown rectal mucosa with an inflammatory infiltrate, goblet cell depletion, glandular distortion and crypt abscesses (the latter two are not usually seen with an infective process). Stool cultures have been negative and microscopic examination of a fresh stool specimen did not show any ova, cysts or parasites.

Question 1.7: He is seen by the Consultant who agrees with the diagnosis. What treatment do you want to start immediately?

After 3 days, he is still opening his bowel 8 times per day and passing blood. His CRP is 75.

Question 1.8: What are the treatment options at this point?

Question 1.9: If the patient had presented with a mild or moderate flare of UC, what treatment would you recommend?

As an undergraduate, you do not need to know a great amount about the surgery for ulcerative colitis. However, you should be able to answer the following questions so that you can inform your patients as a House Officer or a General Practitioner.

Question 1.10a: Draw the operation of 'panproctocolectomy' and write below in a few words what the operation consists of.

Question 1.10b: Draw the operation of 'total proctocolectomy and ileo-anal pouch anastomosis' and write below in a few words what the operation consists of.

Question 1.10c: What are the indications for total procto-colectomy and ileo-anal pouch anastomosis?

Question 2: Case scenario

You are attending a surgical outpatient clinic. You see a 34-year-old Australian lady. The GP referral letter is shown below:

Dear Surgical Team,

Please could you see this 34-year-old lady in your surgical clinic? She presented to me with a history of intermittent diarrhea for 4 years. When her symptoms are bad she may open her bowels up to 6 times per day and once or twice overnight; this may last for a month before settling down. She does not pass any blood. When her diarrhea is bad she also suffers from abdominal pain. This is on the right side and is crampy in nature, she sometimes feels bloated with it. She does not have any nausea or vomiting but recalls one episode when she did vomit.

Recently, she thinks she may have lost weight and her partner thinks she looks pale.

Thanks for you advice on further investigation and management.

Yours

Dr G Peel

Question 2.1: What other questions will you ask her in the history?

On examination, you find her to be very thin. Her abdomen is soft with mild tenderness in the right iliac fossa. On rectal examination you notice fleshy external skin tags and a perianal abscess.

Question 2.2: What extra gastrointestinal signs would you look for on examination?

Question 2.3: What is the differential diagnosis? List at least 4.

Question 2.4a: Which parts of the gastrointestinal tract can Crohn's affect?

Question 2.4b: What 3 sites in the GI tract are most commonly affected in Crohn's disease.

Question 2.5: What investigations would you request (include one endoscopic test and one radiology test)?

The patient goes on to have a colonoscopy which shows a normal colon. Multiple small aphthous ulcers are seen in the terminal ileum. A biopsy is taken.

Question 2.6: What are the features of Crohn's disease on histology? Compare the changes to those seen in ulcerative colitis.

The biopsies from the terminal ileum confirm Crohn's disease. At the next clinic appointment, you are with the Consultant when he tells the patient she has Crohn's disease. The patient is very upset. The Consultant asks you to talk to her to find out what is concerning her and to try to calm her down.

Question 2.7: How will you approach this situation, what questions will you ask her, what will you say to reassure her?

You successfully manage to calm her down and reassure her. She has a lot of questions about what treatments she will need.

Question 2.8: Outline the treatment options for Crohn's disease; bear in mind the different patterns of presentation.

Use contents of Table 16.2 to help you remember the differences between Ulcerative Colitis and Crohn's disease.

To finish with here are a few 'photo quiz' questions on IBD:

Question 2.9: What disease process is shown in Figures 16.3 and 16.4 and why?

Question 2.10: What pathological processes are illustrated on these images (Figs 16.5A to C) of a female perianal area? What is your differential diagnosis?

Question 2.11: This is a view of the sigmoid colon on colonoscopy (Fig. 16.6). Describe what you see and give a differential diagnosis.

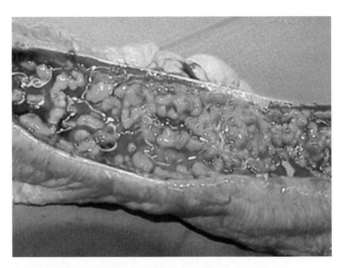

Fig. 16.3 Segment of diseased ileum (opened)

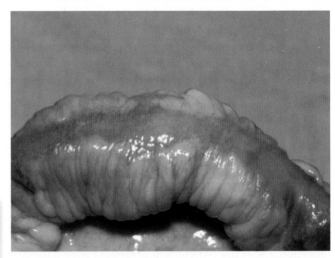

Fig. 16.4 Segment of diseased ileum (unopened) Courtesy ACPGBI

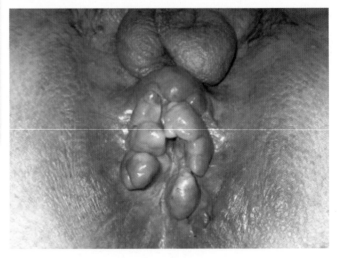

Fig. 16.5A

Table 16.2	Distinguishing features of ulcerative colitis and Crohn's disease	
	Ulcerative colitis	*Crohn's disease*
Involvement of GI tract	Confined to colon and rectum	Mouth to anus
Continuity	Continuous from rectum	Skip lesions
Rectal involvement	Always	Rectal sparing common
Histology	No granulomas	Granulomas are diagnostic
Histological extent	Mucosal involvement only	Full bowel wall thickness
Smoking	Protective	Worsens prognosis

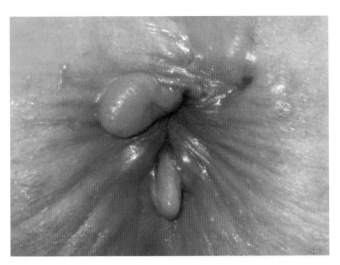

Fig. 16.5B Reproduced from Seminars in Colon and Rectal Surgery, 23, 3, Perianal Crohn's Disease, Krieger B and Steinhagen R, p126-9, 2012, with permission Elsevier

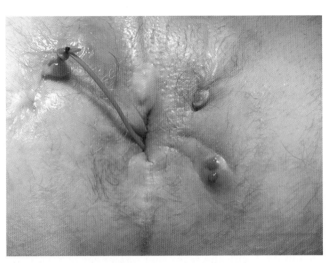

Fig. 16.5C Courtesy of ACPGBI

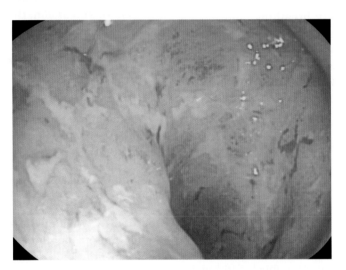

Fig. 16.6 Colonoscopic view of sigmoid colon

TUTORIAL 17: Multiple Trauma

Please note that this final segment of the tutorials is again 'set-up' as an MEQ (Modified Essay Question). The MEQ format is frequently used in the summative examinations of the undergraduate course (end of module or course assessment). Much of the answer of each question is given in the next stage of the continuing case scenario. Please do not look at the next page before you have answered the questions, if you do this you are defeating the purpose of the scenario, both as a learning tool or an 'assessment' of your knowledge.

Question 1: Case scenario

It is the early hours of Monday morning (3 am) and very quiet in the Accident and Emergency Department. You are the Casualty Officer on call. The triage nurse tells you that the ambulance service has phoned to say, they are bringing three people in with multiple injuries from a motor vehicle accident (ETA 5 min).

The driver of the vehicle has a head injury, chest injuries and a broken leg, he is not intubated but has an IV line running and is being monitored. The front seat passenger is unconscious, may have abdominal injuries, but is stable at present; the third person is a young boy who appears to be in satisfactory condition.

One of the A and E Consultants is on call and is at home. The hospital has a trauma team consisting of the Surgical Specialist Registrar, the Orthopedic Specialist Registrar and the duty Anesthetist. The former two are in theater operating and the latter is sorting out a case on the ward.

Question 1.1: What will you do before the ambulance arrives?

The Senior Triage Nurse, who is experienced, says he will deal with the front seat passenger and you will be responsible for the driver. The other senior nurse will assess the young boy.

The driver is a man of about 40 years of age. He is conscious but having difficulty breathing, and has an obvious open fracture of his right leg. He is on oxygen, has a neck support in place and an IV line running in his right cubital fossa. The ambulance crew tell you the victims were all in the same car which had skidded off the road and went head on into a tree. The driver's conscious status has not altered but he has remained hypotensive through the short journey to A and E.

You proceed to assess the driver.

Question 1.2: Describe exactly what you will do.

You ask the nurse to cut-off the patient's clothes. While you are doing this the paramedics tell you what has happened and at the same time you carry out a very quick primary survey of the patient. You shout at the patient and ask him his name—he tells you it is Russell Young and says he is having a lot of trouble breathing. He has no obvious signs of bruising or bleeding on his head. His neck is in a head support. He has multiple abrasions over his left chest, is slightly cyanotic and is breathing at about 30 breaths per minute. His airway is not occluded. His abdomen does not show any external signs of trauma. He has a sterile pad over his right lower limb which you remove and see an open fracture which is not obviously bleeding excessively. You ask him to move his other arms and legs as you quickly look at them, which he does-no obvious signs of injury. With the aid of the paramedic and nurse you roll him on his side and inspect his back from top to bottom, no signs of injury.

The nurses have connected him to a dinamap and tell you his systolic blood pressure is 80/60, pulse 100 per minute and oxygen saturation 87%. He has a wide bore cannula in his right cubital fossa put in by the paramedics which is running well with Hartmann's solution.

Question 1.3: What do you think are his most IMMEDIATE problems. IN ORDER OF PRIORITY, list below what you are going to do about them?

You think he is hypovolemic from blood loss from his left lower limb fracture and possibly his chest injury. You ask the paramedic to put another IV cannula into his left cubital fossa and while he is doing so to collect blood for FBC/U&Es/group and crossmatch 4 pints. You ask him to run in 500 mL of gelofusine as quickly as it will go.

You decide his chest injury is the next most important problem and examine his chest in detail.

His lips are cyanotic and he has a tachypnea. His trachea is central.

His left chest shows multiple abrasions and has markedly reduced expansion.

There is no surgical emphysema, but he is very tender over ribs 7/8/9 laterally.

There are no breath sounds over his left chest and it is resonant to percussion. His right chest is expanding and has breath sounds present on auscultation.

Question 1.4: What is surgical emphysema and how do you know it is present?

Question 1.5: What do you think is wrong with his chest?

You diagnose fractured ribs with either a pneumo- or hemothorax on the left side. You do not think it is a tension pneumothorax.

Question 1.6: What exactly are you going to do next? List your actions.

Question 1.7: What physical signs would make you think it is a tension pneumothorax and how would this alter your management?

Once the chest drain is in place, the patient's condition improves and he is much less distressed. His systolic BP has come up to 120 mm Hg in response to the IV fluids and he has passed 30 mL of urine in the past hour.

The Orthopedic Specialist Registrar and Anesthetist arrive and you tell them your assessment and actions. They compliment you on what you have done and take over.

Question 1.8: With this patient what will they now do?

The secondary survey is carried out by the Surgeon. The detailed head-to-toe examination does not identify any serious head/spine/abdominal/pelvic injury.

He identifies the open fracture of the right leg and asks the orthopedic surgeon to assess this.

Question 1.9: What will the orthopedic surgeon do?

He identifies an open fracture of the right tibia and fibula without any vascular or neurological deficit.

Question 1.10: What will be the orthopedic surgeon's IMMEDIATE management?

The patient is taken to the high dependency unit of the orthopedic ward. The X-rays taken in A and E before he goes to the ward show a transverse fracture of the right tibia and fibula in the lower third of the leg.

Question 1.11: How will the injury be managed now (Remember it is an open fracture)? If you consider intervention to be necessary please indicate the timing of such intervention(s).

Back to the A and E:

The surgical specialist registrar is assessing the women passenger and you go to help.

This is the situation so far: the quick primary survey has shown the following:

Head injury with altered level of consciousness/ bleeding scalp laceration.

Hypotensive/seat belt marks across abdomen.

Question 1.12: What is a '"Primary Survey" and what is its purpose? This is a very important part of your knowledge. Describe in detail all parts of the primary survey and your immediate management. In assessment of the conscious level describe not only the Glasgow coma score but *exactly what you would do.*

In this patient, the primary survey has identified these problems:

Bleeding scalp laceration.

Hypotensive.

Seat belt marks across abdomen with generalized abdominal tenderness.

Level of consciousness: opens eyes when shouted to (GCS 3).

Garbled response when asked name (GCS 4).

Moves both limbs and arms when commanded (GCS 6) total GCS score =13.

Question 1.13: How will you prioritize these potential problems and list exactly what you will do before you carry out your secondary survey?

You are now in control of the situation, so you carry out a speedy 'secondary survey'.

Question 1.14: What does the secondary survey consist of and what is its purpose?

The surgical Specialist Registrar has completed his primary and secondary survey of the woman passenger—and identified the following:
1. **Pulse 100/min, BP 100/60 peripheries cold.**
2. **She has had a head injury and has a current GCS of 13.**
3. **She has a bleeding scalp laceration which is controlled by pressure.**

4. **There is a seat-belt bruise across her abdomen, which is tender in all four quadrants. There are no bowel sounds present. Bladder not palpable.**
5. **No other abnormalities in head and neck/chest/limbs.**

Question 1.15: What do you consider he thinks is the main problem/diagnosis now?

Question 1.16: What will he do now?

The A and E Consultant arrives and carries out a bedside abdominal ultrasound (FAST) in the Resuscitation Area (FAST—Focused Assessment with Sonography in Trauma). This shows a lot of free fluid in the abdomen suggestive of hemoperitoneum. He thinks the spleen is ruptured.

You should be aware that there is a growing trend towards conservative management of splenic injuries with close clinical and radiological monitorings. If operation is necessary, splenic conservation by partial splenectomy should be considered if appropriate.

The patient's blood pressure is now 110/60 but is maintained only with haemaccel in one line and Hartmann's in the other. Urine output only 20 mL in 30 minutes.

The Neurosurgical Registrar says he would like some skull X-rays and a CT, if the patient is going to X-ray—the Surgical Registrar says she is going up to theater—so the Neurosurgical Registrar says he will come and deal with the scalp laceration and delay X-rays. The Anesthetist says they are set to go and will insert a CVP line in theater.

She has contacted the blood bank and they have blood on the way over (packed cells from 3 pints).

The patient goes to theater and a laparotomy is carried out through a long mid-line incision. The hemoperitoneum is confirmed. The patient has a ruptured spleen which is removed.

No other injuries are identified intra-abdominally. The scalp laceration is cleaned and sutured. No fracture is identified below it.

The patient remains stable throughout the procedure. Her PCV is low so the anesthetist gives her 3 packets of packed cells, and 2 packets of FFP. The patient is extubated and managed in the high dependency unit.

Question 1.17: What routine readings will she be on?

Question 1.18: What prophylaxis will you, as the House Officer have to arrange because she has had her spleen out and why?

Question 1.19: Make a list of what you will be looking for when you examine this patient with your Specialist Registrar on the routine rounds.

Now back to the Resuscitation Area in A and E:

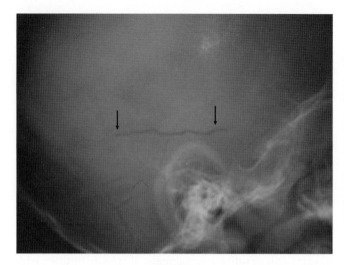

Fig. 17.1

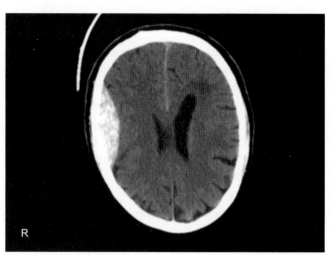

Fig. 17. 2

The Triage Nurse has been dealing with the second passenger in the car. He is a 5-year-old boy and was traveling in the back seat of the car but was not wearing the seat-belt. He is alert and conscious but is crying for his mum. The paramedics do not know if he had a period of loss of consciousness at the scene. He says he banged his head and it hurts. He does not complain of any other injuries. The nurse examines him fully from head-to-toe (secondary survey). He has a bruise and tenderness over his right parietal area, but no other injuries. His Glasgow Coma score is 15, his pupils are equal and react normally to light.

She arranges for him to have skull X-rays.

The skull X-ray is shown in Figure 17.1

Question 1.20: What do you see?

The nurse asks the Neurosurgical Registrar to look at the child (he is in the department looking at the mother).

He arranges for the boy to be admitted to the pediatric surgical ward and says he will keep an eye on him.

The ward nurses are instructed to place him on standard pediatric head injury chart.

Question 1.21: What will be recorded and how often?

His initial GCS is 15 and pupils of normal size and reaction.

Eight hours later, the Neurosurgey Registrar is called to see the child because he has been complaining of a headache and has vomited and the nurses think he is a bit drowsy—GCS down to 12; Pupils equal and reacting to light.

The Neurosurgical Registrar is worried about him and organizes an urgent CT.

One of the films is shown in Figure 17.2

Question 1.22: What does it show?

The child is taken to the operating theater.

Question 1.23: Write in bulleted form:
a. Etiology of extradural hematoma.
b. Mode of presentation (symptoms and signs).
c. Management.

Answers

TUTORIAL 1: Neck Swellings

CASE SCENARIOS

Answer 1.1:
- Dominant nodule of a multinodular goiter (MNG)
- Benign cyst
- Benign tumor—follicular adenoma
- Malignant tumor.

Answer 1.2:
- *Thyroid function tests:* TSH, T3/T4 and thyroid antibodies
- Ultrasound scan of neck
- Fine needle aspiration cytology (FNAC)
- Full blood count (FBC), bioprofile
- Chest X-ray.

Answer 2.1:
- Multinodular goiter (MNG)
- Query malignant change because of recent size increase.

Answer 2.2: Tracheal compression and thoracic inlet obstruction.

Answer 2.3: Mixed cystic and solid nodules.

Answer 2.4: Yes, will confirm the tracheal compression, any retrosternal extension, may help in excluding malignancy.

Answer 2.5:
- CT scan of neck
- Enlarged R lobe of thyroid (septated)
- Tracheal compression.

Answer 2.6: Total or near total thyroidectomy.

Answer 2.7:

FBC—to exclude anemia.

Bioprofile including calcium level—basic renal profile and to make sure serum Ca is normal preoperatively (because parathyroid problems may be a complication of the surgery).

Chest X-ray: Exclude obvious lung disease, exclude metastases.

AP and lateral X-ray of neck-if CT has not been done—may show tracheal compression.

Indirect laryngoscopy (by ENT department)—to confirm both chords moving normally preoperatively (possible RCLN injury at operation is a rare complication).

Group and save: Major operation with chance of bleeding at operation.

Answer 2.8: Tracheal compression.

Answer 2.9: Tell the patient who you are and that you have come to explain about her operation and to get her consent to have it carried out.

Ask her first what she knows about what is wrong with her and what she is going to have done (let us assume she says 'nothing').

Tell her that she has a big enlargement of one half of her thyroid gland and that is pressing on her wind pipe and affecting her breathing. Tell her the tests have shown that it is probably not a cancer but needs to be removed because of the breathing problems.

The operation will be done under general anesthetic so she will not know anything about it. There will be a scar across her neck (show her). The thyroid gland will be almost all removed. Afterwards, the wound will be closed with either an absorbable suture or clips (explain).

Tell her that it is a very safe operation—very occasionally there are problems with bleeding, nerve damage and sometimes with the removal of the little glands within the thyroid called the *parathyroids*. Tell her that there will almost certainly be a little tube in her neck to drain excess blood away and that this will be taken out about 24 hours after the operation.

Tell her that she will be able to drink as soon as she is fully recovered from the operation. Her throat may be sore. She will be able to eat the next day, and if all goes well she will be able to go home in 2 or 3 days.

She will be seen for follow-up at the outpatient clinic in 10 days' time when the results of examining the tissue removed under the microscope will be available.

If she has clips in the skin, the nurse will remove these at the GP surgery in 5 days.

Ask if she has any questions and if she would like you to speak with her relatives.

Answer 2.10: Bleeding into the pretracheal space (just possible a tracheal collapse, if the thyroid has been very big).

Answer 2.11: Ask the nurse to page the on-call anesthetist urgently.

Remove the clips from the neck incision and divide the platysma and midline sutures.

Intubate and take back to theater.

Answer 3.1: He may be hypocalcemic due to parathyroid damage.

Perform Chovestek's test.

Examine for Trousseau's sign, 'La main de Coucheur' - due to carpopedal spasm.

Send off an urgent serum calcium level or better, corrected ionized calcium (venipuncture done without tourniquet).

Give oral calcium supplement, if diagnosis confirmed.

(if you do not know how to perform Chvostek's test or elicit Trousseau's sign, look them up, you will be more likely to remember them).

en.wikipedia.org/wiki/Trousseau_sign_of_latent_tetany or look at the videos: www.nejm.org/doi/full/10.1056/ NEJMicm1110569

Answer 3.2: Calcium Sandoz syrup 5 mL orally daily or bd or calcichew tablets 1–2 daily.

Answer 3.3: 10% calcium gluconate—10 mL by slow IV infusion with ECG control.

Answer 4.1:
- How did you notice the swelling?
- How long have you had it?
- Has it altered recently?
- Is it painful?
- Any other symptoms in mouth/neck?
- Are you otherwise well?

Answer 4.2: A swelling such as this at the angle of the mandible is a parotid swelling until proven otherwise!

In differential diagnosis, decide is it superficial, i.e. skin/ subcutaneous—in which case could be a sebacious cyst or a lipoma.

If deep, could be parotid tumor, lymph node, cold abscess.

Answer 4.3:
1. Examine the oral cavity.
2. Test the 7th nerve function.

Answer 4.4: Bimanual palpation is there any evidence of extension to parapharyngeal space—deep lobe parotid. Also examine the opening parotid duct.

Answer 4.5: 7th nerve function—ask patient to:
- Wrinkle forehead
- Close eyes tight
- Wrinkle nose, show teeth, and blow out cheeks with mouth shut.

Answer 4.6:
- Pleomorphic adenoma (mixed parotid tumor—rubbery and firm).
- Adenolymphoma (Warthin's tumor—soft cystic consistency).
- Carcinoma (hard, fixed, 7th nerve signs).

Answer 4.7:
- US may confirm diagnosis.
- CT to stage, if think malignant.
- FNAC is not always diagnostic of malignancy.

Answer 4.8: Superficial parotidectomy.

Answer 5: Stone at anterior opening of the right submandibular duct.

Answer 5.1: Swelling and pain in the submandibular gland especially after eating. May feel the stone with tongue.

Answer 5.2: Removal of stone under local anesthetic. If the stone lies anywhere more proximally, then should excise the submandibular gland because of the risk of stricture.

Answer 6: This swelling lies in the left anterior triangle of the neck, below the ramus of the mandible.
Differential diagnosis is:
- *Skin:* (sebaceous cyst)
- Subcutaneous (lipoma)
- Lymphatics (lymph node)
- Salivary tissue (submandibular gland)
- Younger group (branchial cyst).

Answer 6.1: Submandibular sialogram with stone far back in the duct.

TUTORIAL 2: Breast Diseases

CASE SCENARIOS

Answer 1.1:
- When did she notice it?
- How did she notice it?
- Has it changed since she noticed it?
- Is it painful?
- Does the lump change with period times?
- Is it painful?
- Has she had a lump before?
- Any nipple discharge?
- Any other changes in breast noticed, e.g. nipple retraction/ skin tethering?

Answer 1.2:
- Age?
- FH of breast cancer?
- Menarche?
- Age of menopause?
- Any children, and if breastfed?
- Late age of 1st childbirth?
- Level of fat consumption?
- Obesity?

- Hormone replacement therapy (HRT)?
- Radiotherapy (DXR)?
- Oral contraceptive pill (OCP)?

Answer 1.3:
- Irregular lump visible
- Overlying skin changes—tethering/Peau d'orange
- Nipple in-drawing
- Hard irregular swelling
- Skin or deep fixity
- Enlarged abnormal axillary glands/supraclavicular glands
- Liver enlargement/ascites on abdominal examination.

Answer 1.4: Figure 2.1

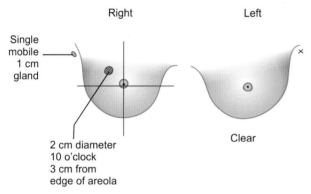

Fig. 2.1 How to record clinical findings of a breast lump?

Answer 1.5:
- Mammograms
- FNAC
  (i.e. complete her triple assessment).

Answer 1.6: The surgeon would tell her that she has a worrying lump in her right breast which may be malignant (a cancer). He would tell her that she needs some investigations performed which will show whether it is definitely a cancer. He should explain these in detail. He should say to her that at this stage, if it is cancer, then there is no reason to believe that it cannot be treated.

Answer 1.7: T2, N1, M0

Answer 1.8: Breast conserving treatment—Lumpectomy (wide local excision) + axillary sampling.

Answer 1.9: Simple mastectomy + axillary clearance is still often used in some countries where patient compliance is poor (i.e. will not come for follow-up) or where the chemoradiotherapy services are poor. This is a "best option" policy as all the breast tissue is removed (so no local DXR needed) and the axilla is cleared (no further surgery or DXR needed).

Answer 1.10: By one of the following which are all 'operative'
1. Axillary clearance (all nodes at levels 1, 2 + 3).
2. Axillary sampling (4 nodes from lower axilla).
3. Sentinal node biopsy (identification and removal of first node or nodes draining the tumor—this is done by injecting a blue dye or radioactive marker adjacent to the tumor).

Note: If facilities available: the patient has an ultrasound scan of their axilla preoperatively (in addition to the tissue diagnosis) and then has either a sentinel node biopsy, sampling or full clearance depending on the result of the axillary US scan.

Answer 1.11: Tell the patient that you have come to explain to her the treatment she needs and to obtain her consent for the operation. It is best to ask her first what she knows about her diagnosis and the results of her investigations. If she does not know she has cancer, then you will have to explain this to her. Tell her that the cancer is small and that she may have one gland in her axilla involved. What she needs is the lump removed with a good margin of normal tissue around it—this is called a *lumpectomy*, this means that the entire breast will not have to be removed. To make sure, there is no cancer left in her armpit (where the lymph nodes lie) the surgeon thinks she should have all the glands removed from that axilla (called axillary clearance). After the operation, she will need to have a course of radiotherapy to the breast but not to the axilla. She may need to take some anti-hormone tablets called *Tamoxifen* and some chemotherapy but this will depend on what the tissue looks like under the microscope after the operation.

Explain that she will need to be put to sleep (general anesthetic). When she wakes up the breast and under her arm will be sore but she will be given painkillers. If all goes well she will be in hospital for 24 hours after the operation and will need to see her doctor to get the stitches removed and to come back to the clinic in 2 weeks for her results and to make arrangements for her radiotherapy.

Explain to her about the complications—hematoma and infection are uncommon (<5%). Sometimes, the nerves in the axilla can be damaged but this is uncommon. Full axillary clearance can cause some loss of shoulder movement to start with and occasionally causes long-standing swelling of the arm.

Ask the patient, if she has any questions and do your best to answer them. If you cannot do so, or if the patient is still worried, or if you do not think you are able to explain the operation and treatment, then arrange for the consultant to see her. Finally, ask if the patient would like you to speak to her relatives, and, if so, how much she wants you to tell them.

Answer 1.12: Yes.

Answer 1.13: To the lumpectomy breast only.

Answer 1.14: Because all the lymph nodes have been removed.

Answer 1.15: She will need an estrogen receptor blocker (Tamoxifen), because she is receptor positive. There is evidence that Tamoxifen will reduce recurrence rate and improve survival.

Answer 1.16:
- The surgeon
- The radiologist
- The pathologist
- The oncologist
- The breast nurse
- Other members of the support team involved in the patient's care.

Answer 1.17: The patient's clinical and investigatory findings can be reviewed and discussed. A joint decision on the correct scheme of management can then be decided with input from all those experts involved in her care. Better care, better outcome, less medical errors.
- If you want to read more go to *www.patient.co.uk/doctor/breast-cancer-pro*
- Excellent review.

Answer 2.1: Yes, the tethering of the skin adjacent to the tumor indicating skin involvement, this will be confirmed on palpation.

Answer 2.2: An operation removing all of the breast tissue including the axillary tail together with an ellipse of skin overlying the tumor.

Answer 2.3: It may be technically difficult to remove this tumor and the involved area of skin.

Answer 2:4: This lady will require preoperative systemic chemotherapy followed by either surgery and radiotherapy or radiotherapy alone.

Answer 2.5: If the whole breast is to be removed, then the patient should be offered the option of breast replacement—either at the time of the mastectomy or at a later date.

Answer 2.6: Either by a silicone implant or a plastic procedure such as a TRAM flap. If you want to know more about breast reconstruction look at *www.cancerresearchuk.org/about-cancer/type/breast-cancer/treatment/surgery/reconstruction/breast-reconstruction-using-body-tissue*

Answer 2.7: Involves the provision of appropriate therapeutic, psychological and physical support for the patient with incurable terminal disease. This may be on a home basis or at a Hospice. It must be carried out by doctors, nurses and support staff who have been specifically trained to deal with the problems associated with this situation.

Answer 3.1: Chemoradiotherapy, if result is satisfactory followed by toilet mastectomy.

Answer 4.1: Second line chemotherapy.

Answer 5.1: Chemoradiotherapy.

Answer 6.1: Lymphedema of her arm.

Answer 6.2: Usually, the result of a combination of surgical lymph node clearance and radiotherapy (which is inappropriate). Sometimes due to tumor recurrence in the axilla.

Answer 6.3: If not due to recurrence: compression bandaging or a compression armlet and the frequent use of physiotherapy involving a compression pump.

TUTORIAL 3: Upper Gastrointestinal Cases

CASE SCENARIOS

Answer 1.1: Barium swallow.

Answer 1.2: A long stenosing lesion of the esophagus (apple core deformity) suggestive of a carcinoma of the esophagus.

Answer 1.3: An elevated, ulcerating lesion arising from the mucosa—the features of a carcinoma.

Answer 1.4: Squamous cell (on the X-ray, it is higher than the gastroesophageal junction, and therefore more likely this than an adenocarcinoma).

Answer 1.5: This is an endoscopic ultrasound.

Its main use is in staging the carcinoma. It will provide the T-staging for the TNM classification and may also identify lymph node enlargement.

Answer 1.6:
1. Radical surgery is advised for disease localized to the esophagus—as shown on CT scan and esophageal US. It might also be advised for resectable disease also involving the lymph nodes—usually preceded by neoadjuvant chemoradiotherapy.
2. The patient must be fit for surgery—in particular their cardiorespiratory status must be adequate.

Answer 1.7a: Total gastrectomy + Roux-en-Y (transhiatal or thoracoabdominal) See Addendum re-Minimally invasive Surgery.

Answer 1.7b: Ivor Lewis 2 stage gastric pull up (laparotomy + R-thoracotomy) or 3 stage McKeown—laparotomy/thoracotomy/neck incision.

Answer 1.7c: Three stage operation with either stomach or colon brought up.

Answer 1.8a: Figure 3.4

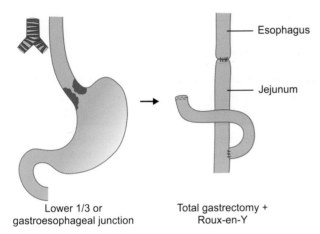

Fig. 3.4 Cancer of esophagus in lower third or at gastro-esophageal junction. Total gastrectomy and Roux-en-Y performed

Answer 1.8b: Figure 3.5

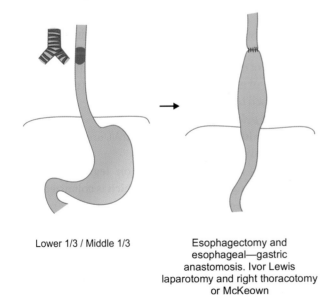

Fig. 3.5 Cancer of esophagus in lower/middle third of esophagus. Esophagogastric resection with esophagogastric anastomosis performed. It is called Ivor Lewis operation using laparotomy and right thoracotomy. The alternative is McKeown operation

Answer 1.8c: Figure 3.6

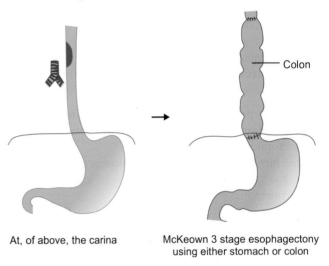

Fig. 3.6 Cancer of esophagus at or above the carina McKeown 3 stage esophagectomy performed using either stomach or colon interposition

Answer 1.9: List the complications as:

1. The general complications of any major surgery, and
2. The complications specific to that operation.

> *Note:* You can use this format to describe the complications of any operation.

If you wish you can divide each group into:
- Perianesthetic
- Early or
- Late.

Hence for esophagectomy:

1. *Complications of any major operation would include:*
   - Respiratory problems, e.g. atelectasis
   - Wound problems, e.g. wound infection
   - Deep venous thrombosis
   - Urinary tract infection (if catheterized).
2. Complications specific to gastroesophagectomy:
   - Pulmonary—atelectasis/consolidation/pleural effusion
   - Anastomotic leak (approximately 10%)
   - Chylothorax
   - Right recurrent laryngeal nerve damage.

Answer 1.10: Recurrent laryngeal nerve involvement by the cancer.

Answer 1.11: He may have developed an esophagotracheal fistula from extension of the tumor or chest infection from inhalation because of tumor obstruction.

Answer 1.12:

- Resection, if possible, is the best means of palliation
- Chemoradiotherapy
- Laser
- Photodynamic therapy
- Stenting (Celestin or Mousseau Barbin tube).

Answer 2.1:

- Tell the patient who you are and that you are going to explain the investigation, the consultant has recommended.
- Tell him that we think he has an ulcer at the outlet of the stomach and that the doctors want to look at this area with a camera to confirm the diagnosis.
- The investigation will be performed in the hospital endoscopy unit as an outpatient and he should not eat for about 4–6 hours before the procedure. He may drink small amounts of water until about 2 hours before the test.
- Explain that the examination is called an endoscopy and that it involves putting a narrow flexible tube with a camera attached through his mouth and down the food tube into his stomach.
- Explain that it will be a little uncomfortable but that his throat will be anesthetized by an anesthetic spray or that he will be given a little sedation through a vein.
- If an ulcer is found the doctor may wish to take a tissue sample and this is easily done through the endoscope.
- The patient may be able to see the investigation as it goes along on the television monitor.
- The investigation takes about 10–20 minutes. Afterwards he will have to stay in the recovery area for about an hour while the anesthetic wears off and to make sure there are no problems.
- He will need someone to take him home and should not drive or operate machinery for 24 hours if he has had sedation.
- Explain that the 'endoscopy' is a very common test nowadays with very few problems or complications, however very rarely the esophagus or stomach can be perforated and sometimes there may be some bleeding.

Answer 2.2: Urease test to see if he is positive for *Helicobacter pylori* (HP).

If the ulcer is gastric in site he will have a biopsy for histology taken as well.

Answer 2.3: The mucosal biopsy specimen is placed on a strip containing a urea solution and an indicator such as phenol red. *Helicobacter pylori* (HP) split the urea because it contains a urease enzyme—the indicator turns from yellow to red, if positive (see CLO test in Figure 3.8).

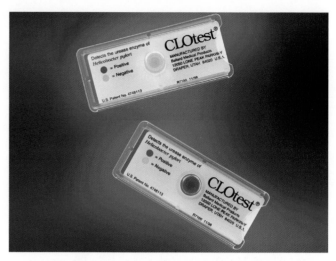

Fig. 3.8 Courtesy of Kimberly-Clark Worldwide, Inc., 2001 Marathon Avenue, Neenah, WI 54956

CLO stands for '*Campylobacter* like organism'

Remember also that the *H. pylori* may be seen by the pathologist on the mucosal biopsy specimen, if sent for histology.

Answer 2.4: Factors associated with duodenal ulcer are:

- Increased acid production (e.g. from stress)
- Smoking
- Genetics
- Increased acid load in duodenum—precipitates bile salts which normally inhibit growth of *H. pylori*.
  - 90% of duodenal ulcers are infected with *H. pylori*.
  - 70% of gastric ulcers are HP positive (rest [30%] are caused by NSAIDs)

How does *H. pylori* cause a duodenal ulcer?

- Query produces toxins (Vac A + Cag A), urease production and adhesive factors.
- Decreases bicarbonate secretion leads to mucosal damage with gastric metaplasia which is colonized by HP with local release of cytokines and damage.

GU: Associated with gastritis

Parietal cell damage occurs with decreased acid production

Ulcer occurs because of local damage by cytokines from HP and abnormal mucin production.

Answer 2.5:

- Combination of a proton pump inhibitor and 2 antibiotics which eradicate *H. pylori*.
- Use omeprazole or lansoprazole + clarithromycin and either amoxicillin or metronidazole.

Answer 2.6:

> Dr PM Boggs MB CH B MRCGP
> Riverside Surgery
> Riverside Rd
> HUMBER

Rx:

> Omeprazole 20 mg O BD 7 days
> Clarithromycin 500 mg O BD 7 days
> Amoxicillin 1 g O BD 7 days

> Signed ....
> Qualifications ....
> Date ....

Note: Take my advice and start now PRINTING all your prescriptions in CAPITAL letters—sooner or later this will save you from a serious medical error.

Answer 2.7:
- Stop smoking.
- 3-4 weeks of proton pump inhibitor then reassess.

Answer 2.8:
1. Put up an IV line—start with Hartmann's solution.
2. When you put in the cannula take off blood for:
   - FBC
   - U and Es
   - Serum amylase   *Note:* As you are doing all this
   - LFTs   explain it to the patient
   - Group and Save
3. Put in a urinary catheter
4. Ask the nurses to start him on:
   - Half hourly pulse and BP, hourly RR, 4 hourly temperature (or dinamap in HDU)
   - Nil by mouth
   - Input and output chart including 1 hourly urine output.
5. Write-up his IV fluids for the next 6 hours.
6. Write-up his drugs: Give him, say, 100 mg pethidine and 25 mg stemetil IM stat.
7. Arrange for an erect chest X-ray and erect and supine abdominal film (if available in emergency situation CT more accurate).
8. Ring-up the MO/Registrar and tell him what you have done and ask him to come and see Mr F urgently.

Answer 2.9:
Normal values:

Hb	M = 13.5–17.5 g/dL
MCV	76–98 fl
PCV	35–55%
WCC	$4–11 \times 10^9$/L
Neutrophils	$2.5–7.58 \times 10^9$/L

Lymphocytes	$1.5–3.5 \times 10^9$/L
Platelets	$150–400 \times 10^9$/L

His Hb is normal—shift towards the high side reflecting dehydration.

WBC count up with neutrophil shift indicating sepsis.

Platelets = Normal (why is this important?—may indicate severe sepsis).

Answer 2.10:
Normal values:

Na	= 135–145 mmol/L
K	= 3.5–4.5 mmol/L
Cl	= 98–108 mmol/L
Urea	= 2.6–6.5 mmol/L
Creatinine	= 0.05–0.12 mmol/L

His urea is raised which would reflect his dehydration.

His K is low—in keeping with vomiting.

Answer 2.11: Within normal limits, so he does not have acute pancreatitis.

Answer 2.12: This shows a large amount of air under the right diaphragm and possibly under the left also.

This indicates a perforated viscus—in this case likely due to a perforated duodenal ulcer.

Answer 2.13: This is an abdominal X-ray taken with the patient lying on his left side. If a perforated viscus is suspected and the patient is too ill to stand or sit erect, a decubitus X-ray may help show free gas.

Answer 2.14: At least dehydrated and probably septic.

Answer 2.15:
1. Run in 500 mL of Hartmann's over 20 minutes, see if his urine output increases and his tachycardia and BP improve and his peripheries warm up.
2. May be necessary to put in a CVP line.

Answer 2.16: Start him on a broad-spectrum antibiotic which will cover gastrointestinal aerobes: 2nd or 3rd generation cephalosporin 1 gram IV 8 hourly, e.g. cefotaxime (2nd gen) or cefotaxime (3rd gen), and metronidazole (flagyl) 500 mg IV 8 hourly to cover anaerobes.

Answer 2.17:
- Checked the blood results and acted on them.
- Made sure he has had his antibiotics and DVT prophylaxis.
- Checked on his routine readings and clinical status regularly.
- Booked the operating room.
- Phoned the emergency anesthetist and asked her to come and see the patient.
- Consented the patient for operation.
- Spoken with the relatives.

Answer 2.18: The patient has peritonitis and therefore requires a laparotomy. What the procedure is performed obviously depends on the findings—in this case, it seems likely that he has a perforated duodenal ulcer.

If confirmed, he will require a washout of his abdomen and oversowing of the ulcer with an omental patch.

If facilities and skill available the operation may be carried out laparoscopically.

Answer 2.19:
- Tell the patient that you are the house officer who will be looking after him.
- Explain that the investigations suggest that he has 'burst' something in his abdomen and that he has 'peritonitis'—you may need to explain this. Say that the surgeons think it is most probable that he has burst his stomach ulcer.
- Explain that if this is confirmed he will need the ulcer repaired.
- The operation will be done as soon as possible under general anesthesia and the anesthetist will be coming to see him.
- Ask him, if he has any questions and answer them. Ask his permission to explain the situation to his relatives, if he agrees, go and see them. Explain that he has almost certainly perforated his ulcer; explain that he is quite ill but that he is responding to treatment and that with the operation he should recover well although he will be in hospital for quite a few days.

Answer 2.20: This is a central venous pressure line (CVP).

Answer 2.21: There are three routes of insertion:
1. Via the subclavian vein
2. Via the internal jugular vein
3. Via a peripheral arm vein.

Whichever, route is used the catheter tip is passed into the SVC and ideally should lie in the SVC just above the right atrium.

In the emergency situation, the line is usually inserted via the subclavian or internal jugular route.

Answer 2.22: A chest X-ray must always be performed to make sure the catheter is correctly positioned—it may be too far in (i.e. in the RA and flapping against the atrial wall) or it may have passed up the jugular vein).

Answer 2.23:
1. To determine right atrial pressure—which reflects venous return to the right side of the heart and therefore is a guide to the patient's state of hydration, i.e. if hypovolemic his CVP will be low, if fluid overloaded it will be high.
2. To provide total parenteral nutrition—usually as a subclavian or peripheral line.
3. For long-term chemotherapy—usually as a tunnelled subclavian line.

Answer 2.24:
- Incorrect positional placement
- Pneumothorax and hemothorax
- Cardiac arrhythmias
- Carotid artery puncture
- Air embolism
- Bleeding
- Catheter sepsis.

Answer 2.25: This is a simple fluid pressure manometer for measuring the CVP in the ward situation.

It has largely been replaced by electronic measuring as part of continuous measurement of the pulse, BP, oxygen saturation and ECG (e.g. dinamap) as used in all high dependency units and ICUs.

However, these manometers are still used in some wards, as the house officer you will be responsible for the functioning of the CVP line and the readings so you must understand the principles, how to set it up and how to read it.

This is a simple fluid manometer in which the pressure in the RA is balanced against a column of water. It consists of a central measuring scale with a long pointer attached for 'zeroing' the line together with a T-shaped tubing with a 3-way tape in the center. One end of the horizontal tubing passes to the IV line and the other end is connected to the CVP line. The vertical limb of the tubing passes up the measuring scale (see Fig. 3.14).

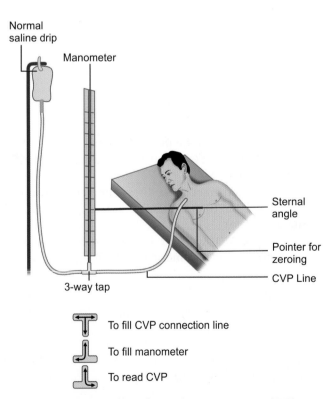

Fig. 3.14 Recording of central venous pressure (CVP)

Instructions for connecting and reading CVP:

1. Fill the line for connection to the patient with N saline by correct alignment of the 3-way tap.

   Note: Must be done before connection to CVP line, i.e. no air.

2. Partially fill the manometer line.

3. Connect up to CVP line.

4. Zero the manometer gauge, note the manubriosternal angle is 5 cm above the right atrium. You can either position the pointer on the patient's manubriosternal angle with him lying flat and align the measuring column to 5 cm or zero at the level of the RA in mid-axillary line (zero to 0). All measurements are best taken with the same zeroing position.

5. Turn the 3-way tap to the position for reading CVP—allow the fluid column to settle and read.

Note: Normal is 5–10 cm water above RA.

Answer 2.26: Run in a 'test' amount of Hartmann's solution— say 200 mL and recheck the CVP, if it has gone up, then the patient is hypovolemic and the appropriate quantity of fluid can be written up.

Answer 2.27: This would indicate the patient is normovolemic and therefore just needs maintenance fluids.

Answer 2.28: He is either overloaded with fluid or has right heart failure; slow down the IV fluids and reassess with senior help.

TUTORIAL 4: Hepatobiliary

CASE SCENARIOS

Answer 1.1: Although the stones have been removed from her common bile duct (CBD), she still has multiple stones in her gallbladder and needs to have this removed. It is better to do this as soon as she is fit and well before she has further problems. She may have either: laparoscopic cholecystectomy or open cholecystectomy.

Answer 1.2: *Laparoscopic cholecystectomy:*

- This is now the procedure of choice provided the patient agrees.

- The operation is carried out under general anesthesia often with prophylactic antibiotic cover. (Evidence-based medicine would suggest in uncomplicated laparoscopic cholecystectomy prophylactic antibiotics are not necessary—why not carry out a search on this—good practice.)

- The patient's abdomen is distended with CO_2 gas using an open 'Hassan' technique to insert the umbilical port (safer than Veress Needle).

- The laparoscope is then inserted via a small incision below the umbilicus and the rest of the procedure is carried out under camera vision displayed on the video monitors.

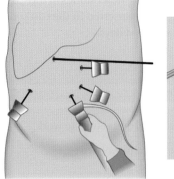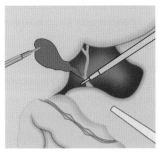

Fig. 4.1 Laparoscopic cholecystectomy

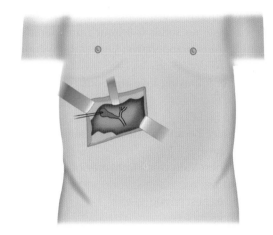

Fig. 4.2 Open cholecystectomy using Kocher's incision

- Three small, approximately 1 cm incisions are made in the epigastrium and right hypochondrium through which the operating instruments are inserted (Fig. 4.1).

   The surgical anatomy is defined and the gallbladder removed—clipping the cystic duct and artery. Hemostasis is obtained with diathermy.

   The CO_2 pneumoperitoneum is then removed and the port sites closed with subcuticular sutures. The patient may go home the same or the next day. It is common for the patient to have some mild abdominal pain postoperatively because of the pneumoperitoneum. They should be warned of this and provided with appropriate analgesia.

Open Cholecystectomy:

- This operation is still used when laparoscopic experience is not available, or when the laparoscopic procedure has to be converted to 'open' because of a difficult gallbladder or operative problems.

- An upper midline incision is used (or sometimes a subcostal one—Kocher's incision as shown in Figure 4.2).

- The cystic duct, artery and CBD are identified and the gallbladder removed after an operative cholangiogram has been performed. If the latter shows stones in the CBD, these are removed and a T-tube inserted in the CBD. The patient may be in hospital for 3–4 days.

Answer 1.3:
1. Short hospital stay
2. Cosmetic (small incisions)
3. Less pain
4. Quicker postoperative recovery and return to work.

Answer 1.4: Ask nurses to put on routine charts:
P BP RR Temperature
Input and Output

Instructions to put on nil-by-mouth before surgery. Note this should be according to hospital/anesthetic department policy. Conventional is 6–8 hours before surgery. Newer guidelines advise: no solids 6–8 hour's preoperative; free fluids until 2 hours preoperative; high carbohydrate drink preoperative.

Arrange the following investigations (and look at the results!!):
• FBC, U and Es, LFTs
• Clotting screen because she has been jaundiced
• Group and save
• Check the chest X-ray result from previous admission.

Make sure she has:
1. Preoperative chest physio
2. TED stockings
3. Informed consent.

Write up her medications:
1. *Subcutaneous heparin:* Clexane 2500 IU subcutaneous daily X1 [(low molecular weight heparin (LMWH)] or unfractionated calcium heparin 5000 IU subcutaneous BD.
2. *If surgeons practice is to use prophylactic antibiotics:* 3rd generation cephalosporin either IM with premed or IV at induction (e.g. cefazolin 1 gram).

Answer 2.1: Charcot's triad.

Answer 2.2: Acute obstructive cholangitis, i.e. infection in the common bile duct—usually (but not always) due to stone disease.

Answer 2.3:
1. Ascending cholangitis—probably due to stones in CBD.
2. Clinically 'shocked'.
3. Diabetes—probably uncontrolled.

Answer 2.4:
1. Insert IV line and start with Hartmann's solution (dehydrated—always worry about low urine output in jaundiced patient—hepatorenal syndrome).

2. While putting up IV line send off urgent blood investigations for:
   • FBC (Hb WCC platelets)
   • U + Es (dehydrated)
   • LFTs (diagnosis)
   • Amylase (diagnosis—could have pancreatitis)
   • Blood glucose (diabetic)
   • Clotting screen (jaundiced)
   • Group + Save (may need intervention).
3. Put in urinary catheter (shocked—need to know hourly urine output).
4. Arrange for her to be admitted to the high dependency ward with dynamap monitoring of P/BP/O_2 sat/ECG—you may need to speak to your chief first. If not in ICU/high dependancy needs 1 hourly pulse, etc. pulse BP RR 4 hourly temperature.
   Nil-by-mouth + input/output chart.
5. Put on high flow O_2 mask (shocked).
6. When all above is arranged ring your registrar or consultant, tell him about the patient and ask him to come and see her.
7. Then send off blood gases and blood cultures (shocked—need to know organisms).
8. Dipstick test urine on ward (looking at glucose, ketones, bile, urobilinogen).
9. Obtain the U and electrolytes and blood glucose results (to decide IV fluids and diabetic management).
   Discuss with senior:
   • Antibiotics and analgesic
   • Need for CVP line
   • Management of diabetes
   • Need for inotropic support.
10. When treatment underway arrange for urgent ultrasound scan (help to confirm diagnosis).
    When clotting screen results are available think about prophylactic heparin and arrange antiembolic stockings (TEDS).

Answer 2.5:
1. Organism associated with stone disease are gram +ve, gram –ve and anaerobes (*E. coli, Streptococcus, Salmonella, Klebsiella, Bacteroides*).
   So, use broad-spectrum antibiotics, e.g. cephalosporin - 3rd generation
   1 gram IV 8 hourly plus metronidazole (flagyl) 500 mg IV 8 hourly to cover the anaerobes).
2. Analgesic—give with antiemetic
   e.g. diamorphine 5–10 mg IM 6 hourly PRN
       prochlorperazine (stemetil) 12.5 mg IM 6 hourly.

Answer 2.6: ERCP with removal of stones or stenting.

Answer 2.7:
- Yes, clotting is likely to be deranged and ERCP is interventional.
- Vitamin K 10 mg IM daily for 2–3 days.

Answer 2.8:
- She is ill and her diabetes will be out of control due to the sepsis.
- She will almost certainly require conversion to insulin.
- In the high dependency setting, this is usually administered as a GKI or VRIII regime (this is discussed later in Module 3, Tutorial 8 answers).

TUTORIAL 5: Jaundice and Weight Loss (Pancreas)

CASE SCENARIOS

Answer 1: Older patients with progressive obstructive type jaundice which initially is painless but by the time the patient presents is usually accompanied by pain (epigastric or back); accompanied by loss of appetite and weight.

Answer 2:
- 70% occur in the periampullary region and the head
- 30% occur in the body and tail
- 70% are adenocarcinoma of duct cell origin.

Answer 3: Periampullary cancer arises from the wall of the duodenum at the Ampulla of Vater. It presents with a short history of progressive obstructive jaundice, usually painless. It is diagnosed at endoscopy because the ulcerated lesion can be seen. Because of the short history, these are the most likely pancreatic neoplasms to be operable.

Answer 4:
- History and clinical examination—Courvoisier's law.
- *LFTs*—picture of obstructive jaundice.
- Tumor markers—CA 19-9.
- US scan may show dilated ducts (extrahepatic +/– intrahepatic).
- CT may show mass in pancreas. With IV contrast can show involvement of portal vein, obliteration of fat plane between tumor and superior mesenteric vessels, involved lymph nodes and metastases in liver.
- MRI with vascular enhancement can give diagnosis and predict operability.
- Endoscopy can show periampullary tumor.
- ERCP—with side viewing scope can cannulate ampulla of Vater and fill up the pancreatic and biliary systems.

Answer 5.1a: Hb is at low side of normal.

Answer 5.1b: Suggests obstructive jaundice; albumin suggests nutritionally deficient/hepatic dysfunction.

Answer 5.1c: Suggests a pancreatic cancer.

Answer 5.2: MR cholangiohepatogram (if available);

    If not, contrast enhanced CT.

Answer 5.3: The radiologist says there is a 3 cm mass in the head of the pancreas.

Answer 5.4: Whipple's operation or pancreaticoduo-denectomy—removing the tumor and part of the duodenum.

Answer 5.5: Figure 5.3

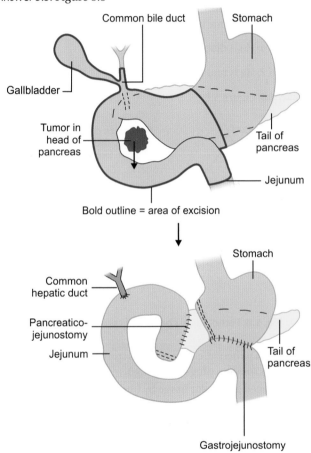

Fig. 5.3 Whipple's procedure

Chronic Abdominal Pain (Pancreas)

Answer 6.1:
- Upper GI malignancy
- Acute pancreatitis
- Chronic pancreatitis.

Answer 6.2:
- FBC
- U and E
- LFTs
- Serum amylase
- CA 19-9
- Urine dipstick
- Chest X-ray
- Plain film of abdomen.

Answer 6.3: Pancreatic calcification.

Answer 6.4: Chronic pancreatitis.

Answer 6.5:
- Glucose tolerance test
- 3-day stool fat collection*
- CT scan of abdomen.

*This is the most accurate test for fat malabsorption and involves a 3-day collection of the feces while on a high fat diet (100 g/day). The feces are dried and the fat extracted.

Answer 6.6: He is diabetic.

Answer 6.7: He is malabsorbing.

Answer 6.8: Figure 5.6

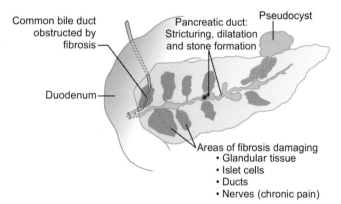

Fig. 5.6 Pathological changes of chronic pancreatitis

- Dilated pancreatic duct with strictures
- Stones/protein plugs in the duct
- Damaged glandular tissue by fibrosis
- Early pseudocyst formation.

(Calcification in parenchyma and a shrunken pancreas also occur but are not shown. The common bile duct may also be dilated because of fibrotic stenosis.)

Answer 6.9:

Medically:
- Pain relief with non-narcotic analgesics, and if necessary splanchnic nerve block
- Pancreatic supplements
- Low fat diet
- Vitamin D supplements
- Control his diabetes
- Try and stop him drinking alcohol.

Answer 6.10: Sometimes: depending on the pancreatic ductal changes:
- Changes involving tail—consider distal pancreatectomy
- Stricture to the L of Ll with distal dilatation can be considered for either endoscopic stenting and ESWT

(shock wave therapy) for the stones or splitting of the duct with a Roux-en-Y small bowel anastomosis along the duct (Puestow procedure)
- Changes involving the head require either coring out of the head (Frey's procedure) or a Whipple's operation +/- pancreatic transplant.

Severe Abdominal Pain (Pancreas)

Answer 7.1: She has peritonitis.

Answer 7.2:
1. Insert an IV line with Hartmann's solution running.
2. As you put up the line take-off bloods for urgent investigation: FBC, U+E, LFTs amylase, CRP, blood cultures and group and save.
3. Give her appropriate analgesia, e.g. 50 mg of pethidine and 12.5 mg of stemetil slowly IV (if you are not happy to do, this contact the MO straightaway).
4. Put her on NBM and arrange routine readings and input/output chart (she is clearly ill and would be better in HDU with continuous monitoring) if not available then one hourly P, BP, urine output.
5. Write out and send down request for urgent chest X-ray and erect and supine abdominal X-rays.
   (If available and agreed by senior staff member, then a CT with scout films will be better.)
6. Put in a urinary catheter.
7. Contact MO/Specialist/Registrar and ask him to come and see her as soon as possible.
8. Explain everything you are doing to the patient as you go along and when above done find time to speak to relatives.

Answer 7.3: Acute pancreatitis.

Answer 7.4: Mild or severe.

Answer 7.5: By ordering the blood tests necessary to complete either Imrie's (Glasgow) or Ransome's Criteria.

Answer 7.6:

Albumin (you already have WCC, urea, age)
Serum calcium
Blood glucose
LDH
AST/ALT
PaO_2

You should also order an urgent US scan (looking for stones in gallbladder). If there is any doubt about the diagnosis an urgent CT scan of abdomen may help. A CT should be performed at day 5 looking for the complications of pancreatitis (necrosis or pseudocyst).

Answer 7.7: The patient should immediately be put in a high dependency unit or in the ICU—with full monitoring.

Answer 7.8:
- *Respiratory:* ARDS
- Renal failure
- Sepsis: Local and systemic
- Pancreatic necrosis.

Answer 7.9:
1. *Supportive:*
   - If possible continue eating and drinking orally— if patient cannot tolerate consider early enteral nutrition
   - Analgesia for pain—avoid morphine
   - IV fluids for replacement
   - Continuous bladder drainage for urine output
   - Correct electrolytes, if abnormal
   - Antibiotics, if indicated, e.g. +ve blood cultures, fever, or if necrotizing pancreatitis present
   - Respiratory support/ventilation
   - Inotropic support, if required.
2. Specific if indicated
   - ERCP and sphincterotomy (stones in CBD)
   - Necrosectomy/abscess drainage
   - Hemofiltration/hemodialysis
   - Nutrition—TPN or enteral feeding.

TUTORIAL 6: Lower Gastrointestinal Tract

Answer 1.1a: Dark red or purple.

Answer 1.1b: Bright red.

Answer 1.1c: Incomplete emptying is the feeling or desire to have your bowels open again soon after completing a bowel action.

This may be a symptom of a large rectal polyp or a carcinoma of the rectum but is also a common symptom in the elderly who have a problem with pelvic floor descent (weakness of the pelvic floor muscles causes the floor to descend on defecation and 'obstruct' evacuation).

Tenesmus is often used by clinicians to describe 'incomplete evacuation or emptying' but strictly speaking tenesmus is a painful desire to evacuate on a persistent basis.

It is the anorectal equivalent of strangury (painful desire to pass urine) and indicates either an inflammatory or malignant involvement of the anorectal sphincters.

Answer 1.2a: Need a chest X-ray and a CT scan of the abdomen.

Answer 1.2b: Need a chest X-ray and an MRI of the abdomen and pelvis.

Answer 1.3: Dukes Classification (this can only be decided after the resected specimen pathology is available) and/or TNM.

(Note the MRI of the pelvis will give you the T-staging of a rectal tumor preoperatively and will serve as a guide as to whether or not neoadjuvant therapy is required).

Answer 1.4a: This is additional therapy used before the definitive surgery is carried out (in colorectal cancer— Radiotherapy (DXR) +/– chemotherapy or chemotherapy alone).

Answer 1.4b: This is additional therapy which is carried out after the definitive surgical procedure.

Answer 1.4c:
1. T3/T4 tumor of rectum requires long course chemo-radiotherapy.
2. Short course preoperative DXR with enhancing chemotherapy is under trial for all rectal cancers.
3. Preoperative chemotherapy for potentially resectable liver metastases.
4. Postoperative chemotherapy for Dukes C cases of colorectal cancer.
5. Postoperative DXR for resected rectal lesions with +ve CMR (circumferential margins on histology).

CASE SCENARIOS

Answer 2.1:
1. CEA level.
2. Group and X match or group and save (according to hospital policy).

Answer 2.2:
- A laxative to empty the large bowel the day before the operation (usually Picolax, which is sodium picosulfate 10 mg with magnesium citrate).
- A single disposable enema to empty the rectum (usually few hours after the Picolax).
- Oral enteral nutrition for 24 hours preoperative (low residue).
- Nil-by-mouth 6–8 hours preoperative.
- However, please note the place of routine mechanical bowel preparation in colorectal resections is currently under review (see Module 2 Tutorial 11 on Fluid and Electrolyte balance).

Answer 2.3:
1. *DVT prophylaxis:* Subcutaneous heparin and TED stockings.
2. Preoperative physiotherapy for chest.
3. Antibiotic prophylaxis—usually Flagyl and a cephalosporin given IV on anesthetic induction.
(Some protocols continue to use x 2 postoperative doses at 8 and 16 hours.)

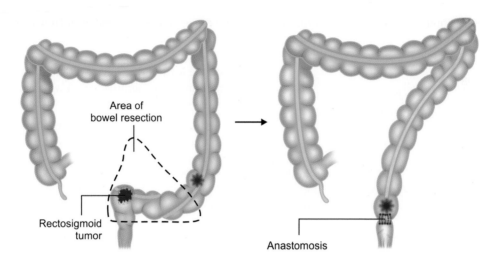

Area of
bowel resection

Rectosigmoid
tumor

Anastomosis

Fig. 6.1 Anterior resection of rectum

Answer 2.4:

Heparin: Enoxaparin (clexane) 20 mg (2000 units) or
dalteparin (fragmin)
2,500 units daily subcutaneously
(Low Molecular Weight Heparin)
or unfractionated heparin 5000 IU bd
subcutaneously.

Antibiotics: • Cefuroxime 2nd generation cephalosporin
1 g and metronidazole (flagyl) 500 mg IV with
induction.
• Cefuroxime 1 g and metronidazole (flagyl)
500 mg IV at 8 and 16 hours postoperative.
• There is some evidence that a single
preoperative dose is adequate.

Answer 2.5: Figure 6.1.

Answer 2.6: Figure 6.2.

Answer 2.7: Figure 6.3.

The ileostomy should be in the right iliac fossa—at level
of McBurney's point, but within the lateral margin of the
rectus sheath. Once you have decided the provisional site put
an ileostomy bag on the position you have chosen and ask
the patient to sit forward and stand up. It must not abut onto
any skin fold, scar or the ASIS. Then mark the appropriate site
with an indelible marker.

Answer 2.8: Until proven otherwise he has leaked from his
anastomosis.

Answer 2.9:

1. Put him onto a dinamap with P/BP/ECG/O_2 sat
continuous monitoring.
2. Put him on an oxygen mask at full flow.

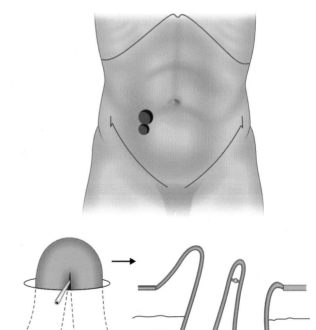

Fig. 6.2 Formation of loop ileostomy over bridge

3. Restart his IV line and run in Hartmann's solution, or
if indicated a volume expander. Send off urgent bloods
(FBC, bioprofile and regroup and save).
4. Give him IV antibiotics—cephalosporin and flagyl.
5. Catheterize him and put on hourly urimeter.
6. Give appropriate analgesia, if necessary.
7. Ask the Registrar/MO to insert CVP line and monitor his
fluid replacement.
8. Inotropes may be necessary.

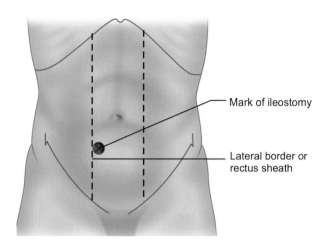

Fig. 6.3 Preoperative marking of loop/end ileostomy stoma

Answer 2.10: He arranges for a laparotomy as soon as possible—this must not be delayed, i.e. immediate resuscitation only.

Answer 2.11: Provided it is confirmed that he has leaked, the safest operation will be to take down the anastomosis, bring the upper end out as end colostomy and close the lower end (+ washout + drains).

Answer 3.1: Fissure in Ano.

Answer 3.2: Local cream or suppositories containing local anesthetic +/– steroid. Give bulking agent or mild irritant laxative.

Answer 3.3: Either to continue medical management with 0.3% GTN paste or to advise a lateral subcutaneous sphincterotomy.

Answer 4.1: Hemorrhoids.

Answer 4.2:

Table 6.1 Classification of hemorrhoids and management according to classification

Classification	Treatment
1st degree (symptoms but seen only on protoscopy)	High fiber diet +/– injection with 5% phenol in almond oil
2nd degree (come down on straining and retract)	Small = Inject + fiber Large = Band + fiber
3rd degree (come down on straining—able to reduce)	No external component = band Significant external component = hemorrhoidectomy
4th degree come down and stay down	Hemorrhoidectomy

Answer 4.3: The technique of stapled hemorrhoidectomy.

Answer 4.4: Ligation and excision hemorrhoidectomy (Milligan-Morgan operation).

Answer 4.5:
1. Postoperative pain and its control
2. Hemorrhage
3. Urinary retention
4. Difficulty in achieving bowel evacuation.

Answer 5.1:
• Perianal/ischiorectal abscess
• Treatment—incision and drainage of abscess
• Identification of an accompanying fistula, if it exists—either at primary operation or at EUA in one week (depends on operator experience).

Answer 6.1:
• Fistula in ano.
• The opening of the fistula is shown in the 10' o'clock position about 1 cm from the anal verge. Shown in Figure 6.10 with probe inserted at operation.

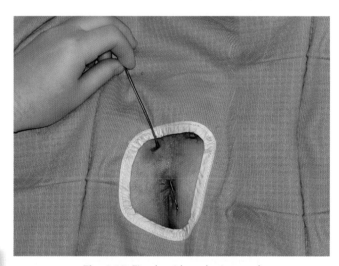

Fig. 6.10 Fistula with probe inserted
Copyright RCSI with permission

Answer 6.2: If the fistula crosses only a small amount of the sphincter muscles, it is usually treated by simple laying open. If more complex, it may require the use of a seton (rubber sling) or an advancement flap. You are not required to know details of these as a medical student.

Answer 7: Figures 6.11, 6.12 and 6.13.

Ileostomy • Usually on R side of abdomen
• Everted 'spout'
• Bag content will usually be liquid and have appearance of small bowel content

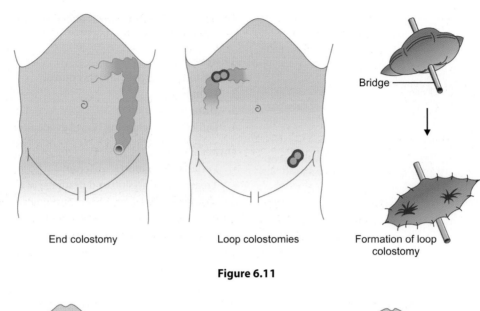

End colostomy   Loop colostomies   Formation of loop colostomy

Figure 6.11

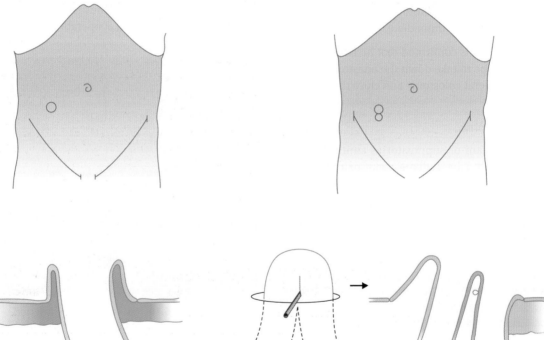

Fig. 6.12 End and loop ileostomy

- End ileostomy will have one opening, loop ileostomy will have two. Distal opening may be difficult to see.

Colostomy
- Usually end colostomy in LIF or loop in RUQ
- 'Flat' to skin
- Solid fecal content
- End = one lumen, loop = two.

Ileal conduit
- Usually in RIF everted spout, single lumen and bag contains urine.

Answer 8:
1. Retraction
2. Prolapse
3. Necrosis
4. Stenosis
5. Skin problems
6. Appliance adhesion
7. Parastomal hernia
8. High output (ileostomy).

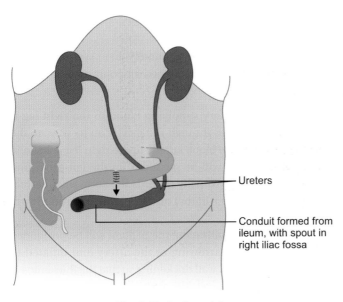

Ureters

Conduit formed from ileum, with spout in right iliac fossa

Fig. 6.13 Ileal conduit

Answer 9a: Loop colostomy.

Note: In the operating theater, the loop colostomy is formed over a 'bridge' before the 2 barrels are opened and sutured back to the skin. The bridge is usually removed at day 7 postoperatively.

Answer 9b: Prolapsed thrombosed 4th hemorrhoids.
Treatment: Acute hemorrhoidectomy.

Answer 9c: Ileostomy—note the 'spout' to protect the skin from effluent.

Answer 9d: Full thickness rectal prolapse.
Treatment:
- Transabdominal rectopexy (+/– sigmoid excision)
- Per anal approach—Delorme's procedure or a sigmoidectomy.

Answer 9e: Pilonidal sinus.
Treatment: Lay open and marsupialization or excision or plastic procedure.

Answer 9f: Pruritus ani.
Treatment: Depends on cause. Majority are caused by mucus leakage from hemorrhoids of which the patient may be unaware—in this case treat the hemorrhoids. Use protective skin cream, e.g. calamine lotion and improve anal hygiene.

Other specific causes and treat cause, e.g. diabetes, fungal, anorectal pathology.

Answer 9g: Anal carcinoma.
Treatment: Usually now chemo/radiotherapy, sometimes APER.

Answer 9h: Condylomata accuminata.
Treatment: Local creams (podophyllin) or cryosurgery or surgical excision.

Answer 9i: Parastomal hernia.
Treatment: Requires further surgery if causing the patient problems—often involving resting the stoma.

Answer 9j: Stomal prolapse.
Treatment: If not causing problems, leave alone otherwise needs refashioning.

TUTORIAL 7: Vascular Disease (Arterial)

CASE SCENARIOS

Answer 1.1:
- Intermittent claudication
- Spinal stenosis
- Venous claudication
- Prolapsed intervertebral disc
  (Acute limb ischemia usually occurs spontaneously with pistol shot pain usually felt in the foot.)
- Arthritis.

Answer 1.2:

General:	Face/hands.
Vital Signs:	Pulse, blood pressure, respiration rate, temperature
Specific:	Peripheral arterial system
	Abdomen for AAA
	Cardiovascular and respiratory systems
	Neurological examination back and legs

Answer 1.3: Intermittent claudication from peripheral arterial disease.

Answer 1.4:
- The cramping calf pain is due to inadequate blood supply to the calf muscle because of underlying atherosclerosis (hardening of the arteries).
- The pain is felt in the calf during fast walking because the calf is the predominant muscle working during walking.
- Pain occurs due to oxygen deficiency and the abnormal accumulation of products of anaerobic metabolism.

Answer 1.5: Risk factors including hyperlipidemia and hypertension. Arterial injury leading to endothelial cell (the lining cells of the arteries) injury. Lipids from the arterial blood get into and accumulate in the arterial wall. In response to this insult, inflammatory cells and smooth cell muscle cells accumulate in the arterial wall. The lipid accumulation and accumulation of inflammatory and smooth muscles in the arterial wall result in the thickening of the arterial wall.

Answer 1.6: PVD is progressive and is a manifestation of generalized artherosclerosis. It becomes worse with time. Symptoms may become less severe because collateral blood vessels (alternative pathways of blood supply) develop and this temporarily may improve the blood supply. When the disease progresses, collateral vessels are affected, symptoms then become worse again.

Answer 1.7:

Blood Tests: FBC, ESR, CRP, renal function, creatinine, lipid profile, glucose.

Noninvasive Tests: Ankle brachial index, duplex scanning of the arteries, CT angiograph or MR angiography.

Answer 1.8: Age, hyperlipidemia, smoking, hypertension, diabetes, sedentary lifestyle, obesity and the metabolic syndrome.

Answer 1.9: Table 7.1

Table 7.1 Risk factors of peripheral vascular disease and their management	
Risk factor	*Management*
Hypertension	(medication)
Cholesterol raised	(medication—statins)
Obesity	(lose weight)
Diabetes	(control)
Sedentary	(exercise)
Smoking	(stop it)
	Antiplatelet therapy
	Structured exercise program

Note: This is an easy way of remembering the management!

Just to remind you about serum cholesterol levels:

Total cholesterol (TC) should be 5 mmol/L or <

Low density cholesterol (LDL): 3 mmol/L or < (bad cholesterol)

High density cholesterol (HDL): above 1 mmol/L (good cholesterol)

TC/HDL ratio 4.5 or <

Answer 1.10:
- Foot pain at rest
- Foot ulcers especially toe ulcers
- Toe gangrene
- Non-healing and/or infected cuts and scratches in the foot or toes
- Any ulcer or lesion on lower limb especially, if non-healing.

Answer 1.11: Rest pain and perhaps impending tissue loss.

Answer 1.12:

Critical limb ischemia: If feasible a procedure to improve blood supply to his foot should be considered.

Answer 1.13:
- Percutaneous angioplasty
- Arterial bypass using autogenous vein or synthetic graft
- Combination of percutaneous angioplasty and arterial bypass.

Answer 1.14: The artery supplying blood to the right leg is narrowed as it passes through the pelvis "on its way" to the right leg. To improve blood supply to the right leg, a balloon attached on a wire will be passed from the left groin into the left leg artery proximally towards the aorta (main artery supplying both lower limbs) and then into the right lower limb artery.

Under X-ray visualization, the balloon will be positioned at the area of the narrowing of the artery and inflated to compress the arterial wall thickening so that the thickening is compressed and reduced. The arterial lumen is widened and blood supply improves. Sometimes a stent or tube is inserted to keep the 'widening' patent.

Answer 1.15: Figure 7.4

Answer 1.16: A bypass which brings blood from a donor artery which does not normally supply blood to the recipient artery and which is not anatomically in continuity with the donor artery.

Examples are right femoral to left femoral artery bypass, and left axillary bifemoral bypass.

Answer 1.17:
1. Severe rest pain in non-revascularizable chronic critical ischemia.
2. Non-reversible acute ischemia.
3. Extensive acute ischemia with high-risk of reperfusion syndrome.
4. Spreading lower limb ischemia, with necrosis and infection.
5. Substantial tissue loss in non-revascularizable ischemia.

Answer 1.18: Figure 7.5

Answer 2.1: No.

Answer 2.2:
- Confluent mottling
- Fixed capillary staining
- Tender muscle
- Blistering
- Swelling
- Paralysis.

Answer 3.1: Acute embolism of left leg.

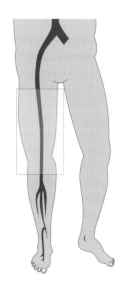

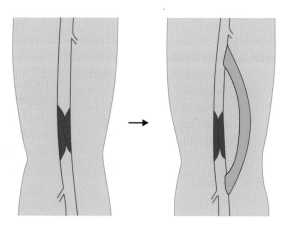

Fig. 7.4 Femoropopliteal bypass operation

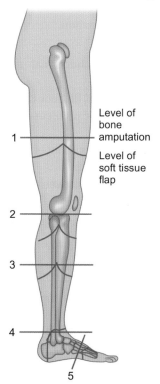

Fig. 7.5 Common sites for amputation in lower limb
1 = Above knee; 2 = Through knee (Gritti Stokes); 3 = Below knee (trans tibial); 4 = Through ankle (Symes); 5 = Forefoot and 6 = Ray amputation (see Fig. 7.6)

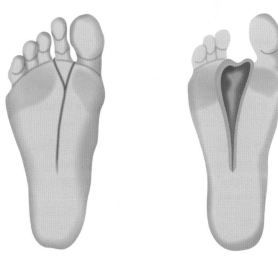

Fig. 7.6 Ray amputation of toe

Answer 3.2:
- He has atrial fibrillation.
- Contralateral limb has no features of chronic ischemia.

Answer 3.3:
- Explain the diagnosis to the patient, its seriousness, potential treatment options and possible outcomes.

- Place him on oxygen, IV fluids for hydration.
- Administer analgesia.
  Send off baseline FBC, ESR, urea, creatinine, electrolytes, LFTs, coagulation profile, lipid profile, glucose, X-match blood 3 units, ECG, CXR.
- Ensure adequate urine output.
- Commence anticoagulation (Heparin IV 5000 IU stat and infusion of 1000 IU/hour and continue with dose adjusted according to serial APTT).
- Prepare for operating theater with informed consent.

Answer 3.4: Explore left femoral artery and perform embolectomy with preoperative and completion on table angiography.

TUTORIAL 8: The Acute Abdomen

CASE SCENARIOS

Answer 1.1: Acute cholecystitis.

Answer 1.2:

Plain X-rays of abdomen	• 10–20% gallstones are radiopaque. May indicate other diagnoses
US scan Abdomen	• may show gallstones thickened gallbladder dilated ducts.

Answer 1.3:
1. Limited fluids orally as tolerated.
2. IV fluids
3. Antibiotics—2nd or 3rd generation cephalosporin, e.g. cefazolin 750 mg to 1 g IV BD.
4. Analgesia—Pethidine 50–100 mg IM q 4–6 hours prn prochlorperazine (stemetil) 25 mg IM q 4–6 hours prn.
5. Routine charts.

Then   Either   Acute cholecystectomy on next list (i.e. within 48 hours)

     or   Continue conservative treatment, allow to settle and then readmit for planned cholecystectomy.

Answer 1.4: Should be done before the operation, if liver function tests are abnormal, amylase is raised or if US scan suggests dilated ducts. All of these may suggest presence of bile duct stones.

Answer 2.1:
Lower abdominal peritonitis:
• Acute diverticulitis
• Large bowel obstruction
• Gynecological cause.

Answer 2.2:
• Yes, raised WCC suggests infection.
• Amylase rules out pancreatitis.
• Abdominal X-rays rule out large bowel obstruction and possibly a perforated viscus.

Answer 2.3: Contrast enhanced CT scan of abdomen.

Answer 2.4: Acute diverticulitis with probable pericolic sepsis.

Answer 2.5:
1. NBM
2. IV fluids
3. *Antibiotics:*
   Cefuroxime 1 g IV BD
   Metronidazole (flagyl) 500 mg IV TDS

4. *Analgesia + antiemetic:*
   Pethidine 50–100 mg IM q 4–6 hours
   Prochlorperazine (stemetil) 25 mg IM q 4–6 hours
   or tramadol 50 mg IM q 4–6 hours
5. Routine readings—1 hourly pulse, 4 hourly BP, RR, temperature
6. Input and output chart
7. Clinical review.

Answer 2.6:
1. Increasing abdominal pain and abdominal signs suggestive of perforation and generalized peritonitis.
2. Increasing 'local sepsis' in the form of an abscess— swinging fever, tender LIF mass, WCC markedly elevated.

Answer 3.1:
• Intestinal obstruction
• Acute exacerbation of ulcer
• Pancreatitis.

Answer 3.2: Intestinal obstruction.

Answer 3.3:
1. Establish diagnosis of abdominal problem (abdominal films ?CT).
2. Diabetes (blood glucose, diabetic medical team).
3. Previous neck anesthetic problem + scoliosis + thick neck (tell anesthetist).
4. Penicillin allergy (write on front of notes, tell surgeon and anesthetist).
5. PH of ulcer—may need cover for this (proton pump inhibitor).

Answer 3.4:
1. Put up an IV line (green 18 gauge) at wrist, cubital fossa or if big vein—back of hand.
2. While putting IV up, take off blood for FBC, bioprofile, serum amylase, group and save, blood glucose.
3. Put him on 'nil-by-mouth'.
4. Put him on routine readings: 'dinamap' if possible, otherwise 1 hourly P/BP/RR/4 hourly temperature.
5. Start input/output chart.
6. Provide appropriate analgesia.
7. Arrange for him to have erect chest X-ray/erect and supine abdominal films or CT (see addendum).
8. Ring up MO and Specialist—tell them your provisional diagnosis and the patient's condition and ask them to see the patient as soon as possible.
9. Sit down with the patient (plus the relatives, if present) and tell him what you think is wrong with him and what you are doing about it. Ask if he has any questions.
10. Obtain his blood results as soon as possible and ACT on them.

Answer 3.5: 1 liter Hartmann's solution over 6 hours to start with.

Answer 3.6:
- FBC bioprofile, serum amylase, glucose, group and save
- Dipstick urine
- Erect chest X-ray, erect and supine abdominal films/CT.

Answer 3.7: Looks normal. NO gas under diaphragm.

Answer 3.8:

Erect X-ray: Multiple air-fluid levels
Distended small bowel.

Supine X-ray: Dilated small bowel loops—centrally placed in step ladder formation with visible valvulae conniventes.

Diagnosis: Intestinal obstrction—small bowel.

Answer 3.9: Intestinal adhesions from his previous surgery.

Answer 3.10:
1. Adhesions.
2. Obstructed hernia—inguinal, femoral, incisional, para-umbilical, internal.
3. Peritoneal carcinomatosis.
4. Others—Much less common:
   - Polyp intussusception
   - Primary small bowel tumors
   - Food bolus
   - Gallstone ileus.

Answer 3.11:
- Conservative
- Operative.

Answer 3.12:
1. Equipment needed:
   - Suitable sized NG tube (adult) = 10–12 Fr
   - Lubricating jelly
   - Lignocaine throat spray, if required
   - Catheter tipped syringe for aspiration
   - Stethoscope.
2. Explain the procedure to the patient, why he needs it and how you will do it. Explain that when he feels the tube at the back of his throat he must swallow at your instruction.
3. Ask him if he has any preference for which nostril the tube goes down.
4. Measure on the tube the approximate distance from nose to earlobe, to upper abdomen and note the appropriate graduation mark.
5. Lubricate the tube.
6. Insert via the chosen nostril with smooth, non-forceful pressure.

7. Ask patient to swallow when he feels it at the back of the throat—he will gag a little.
8. Insert down to chosen mark.
9. Test for correct positioning by aspiration of stomach contents or instil a few mL of air and listen with stethoscope.
11. Fix to nose with sticky tape or fixation device.

Answer 3.13:
1. Check regularly that the patient is not developing local abdominal signs/increasing pain/tachycardia/hypotension—all signs of gut ischemia.
2. Check hydration status, urinary output and volume and type of NG aspirate.
3. Identify electrolytic status and correct as necessary.

Answer 3.14: As a house officer, you must be familiar with the perioperative management of the diabetic patient. You must understand the basic principles and problems of the diabetic patient undergoing surgery and have access to a standard protocol for the management of the diabetic patient or be familiar with the regime in use on your ward. If you are uncertain, always seek advice from your seniors, the anesthetist or the medical diabetologist.

A basic protocol is added as an appendix to this tutorial. This protocol involves the use of a GKI (Glucose/Potassium/Insulin) infusion given through a single infusion line (single bag infusion)—because of which it is safer than the alternative 'Sliding scale' IV insulin infusion (or VRIII), which involves the use of two infusion pumps delivered through a single cannula. The use of sliding scale subcutaneous insulin based on 2 hourly fingerprick blood glucose or 4 hourly urine testing for glucose is no longer recommended in the UK—because of likely poor glycemic control and the unreliability of urine testing. However, in some parts of the world, this may still be the chosen regime.

In this case, the patient is a special situation—a surgical emergency: his management will depend on the state of his diabetic control, his blood glucose and when he last had his subcutaneous insulin.

a. If the patient is significantly hyperglycemic and/or ketoacidotic correct with saline +/– 10% glucose plus 6 units of solute insulin/hour. When corrected use normal GKI regime (in these cases, you must seek advice from diabetologist).

b. If the patient is well controlled, treatment depends on when last dose of subcutaneous insulin was given:
   1. If recent give 10% glucose infusion + monitor blood sugar.
   2. If no recent subcutaneous insulin, use GKI or sliding scale IV insulin.

Answer 3.15: Multiple small bowel fluid levels with a *cut-off point* in the RIF—suggestive of adhesions.

Answer 3.16:

1. A 57-year-old man with intestinal obstruction probably due to adhesions has not settled on conservative management and the Consultant has decided he needs surgery.
2. His problems are:
   - Insulin dependent diabetic now on GKI regime with latest blood sugar of .... (give latest result)
   - Dehydrated when he came in—now corrected—latest U and E are normal
   - Had one anesthetic previously—and had problems—he has short, thick neck and scoliosis.

3. Allergic to penicillin.
4. Patient and relatives know the likely diagnosis and that he needs further surgery.
5. Consultant has requested that you see the patient before surgery because of the diabetes and previous problem with anesthetic.

APPENDIX: GUIDELINES FOR DIABETIC MANAGEMENT IN SURGICAL PATIENT

The alogrithm given in Flow chart 8.1 and the special situation advice are an attempt to give the student/house officer some 'simplified' practical guidelines. The management of diabetes in the surgical patient is, however, a complex and very important subject. A short summary of the currently

Flow chart 8.1 Mangement of diabetes in surgical patient

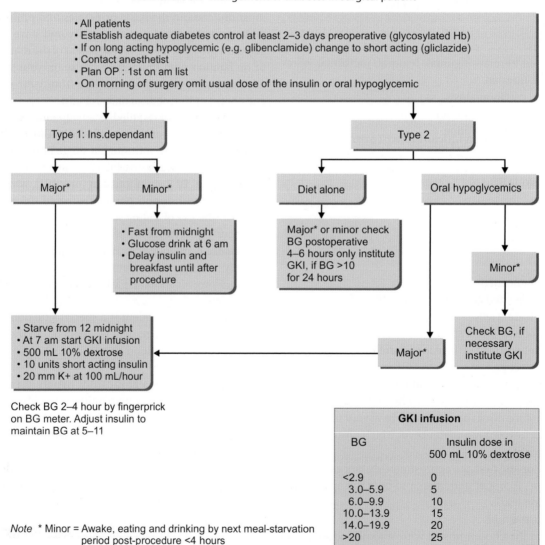

Check BG 2–4 hour by fingerprick on BG meter. Adjust insulin to maintain BG at 5–11

Note * Minor = Awake, eating and drinking by next meal-starvation period post-procedure <4 hours
* Major = If not able to resume full diet > 6 hours post-procedure

GKI infusion	
BG	Insulin dose in 500 mL 10% dextrose
<2.9	0
3.0–5.9	5
6.0–9.9	10
10.0–13.9	15
14.0–19.9	20
>20	25

recommended sliding scale IV Insulin (VR111) is also given together with some essential selected readings for the student/House Officer which will help their understanding.

Special Situations

1. Most diabetologist would say there is *no* longer any place for use of subcutaneous insulin sliding scale and urine testing. However, if the nurses are not familiar with the GKI regime it may be safer to use a sliding scale subcut insulin regime based on 4–6 hourly glucometer/fingerprick testing. This will not however give as good glycemic control as the GKI regime which should always be employed if the patient is in high dependency or ICU where the nurses are familiar with its use.
2. If need to restrict fluids (e.g. renal failure cardiac, elderly) half rate of infusion, i.e. 50 mL/hour.
   Use 20% dextrose and double insulin.
3. Insulin requirements likely to be higher in:
   - Hepatic disease
   - Obesity
   - Sepsis
   - Patients on steroids
   - Bypass surgery.
4. *Surgical emergencies:*
   a. If patient is significantly hyperglycemic and/or ketoacidotic correct with infusion of saline +/– glucose plus 6 units Insulin/hour. When corrected use normal GKI regime.
   b. If well-controlled, treatment depends on when last dose of subcutaneous insulin was given:
   If recent give 10% glucose infusion + monitor BS.
   If not, use GKI regime.
5. If not morning list (i.e. afternoon list):
   Patients on Insulin Therapy:
   Minor Surgery: Fast from 8 am
   - Half morning dose of insulin before early breakfast
   - Glucose drink at 10.30 am
   - Delay lunch time insulin and lunch after procedure.
   Major Surgery: Fast from 8 am
   - Half insulin dose before eating breakfast
   - Start GKI infusion at 11 am.
   Patients on Oral Hypoglycemic (Major Surgery):
   Fast at 8 am
   - Usual tablets with early breakfast
   - Start GKI at 11 am.
6. If having major surgery and on metformin, this metformin regime should be changed (because of renal problem/acute acidosis).

When a glucose infusion is needed, most UK guidelines now recommend the use of an intravenous 'sliding scale' infusion rather than the GKI infusion because better glycemic control is achieved. The insulin solution is delivered via a syringe pump connected to a Y-adaptor. Down the other limb of the Y-adaptor, the dextrose containing crystalloid solution is delivered via a second syringe pump at the same time.

Example of 'Sliding Scale' Insulin (IV) with Infusion of 10% Dextrose (IV)

(After Ward and Gatling Surgery, Oxford, 2005:23:7:243 with acknowledgment)

- Add 50 units of soluble insulin (Actrapid, Humulin S) to 49.5 mL of 0.9% saline in a 50 mL syringe. Infuse via syringe pump. Gives a concentration of insulin 1 unit per mL
- At the same time via a second syringe pump infuse 10% dextrose with potassium chloride (20 mmol) at a rate of 83 mL per hour
- Measure the capillary glucose by fingerprick every hour
- Adjust the rate of insulin infusion according to the capillary glucose according to the Table 8.2.

Table 8.2 Sliding scale insulin infusion (IV) with 10% dextrose (IV)—suggested rates

Blood glucose (mmol/L)	Insulin (units/hour) scale 1	First alteration of sliding scale 2
<3.0	0	0
3.1–3.9	0.5	0.5
4.0–6.9	1	2
7.0–9.9	2	3
10.0–14.9	3	4
15.0–19.9	4	5
> 20	5	6

- Aim for glucose level of 6–10 mmol/L
- If glucose <3 mmo/L stop insulin pump and treat 'hypo' with glucose drink/Hypostop gel or 20 mL 50% dextrose IV Recheck glucose in 15 min and restart infusion if glucose >4 mmol/L.

Note: Scale 1 is the rate the infusion is started at depending on the intial capillary glucose.

Scale 2 is the rate adjusted to, when necessary, on subsequent capillary glucose results.

In the recently published guidelines for **'The perioperative management of the adult patient with diabetes ASGBI May 2012**, the sliding scale is renamed VRIII (Variable Rate Intravenous Insulin Infusion). The following regime is recommended:

Make up 50 mL syringe with 50 units of soluble human insulin and 49.5 mL of 0.9% sodium chloride solution. This gives a concentration of 1 unit/mL.

The initial crystalloid solution to be co administered with the VRIII is 0.45% saline with 5% glucose and 0.15% KCl. This should be administered via an infusion pump.

Subsequently, the crystalloid solution to be used alongside the VRIII should be:

- Either 0.45% saline with 5% glucose and 0.15% KCl
- Or 0.45% saline with 5% glucose and 0.3% KCl
- Depending on the serum electrolytes. The rate of this infusion should be set to deliver the hourly fluid replacement of the individual patient.

The rate of the VRIII is dependent on the patients capillary blood glucose (BG) according to the Table 8.3:

Table 8.3 VRIII: Suggested scales for insulin infusion rate

Bedside BG (mmol/L)	Initial rate of insulin infusion (units/hour)
<4	0.5 (0.0, if long-acting background insulin has been discontinued)
4.1–7.0	1
7.1–9.0	2
9.1–11.0	3
11.1–14.0	4
14.1–17.0	5
17.1–20	6
>20	involve diabetic team/physician

The following important guidelines for setting up the VRIII are given:

1. IV fluid must be administered using a volumetric pump
2. Delivery of the substrate (crystalloid) solution and the VRIII must be via a single cannula with one way and anti-siphon valves.
3. Set fluid replacement rate to deliver the hourly fluid requirement of the patient, this should not be altered without senior advice.
4. Insulin must be delivered via a syringe pump alongside the substrate infusion.
5. Insulin should not be administered without substrate except on senior advice and in an ITU/HDU setting.
6. Insulin must be infused at a variable rate to keep the BG at 6–10 mmol/L acceptable range 4–12 mmol/L.
7. Continue the substrate solution and the VRIII, until the patient is eating and drinking and back on their usual glucose lowering medication.
8. Additional fluid therapy may be required—use Hartmann's.
9. If the insulin or substrate solutions are disconnected recommence with new solutions and giving sets to reduce infection risk.

Authors' Comments

- The sliding scale and VRIII regimes require intensive, knowledgable nursing and should not be used except in the HDU/ITU setting when degree of expertise is available.

- If the appropriate BG measurements and adjustments are not carried out or the infusion sets malfunction or run out, then serious consequences will ensue. The GKI regime is safer but not without dangers if used on a busy ward without trained staff familiar with the insulin regimes.
- The student/intern/house officer is advised to read the following so that they not only acquire the background knowledge required but appreciate the complexities and dangers for their patients.
  1. Perioperative management of endocrine disease (including diabetes). Ward A Gatling, W Surgery. Oxford/Elservier: 2005;23(7): 243-5.
  2. The perioperative management of the adult patient with diabetes, ASGBI publication, May 2012 accessible at *www.asgbi.org.uk/en/publications/ issues_in_professional_practice.cfm*

(Thank you to John MacFie, President of ASGBI for permission to use extracts and for helpful advice)

  3. American Family Physcian: *www.aafp.org/ afp/2003/0101/p93html*, gives a comprehensive and understandable review.

TUTORIAL 9: Patient 1: Varicose Veins
Patient 2: Leg Ulcer
Patient 3: A Swollen Leg

CASE SCENARIOS

Answer 1.1: Figures 9.2A to C.

Answer 1.2:

- I am Professor S's house officer. He has asked me to come and explain to you about your operation and to get you to sign the consent.
- May I ask you what you know about the operation? (Says nothing!)
- The operation is to remove your varicose veins. It will be performed under general anesthesia so you will not feel anything. When you wake up, you will be in the recovery area and will be drowsy, your legs will be firmly bandaged—this is routine. You will have a fluid line in your arm.
- The surgeon will make a short cut in your groins and tie off the problem veins. The cut will be sown up by a self-dissolving suture. He will then remove the large vein from your thigh and a lot of the smaller veins on your calf through small incisions. The same will be done on both sides. The legs will then be firmly bandaged to stop bleeding.
- You will be able to eat and drink as soon as you come round properly. You will be encouraged to get up and

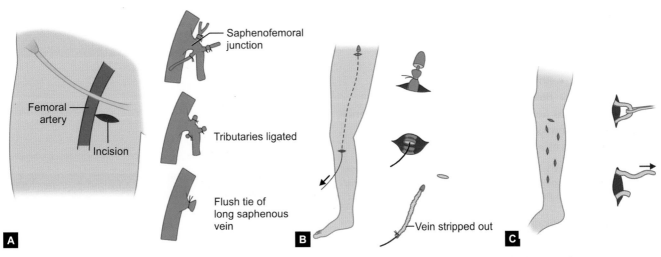

Figs 9.2A to C (A) High ligation of saphenofemoral junction; (B) Stripping groin to knee; (C) Multiple avulsions

walk around as soon as possible. Because you are having both sides done we will probably keep you in hospital overnight. You will be given mild painkillers, if necessary.

- In the morning, the heavy bandages will be removed and an elastic stocking fitted over the dressings.
  There will be some bruising—do not worry about this.
- You should walk about as much as possible—at least a mile per day.
- You will come back to the clinic for review in about a week. You will probably not have any stitches to remove but will have some adhesive strips to soak off.
- The operation is a very safe one with very few complications—rarely is there postoperative bleeding which may mean going back to the theater. Occasionally, there is numbness of the skin to start with. Sometimes, the wounds may become a little red and moist especially the groin incisions.
- Please read this booklet, which explains the operation.
- Have you any questions?
- Would you sign the consent form—it says bilateral high ligation, stripping and multiple ligations which is the description of the operation, I have explained to you.

Answer 1.3: Figure 9.3.

1. Patient stands or sits with leg dependent.
2. Mark perforators with pen.
3. Elastic compression bandage applied at foot.
4. *Start distally:* Inject 1–2 mL STD (sodium tetradecyl sulfate) into vein.
5. Put on foam compression pad and bandage over it.
6. Work upwards applying bandage as you go.
7. Put elastocrepe bandage over bandage when complete - full length.

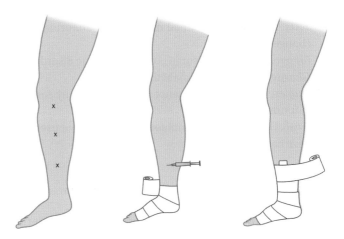

Fig. 9.3 Sclerotherapy of varicose veins

8. Give instruction and complication leaflet.
   Walk at least 1 mile per day.
   Reapply bandages, if work loose.
   Remove at 3 weeks and wear elastic compression stockings for further 3 weeks day and night.

Answer 1.4: Yes, she should not have sclerosant therapy until she has been off the pill for 6 weeks. The same applies for VV operations. This is to reduce the risk of DVT.

Answer 1.5: Yes, treatment is carried out using direct injection of a very small quantity of STD sclerosant using a fine needle.
   Laser has been used.
   The results are variable.

Answer 2.1:

1. Check her peripheral pulses and her ABPI (Ankle Brachial Pressure Index **).

2. Perform
   - FBC
   - U and Es
   - TFTs
   - Lipid profile
   - Rh factor
   - Blood glucose.
3. Duplex scan to her leg for evidence of incompetence above and below knee.
4. Pus swab from ulcer.

If you do not know what this is –look it up *www.nursingtimes. net/home/clinical-zones/assessment-skills/doppler-assessment-calculation- an -ankle-brachial-pressure*

Answer 2.2: No significant evidence of PVD.

Answer 2.3:
1. *FBC:* Checking for anemia.
2. *U and E:* Renal status.
3. *Lipid profile:* Relevant to atherosclerosis.
4. *TFTs:* Myxedema, pretibial myxedema—abnormal skin changes.
5. *Rh serology:* Ulcers occur in connective tissue disorders.
6. *Glucose:* Make sure not diabetic.
7. *Duplex:* If have incompetence may be helped by surgery in future.
8. *Swab:* Usually only use antibiotics if cellulitis but useful to have baseline.

Answer 2.4:
1. Attempt to minimize the venous hypertension:
   a. Bed rest and foot elevation (not practical)
   b. Compression bandaging (technique and material important).
2. Local treatment of ulcer
   - Daily dressing with either iodine-based or water-based solution
   - Non-stick dressing.
3. *Consideration of surgery:*
   - Better when ulcer has healed, if possible
   - High tie and stripping + avulsions, if incompetence and perforators
   - Occasionally—subfascial ligation (Cockett's operation).

Answer 3.1:
1. Post-phlebitic limb (pain in leg and in bed for 6 weeks suggestive of DVT many years ago).
2. Congestive cardiac failure (trouble with heart).
3. Recurrence of her gynecological cancer with pelvic obstruction.
4. Lymphedema—area she lived, long history of problems, more swelling one side.

Answer 3.2: Tables 9.1, 9.2 and 9.3.

Table 9.1 Causes of limb swelling: Bilateral pitting edema
• Heart failure
• Renal failure
• Proteinuria
• Cirrhosis
• Carcinomatosis
• Nutrition

Table 9.2 Causes of limb swelling: Painful unilateral edema
• DVT
• Superficial thrombophlebitis
• Cellulitis
• Trauma
• Ischemia

Table 9.3 Causes of limb swelling: Painless unilatereal edema
• Post-phlebitic limb
• External compression of pelvic veins
• Deep venous incompetence
• Lymphedema
• Immobility

Answer 3.3: Lymphedema.

Answer 3.4: Congestive cardiac failure.

Answer 3.5:

Primary   *Congenital:* 2% adult population
Developmental failure of lymphatics
Classified by age of onset:
l. congenital: at birth,
l. precox: 1–35 years,
l. tarda: > 35 years

Secondary—causes: 1. Lymphatic system obstruction by tumor, recurrent infection or infestation
2. Obliterated by surgery or radiotherapy

Answer 3.6: Gradual painless swelling of one or both legs. To start with is pitting in type and worse with standing; then becomes non-pitting and non-posture dependent; usually only extends to knee, prone to bouts of cellulitis which makes it worse.

First involves the foot
   - Loss of submalleolar depressions, square toes, fullness over dorsum
   - Pits at first
   - If severe may be accompanied by fungal infection of skin and toes.

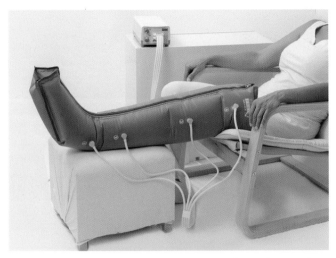

Fig. 9.7 Compression trousers (Courtesy of Lympha-press)

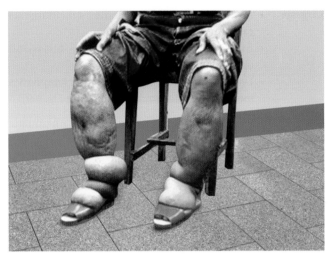

Fig. 9.8 Lymphedema of leg due to filariasis
Courtesy CDC (Atlanta, USA)

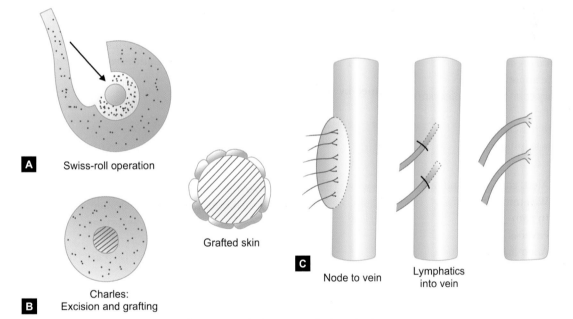

A Swiss-roll operation

B Charles:
Excision and grafting

Grafted skin

C Node to vein   Lymphatics into vein

Figs 9.9A to C Operations for lymphedema

Answer 3.7: Usually on clinical grounds.

Answer 3.8:

1. Elevation, massage, pneumatic pump (Fig. 9.7), compression stockings and bandages.
2. Antibiotics for cellulitis, antifungals for fungal infection.
3. Surgery—only suitable for a small number—either bypass procedures or reduction.

Answer 3.9: Acquired infestation from the worm *Wuchereria bancrofti*—transmitted by mosquitoes.

- Adult worms migrate to lymphatics and lymph nodes.
- Initially, presents with lymphangitis with fever, chills and rigors and red streaks on limb.

- Lymph nodes are swollen and tender.
- Repeated attacks obliterate the lymphatics and the classical signs of lymphedema occur.
- If severe, get the 'elephant leg' with dry, thickened folds (Fig 9.8).

Answer 3.10:

Conservative:
- Bandages, massage, elevation
- Skin care and good hygiene
- Diuretics
- Antifilarial drugs—diethyl carbamazine citrate (DEC)
- Warfarin has been used.

Surgery:
- *Reduction procedures:* Charles subcutaneous excision and skin grafting.
- Excision combined with bypass—Swiss-roll operation.
- Lymphatic bypass—node to vein or lymphatics into vein omental transposition (see Fig. 9.9).

Answer 3.11: Elevation, compression with armlet, pneumatic pump.

TUTORIAL 10: Renal Problems

CASE SCENARIOS

Answer 1.1:
- *Skin:* Herpes zoster
- *Musculoskeletal/Spine:* Trauma, infection, disc problems
- *Kidney:*
  - Renal/ureteric colic
    i. Stone
    ii. Tumor
    iii. Pyelonephritis
- *Abdominal organ:*
  - Acute appendicitis
  - Biliary colic/acute cholecystitis
  - Dissecting AAA in elderly
  - Acute pancreatitis
  - Acute salpingitis.

Answer 1.2:
General:
- Alert, conscious and orientated
- Well nourished
- In pain
- Fevered
- Anemic/jaundice
- Lip/mouth signs
- Signs in hands
- Vital signs.

Specific:
- Chest examination
- Abdominal examination: – Inspection
  – Palpation
  – Percussion
  – Auscultation
- Groins/penis/scrotum
- Rectal examination
- Spinal tenderness/neurological examination, if indicated.

Answer 1.3: Presence of RBCs: Gross or microscopic hematuria is found in 85% of patients with renal/ureteric colic.

Answer 1.4: Opacity(s) over the renal or ureteric area (70% of renal calculi are radiopaque).

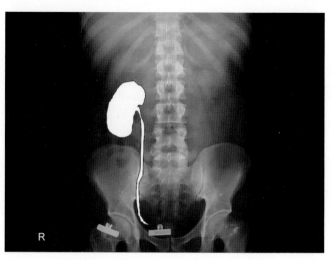

Fig. 10.1 The anatomical line of the ureter

Answer 1.5: It should lie in the line of the ureter, which passes downwards along the line of the tips of the lumbar transverse processes, across the sacroiliac joint, bowing across the pelvis to enter the bladder opposite the tip of coccyx (Fig. 10.1).

Answer 1.6:
1. Conservative
2. Invasive
   - ESWL (External corporeal shockwave lithotripsy) or
   - URSL (Ureteroscopic lithotripsy).

Answer 1.7: Conservative management for urinary tract stone (95% of stones 2–4 mm in diameter will pass spontaneously. 50% of those >5 mm will pass; stones >7 mm are unlikely to pass spontaneously):
- Increase oral fluid intake (at least 3 liters/day)
- Analgesia
- Pethidine IMI at 1 mg/kg (max 100 mg) repeated 4–6 hourly as necessary or
  - Diclofenac IMI 75 mg 4–6 hourly as necessary or
  - Oral diclofenac, if being treated at home—50 mg 6 hourly
- Antiemetics:
  - Metoclopramide IMI 10 mg with pethidine or
  - Prochlorperazine IMI 12.5 mg with the pethidine
- Antispasmodic
  - Hyoscine oral 10 mg TDS.

Answer 1.8:
1. Continued pain.
2. Hydronephrosis with impairment of renal function.
3. Infection.

Answer 1.9: Advise intervention.

Answer 1.10:
- *Advantages:*
  - Noninvasive procedure
  - Does not require general anesthesia
  - Outpatient procedure
  - Effective (overall 80%).
- *Disadvantages:*
  - May be painful
  - May need repeated sessions
  - Large stone—may require secondary procedure like ureteroscopic lithotripsy, insertion of ureteric stent
  - Exposure to X-rays
  - *Complications of the procedure:*
    - Bruising of skin
    - Renal injury
    - Ureteric obstruction due to stone fragments
    - Pyelonephritis
    - Injury to surrounding organs.

Answer 1.11:
- Ureteroscopic lithotripsy
- Open surgery (ureterotomy)
- Laparoscopic removal.

Answer 2.1: Interventional management required: ESWL or PCNL (percutaneous nephrolithotomy).

Answer 3.1: IVP (Intravenous pyelogram/urogram).

Answer 3.2:
- Any history of allergy to contrast?
- Any history of asthma?
- Any history of allergic rhinitis?
- Any history of allergy to food, especially seafood or medications?
- Any history of diabetes? If so, whether the patient is on metformin?
- Any history of renal diseases?
- In female, when was her LNMP?

Answer 3.3: The patient is having an anaphylactic reaction to the contrast.

Management:
- Stop the injection
- Give the patient subcutaneous adrenaline (1:1000) 0.5 mL + 100 mg hydrocortisone IV stat (this is available on all resuscitation trolleys).
Then,
- High flow oxygen, ECG cardiac monitoring, pulse oximeter, large bore intravenous access.
- Immediate assessment of airway, if airway is compromised, immediate intubation.

Cricothyrotomy is an option when orotracheal intubation or bag/valve/mask ventilation is not effective.
- *Intravenous fluids:*
  - 1 L of Hartmann's solution stat
- Drugs, if above does not improve condition
  - 0.5 mL adrenalin 1:1000 SC repeated every 15 minutes if necessary
  - In patient who is on beta-blockers and resistant to adrenalin, add glucagon (in addition to adrenalin) 1 mg every 5 minutes
  - Chlorpheniramine (Piriton) 10 mg IV
  - Ventolin inhalation, if patient has wheezes

Answer 3.4: There is a delay of contrast excretion from the right kidney. The right kidney is hydronephrotic. There are two opacities one probably in the kidney and the second at the pelviureteric junction.

The left kidney and upper ureter appears normal.

Answer 3.5: Yes. The patient might be at risk of developing lactic acidosis, if renal failure occurs as a result of contrast-induced nephrotoxicity (Metformin is excreted mainly in urine. In renal failure, metformin overdosage might develop. *Mechanism of Metformin:* To decrease hepatic glucose production and to increase its peripheral utilization).

Answer 3.6: Perform a urological CT instead or, if necessary, withhold the metformin for 48 hours after IV contrast.

Check renal function 48 hours later, if remains unchanged, the metformin can be resumed.

Answer 4.1:
- *Environmental:*
  - Excessive fluid loss, dehydration
- *Diet:*
  - Excess dietary sodium, oxalate, calcium and purines
  - Low fluid intake
- *Metabolic:*
  - Hypercalciuria
  - Hyperparathyroidism
  - Hyperuricosuria
  - Cystine
- Recurrent urinary tract infection
- *Others:*
  - Inflammatory bowel disease
  - Obstruction of urinary tract
  - Ureteric stricture.

Answer 4.2: Send stone for biochemical analysis. If possible stone analysis is recommended in:
1. All first time stone formers
2. All patients with recurrent stones on preventative treatment

3. Patients with early recurrence after complete stone clearance

4. Late recurrence of stones after a long stone free period (ask patient to strain urine through a sieve, tea strainer, coffee filter or gauze)

5. *Blood:* Check calcium, phosphate and uric acid level

6. *MSU:* Culture

7. 24 hours urine for sodium, uric acid, oxalate, citrate, calcium and phosphate

8. A spot nitroprusside test for cystine in patient with cystine stone.

Answer 4.3: Lifestyle changes

- *Oral fluid:*
  - Increase oral fluid intake sufficient to produce a urine volume of 2–2.5 L per day
- *Diet:*
  - Low sodium intake (< 3 g per day)
  - Moderate restriction of red meat intake
  - Limit oxalate rich food
  - Increase citric fruit intake
  - Moderate restriction of dairy produce intake
  - Restrict refined sugar.

> If you wish to read more about urinary tract stones and their management look at *www. patient.co.uk/doctor/urinary-tract-stones-urolithiasis.* This is an excellent review.

TUTORIAL 11: Testis/Scrotum/Penis

Answer 1: Figure 11.1

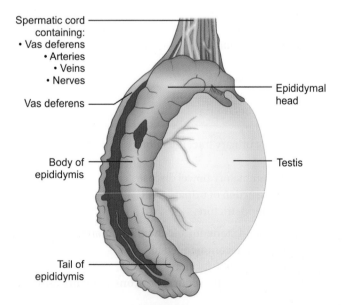

Spermatic cord
containing:
• Vas deferens
  • Arteries
  • Veins
  • Nerves

Vas deferens

Body of
epididymis

Tail of
epididymis

Epididymal
head

Testis

Fig. 11.1 The epididymis and testis

CASE SCENARIOS

Answer 2.1:

- Has he had similar pain before?
- What does he mean by the 'difficulty in passing urine'—when did it start and how does it bother him, i.e. is it suggestive of 'obstructive or irritative' symptoms and is cause suggested, e.g. BPH?
- Has the urine been smelly or cloudy—suggestive of infection?
- Any penile discharge—urethritis?
- Did he have history suggestive of sexually transmitted disease while a sailor?

Answer 2.2: Epididymo-orchitis.

Answer 2.3: Most cases are caused by retrograde infection via the urethra.

Two groups:

1. Occur in men < 35 years: Sexually transmitted (*Chlamydia trachomatis, N. gonorrhoeae*).

2. Bacterial GU infection in men > 40 years.

Answer 2.4:

- FBC
- U and Es
- Urine microscopy and culture
- Ultrasound, if doubt over diagnosis
- STD work-up, if indicated (Sexually Transmitted Disease).

Answer 2.5:

- Analgesics
- Scrotal support and rest
- Appropriate antibiotics
  Older man with GU tract source need broad-spectrum antibiotic to cover Gram –ve and +ve organisms, e.g. trimethoprim or fluoroquinolone.
  Younger man with *Chlamydia*—tetracycline.
  Other STDs, e.g. *Gonococcus*—appropriate tratment.

Note: Do not forget to investigate GU system, if symptoms suggest additional problems.

Answer 2.6:

- Adolescent boys or young adults
- 30% of patients with mumps will develop this complication
- Starts about 3–4 days after the parotitis
- Scrotum becomes red and edematous
- Usually no urinary tract symptoms and little pyrexia
- Differential diagnosis is acute epididymitis, torsion of testis, trauma, tumor, TB
- Treatment symptomatic with reassurance of mother.

Answer 3.1: Scrotal gangrene or necrotizing fasciitis, i.e. involves the subcutaneous fat and deep fascia.

Answer 3.2: Yes, you should be worried

- Can spread very quickly to involve whole of scrotum and onto abdominal wall and be life-threatening
- In scrotum, this problem is called Fournier gangrene. (As opposed to progressive bacterial gangrene/dermal gangrene/Meleney's gangrene which involves skin only.)

Answer 3.3:

- Mixed infection of synergistic aerobes and anaerobes.
- Associated with diabetes mellitus, perianal sepsis, periurethral abscess and poor hygiene.

Answer 3.4:

- Broad-spectrum IV antibiotics, e.g. piperacillin/tazobactam or ticaracillin/clavulanate and an aminoglycoside and metronidazole plus vancomycin, if MRSA suspected.
- Urgent debridement—extensive as necessary.

Answer 4.1: You will tell him that his right testis feels abnormal and that you think he should see a specialist for further investigation and assessment.

Answer 4.2: Tell the truth—say there is the possibility that it might be a cancer, the diagnosis needs to be established—if it is a cancer, then modern day treatment is very effective.

Answer 4.3:

- FBC, U and Es
- *Tumor markers:* Alpha fetoproteins, hCG and LDH
- Ultrasound scan of testes
- CT chest and abdomen.

Answer 4.4: Right-sided orchidectomy—done through groin incision with soft clamp on chord before mobilization.

Answer 4.5a: Table 11.1

Table 11.1 Pathology of testicular tumors	

Germ cell tumors (90%)	Seminoma
	Nonseminoma – Embryonal
	                Teratoma
	                Choriocarcinoma

Stromal tumors	Leydig cell Sertoli cell Granulosa cell
Metastatic tumors	Lymphoma Leukemias

Answer 4.5b: Table 11.2

Table 11.2 Staging of testicular tumors (Royal Marsden Hospital Classification)
Stage 1: Confined to testis *Stage 2:* Spread to retroperitoneal nodes below diaphragm *Stage 3:* Spread to nodes above the diaphragm *Stage 4:* Visceral metastases

Note: Germ cell tumors spread to para-aortic nodes, lungs and brain. Stromal tumors rarely metastasize.

Answer 4.5c: Table 11.3

Management: Orchidectomy via groin incision gives histology (radical orchidectomy taking chord up to deep ring).

Further treatment depends on histology and staging

Table 11.3 Management of testicular tumors		
Staging	Management	
	Seminoma	Non-seminoma-germ cell
Stage 1 Stage 2 Stage 3 Stage 4	DXR to abdo nodes DXR to abdo nodes DXR to abdo + thoracic nodes or chemo Chemo	Observe or RPND* Chemo + RPND* Chemo Chemo

*RPND means Retroperitoneal Node Dissection

Answer 4.6: Stage 1 confined to testis.

Yes, he should have radiotherapy to abdominal lymph nodes.

Prognosis excellent > 90% 5-year survival.

Answer 4.7:

- Tell him that the pathology shows he has a testicular cancer called *a seminoma.*
- Tell him that the investigations show no evidence of spread, which makes it a stage 1 tumor which gives him an excellent outlook.
- Tell him that he needs radiotherapy to cover any 'micro-spread' into the lymph nodes of the abdomen.
- Emphasize that he will be almost certainly cured by his treatment (90% + chance).

Answer 5.1:

- How long has he had this problem?
- Can he retract the foreskin easily? If not, has this always been the case?
- What exactly happens when he gets an erection?
- Has he had any episodes of infection of the foreskin?
- Is he diabetic?

Answer 5.2: Phimosis.

Answer 5.3: Usually from recurrent episodes of balanitis (inflammation/infection of glans penis and skin of prepuce).

Answer 5.4: Circumcision or dorsal slit.

Answer 5.5: See Figure 11.5

1. GA.
2. In adult, usually use 3 forceps technique.
3. Stretch out foreskin; excise the excess back to a line just distal to base of glans.
4. Figure-of-8 suture around frenula artery, 2 layers of prepuce sutured with interrupted absorbable suture. Tie off small vessels.
5. Put on 'Sofra-Tulle' dressing.

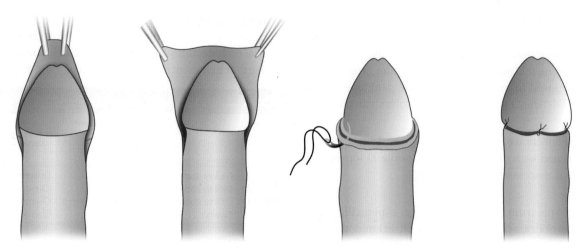

Fig. 11.5 Circumcision

Answer 5.6: Main complication is bleeding—may need to go back to theater. *Ulceration* of the glands may occur from disrupted adhesions, incorrect technique can cause suture line tension and breakdown.

Note: Do not use monopolar diathermy—may lead to conduction injury of penis (safe to use bipolar diathermy).

Answer 6.1: Please stand up.

Answer 6.2: Varicocele—often likened to a "bag of worms".

Note: Most varicoceles are asymptomatic (10–20% only have discomfort). They are said to be caused by venous reflux. On rare occasions, a varicocele can be secondary to lesions involving the left renal vein, e.g. renal cancer.

Answer 6.3: Operation advised only, if:
1. The symptoms are interfering with his life.
2. He is having infertility problems (about 20% of patients with a varicocele have infertility problems)
   Operation • Division of veins in chord at inguinal level (difficult).
   • Embolization has been tried.

Answer 7.1: If a testis is absent from the scrotum, then it may be:
1. Retractile
2. Ectopic
3. Undescended
4. Congenitally absent.
   (just keep these four facts in mind and life is much easier).
   Retractile means, it is in the inguinal canal and can be brought down into the scrotum. Ectopic means it is lying off the normal path of descent—usually in superficial inguinal pouch more rarely in femoral triangle, perineum or root of penis. Undescended means lies somewhere on normal line of descent from abdomen to inguinal canal.
   Congenitally absent—always completely absent.

Answer 7.2:
• Ask mother to hold the child and expose the scrotum and groins.
• Warm environment.
• Put baby powder on groins.
• Gently examine the scrotum and inguinal canals.
• If identify testis see, it can gently slide into scrotum.

Answer 7.3: Retractile testis:
• Tell the mother that it is quite common for the testis to retract into the lower part of the abdomen into the canal there. This is the case with her son.
• It is nothing to worry about as in the next year or two the testis will come down to the correct position, i.e. the same as his other side which is fine.
• She should come back for follow-up each year to check this has happened.

Answer 7.4: Undescended testis.
   Management = orchidopexy by the age of 2 years, i.e. bringing testis into scrotum by mobilizing the chord in inguinal canal and then fixing testis in scrotum.

Answer 7.5: Either testis lies retroperitoneally in abdomen or is absent.

Management: Perform US. If no testis is found perform laparoscopy to ascertain, whether it is congenitally absent or intra-abdominal; if intra-abdominal—remove because of chance of malignant change (usually done laparoscopically).

TUTORIAL 12: Prostate and Bladder

CASE SCENARIOS

Answer 1.1: Obstructive uropathy.

Answer 1.2:

- *Due to bladder outlet obstruction:*
  - Bladder
    - Stone, tumor, bladder neck contracture
  - Prostate
    - Carcinoma, BPH, prostatitis
  - Urethra
    - Stone, stricture, foreign bodies, paraphimosis
- *Due to hypocontractility of the bladder:*
  - Neurological condition
  - Diabetes.

Answer 1.3:

- Ask about lower urinary symptoms
- Obstructive (voiding):
  - Hesitancy
  - Straining
  - Weak stream
  - Terminal dribbling
  - Incomplete emptying
- Irritative (filling)
  - Urgency/urge incontinence
  - Frequency
  - Nocturia
- Other urinary symptoms (e.g. hematuria, dysuria)
- Previous pelvic surgery
- Neuropathy:
  - Any paresthesia or weakness of lower limbs
- Cardiac problems
- Diabetes
- Fluid intake and output.

Answer 1.4:

General:	Any signs of uremia/anemia/jaundice Signs of uremia are: Deterioration of mental status Asterexis (flapping tremor) or tremor Uremic fetor Hyperreflexia and up-going toes Fall in BP, temperature Lemon yellow
Specific:	• Palpable kidneys • Palpable bladder • PR: Anal tone, prostate size, consistency, any nodules • Lower limb neurology.

Answer 1.5: Benign prostatic enlargement.

Answer 1.6:

- *Urine:*
  - Urine dipstick
  - Microscopy, culture and sensitivity
- *Blood:*
  - FBC and bioprofile
  - Serum PSA level
  - Fasting blood glucose.

Answer 1.7: CT urogram or KUB and ultrasound of kidneys and bladder.

Answer 1.8: Cystoscopy to exclude any bladder pathology.

Answer 1.9:

- Flexible cystoscopy is usually performed using a narrow flexible endoscope, which gives a picture on a TV screen.
- It is performed under local anesthesia sometimes with IV sedation.
- You will be asked to lie on the operating table with your legs slightly apart. The surgeon will instil some anesthetic gel into the urethra (center of penis).
- The scope is then gently passed along the urethra into the bladder with the surgeon looking as the 'scope goes along'.
- You may feel a mild discomfort during the procedure.
- If the surgeon sees abnormal tissue in the bladder, he may take a specimen (biopsy).
- When the scope is removed you may feel discomfort when passing urine and pass a little blood. These will pass off, usually within 24 hours.

Answer 1.10:

1. *Mild symptoms:* Watchful, waiting.
2. *Mild-to-moderate symptoms:* Medications.
3. *Moderate-to-severe symptoms:* Surgery.

Answer 1.11: Medical treatment for BPH:

1. Alpha-blockers (terazosin, alfuzosin, and doxazosin)
   - To relax the smooth muscle in the prostate and bladder neck
   - *Common side effects:* Drowsiness, headache, dizziness, postural hypotension, nasal congestion, tachycardia, lethargy.
2. 5-alpha reductase inhibitors (finasteride, dutasteride)
   - Reduction of prostatic volume by inhibiting the conversion of testosterone to dihydrotestosterone
   - Common side effects: Erectile dysfunction, decreased libido, reduced ejaculate volume.

Answer 2.1: MRI of pelvis to exclude any locally advanced disease (the T and N staging). Bone scan to exclude any bone metastases.

Answer 2.2:
- Watchful waiting
- Radical prostatectomy
  - Open
  - Laparoscopic
  - Robotic
- Radiotherapy.

Answer 3.1:
- *Castration:*
  Surgical: With bilateral orchidectomy, or
  Medical: With LHRH agonists
- May need palliative TURP (transurethral prostatectomy) if persistent difficulty in passing urine after castration and radiotherapy to bony metastases if persistent bony pain.

Answer 4.1:
- FBC, bioprofile, clotting screen, PSA
- Urine dipstick and urine microscopy and culture
- CT urogram or IVU
- Flexible cystoscopy.

Answer 4.2: Papillary growth in the bladder suggestive of bladder cancer (transitional cell carcinoma).

Answer 4.3:
- Cigarette smoking (X4 increase in incidence)
- Occupational exposure to benzidine, aromatic amines, nitrosamines and β-naphthylamine
  - Dye and rubber industries, textiles, leather works, printing, aluminum refining and hair-dressing
- *Chronic inflammation:*
  - Chronic infection, catheter, bladder stones
- Pelvic irradiation
- Schistosomiasis (bilharzia)
  - Causes squamous cell bladder cancer
  - Most common cause of bladder cancer worldwide
  - Younger age group, advanced presentation
- Cyclophosphamide
- Old age, male.

Answer 4.4:
- CT urogram/IVU to exclude any upper renal tract transitional cell cancer (TCC)
- EUA and TURBT (transurethral resection of bladder tumor) to stage the tumor
- If histology shows
  - Superficial disease (i.e. Ta, T1) and low grade tumor (Grade 1)
    - Surveillance cystoscopy every 3 month for 2 years, 6 monthly for next 3 years and yearly after that

- Superficial disease (i.e. Ta, T1) and moderate to high grade tumor (Grade 2 or 3)
  - Adjuvant intravesical chemotherapy (thiotepa, mitomycin) or immunotherapy (BCG)
- CIS (carcinoma *in situ*)
  - Adjuvant immunotherapy
- Myoinvasive disease, i.e. T2/3
  - MRI or CT pelvis for staging
  - If organ-confined tumor
    - Total cystectomy with ileal conduit or bladder reconstruction
    - Radical radiotherapy
    - Consider adjuvant chemotherapy for younger patient
  - If locally invasive, i.e. T4
    - Radiotherapy + chemotherapy
  - If metastatic disease
    - Chemotherapy.

Answer 4.5: Description: The bladder is removed; a segment of ileum about 6 inches long is isolated, the ureters are anastomosed to one end of the ileum and the other end of the ileum is brought out through the abdominal wall, usually in the right iliac fossa as a urostomy (Fig. 12.2).

Answer 4.6: TURP stands for Trans-Urethral Resection of the Prostate and is the shortened terminology widely used by urologists to describe a prostatic resection performed via the urethra using a resectoscope (see Fig. 12.3).

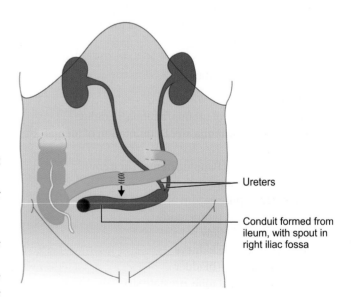

Fig. 12.2 Ileal conduit

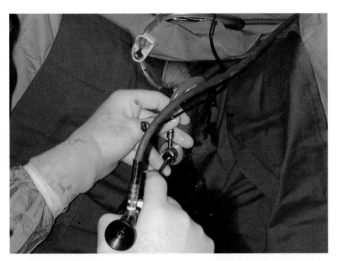

Fig. 12.3 Resectoscope (TURP) (Copyright RCSI with permission)

What Does A TURP Involve?

This is an operation to create a larger channel through the prostate gland. This will prevent or relieve obstruction to the flow of urine. During the operation, a small telescope is passed through the urethra (the tube through which you pass urine) and instruments are passed up the telescope to core out the inside of the prostate gland. There is no wound and no stitches are needed.

The length of stay in hospital varies from 4 to 7 days depending on your recovery and home circumstances.

> Please note that it has become routine practice in most hospitals for patient information leaflets to be made available to the patients—this is 'good' medical practice both from the medical and medicolegal aspects. When consenting the patient they can be asked to read the appropriate leaflet, given the opportunity to ask questions and then be asked to sign the consent.

Below is the patient information leaflet for TURP as provided by the North Devon Healthcare NHS Trust. You will see it is patient friendly (avoiding medical terminology as far as possible), it is comprehensive and includes a description of the common complication and lifestyle answers. You should study it closely because this is the type of information you are now expected to provide to the patient.

Before the Operation

If you regularly take drugs which thin the blood, such as aspirin, warfarin, please contact the Urology Department before you come into hospital.

When you arrive on the ward we will show you to a bed and you will be able to unpack your belongings. There is a small wardrobe to hang up clothes, as well as a locker. The nursing staff will check your details with you. It is **important** to let them know of any changes since your preoperative visit, e.g. illness, different telephone numbers, transport problems for going home, etc.

The anesthetist will visit to discuss the anesthetic with you. This may either be a *General* or a *Spinal* anesthetic.

A *General* anesthetic involves the injection of drugs into a vein in the arm to make you deeply unconscious. When you wake up you may need to have oxygen via a mask for a few hours. If you have any nausea, we can give you some medication to help. It will be a few hours before you can start drinking again, starting with sips of water and building up as tolerated.

A *Spinal* anesthetic involves an injection of local anesthetic into the back, which numbs you from the waist down. You will also be sedated, which means you are asleep throughout and unaware of the operation being done. When you wake up your legs will still be numb, but power and feeling will slowly return over the next few hours. You will experience pins and needles as that happen.

What Special Preparations are Needed?

We will ask you to get ready for theater probably quite soon after coming into hospital. This means changing into a theater gown, and putting on a pair of surgical stockings. These will help prevent a blood clot forming in the legs due to you being less mobile and having anesthetic drugs.

About an hour before going to theater we may give you a tablet, which is taken with a small drink of water to start the relaxation process. We call this a 'pre-med'.

What Happens after the Operation?

You will wake-up either in the recovery room near to the theater, or on the ward. A nurse will take your blood pressure and pulse regularly, and will be available via the nurse call-bell system at any time. You will have a 'drip' in your arm to give you the fluids you need. This is removed when you are drinking normally again.

You will have a plastic tube (catheter) coming out of your penis. This drains the urine into a plastic bag at the side of your bed. Another tube will be attached to the catheter into which water will flow.

During the operation, the prostate tissue has been scraped away, leaving a raw area that heals slowly over the next few weeks. While it is healing, the area will bleed. The catheter acts as a flushing system, allowing fluid to be passed up through the bladder to cleanse it, and to drain the fluid and any blood and urine into the drainage bag. Do not be alarmed to see blood (colored like red wine) in the catheter bag. This is normal. While the catheter is in place, you may feel that your bladder is full. This is also quite normal and you will realize that urine is flowing out of the bladder automatically along the catheter all the time, without any need to strain.

Will it Hurt?

Pain is unusual. Some people find the catheter uncomfortable, whereas many hardly notice it. If you have pain or discomfort, your nurse will give you some painkillers. During the first days, a clot of blood may block the catheter. The bladder will become full and you will have an intense desire to pass water, but urine will be unable to drain out. If you think this has happened please tell the nurse. She/he can then flush the catheter with a syringe to clear it.

The Next Day

The doctor will visit in the morning to check your progress. You will probably be eating and drinking normally by now and the drip will be removed. You will be encouraged to drink about 3 liters (5–6 pints) of fluid each day to continue flushing the bladder. *Please bring a bottle of squash or equivalent with you* to avoid drinking copious amounts of water alone.

If the bleeding is settling down, the bladder irrigation fluid will be stopped, but the catheter will stay in a day or two longer.

If you have not already done so, you will be encouraged to get out of bed and start to walk around.

Catheter Care and Removal

Avoid infection by keeping your catheter clean. Wash your penis under the foreskin and around the catheter where it enters the penis, with soap and water, morning and evening. You may bath or shower while the catheter is in.

Once the doctor is happy with the amount of blood draining into the catheter bag, the catheter will be removed (usually the second or third day, sometimes longer). After removal of the catheter, it may take a while to control your urine flow immediately. You may feel a constant urge to urinate, have leakages, or tend to dribble, or you may have difficulty urinating. Do not worry. These symptoms are all normal and will improve with time. You may experience some burning or stinging when urinating. This will settle down over the next few days.

Once you have gained enough control over your bladder, you will be able to go home.

When I Get Home, what Symptoms may I Still Experience?

Tiredness

When you return home you should take things easy for a fortnight. It is common to feel a bit flat or depressed for a few days. This is natural and will quickly pass. Tiredness is very common and will last longer than you think, e.g. up to a month after leaving hospital.

Bleeding

You will see blood or small clots in your urine but this will slowly settle down over the next few weeks. It will be more noticeable some days than others, and in the morning when you have not drunk for a while. A little extra bleeding is common around the second week after the operation, as the scabs that have formed in the prostate come away.

Leakages on Passing Urine

You may find you leak a little when straining or coughing. This can be managed by wearing a small pad inside your underpants and is temporary. Frequent visits to the toilet and having to get up at night are also common place and will slowly settle down. Many men worry about the possibility of incontinence after the operation. This is very rare indeed.

Difficulty Passing Urine

Sometimes when the bladder muscles have been stretched or strained for a long time, it is necessary to rest them. A small proportion of men are unable to pass urine adequately afterwards and have to be sent home with their catheter in place for about a month. In this case, we will give you full instructions on catheter care. You would then come back to the ward for a day visit to have the catheter removed and progress monitored for a few hours.

Infection

The following symptoms may indicate an infection, which would need treatment from your GP:

- A high temperature.
- It continues to be painful, sting or burn when you urinate.
- Your urine becomes thick, cloudy or smelly.
- Your testicles become swollen or painful.

Exercise

Keep physical activity to a minimum. Short walks (less than a mile) are safe. Anything more active like digging and lifting should be totally avoided. Sports such as golf, cycling and swimming may be resumed after a month or so.

Diet

You can eat normally, but try to ensure a good intake of fruit and vegetables, and other high fiber foods to help avoid constipation. If you do become constipated, it is important not to strain as this puts pressure on the healing wound. Try a mild laxative, or ask your doctor for advice.

Continue to drink 2 liters (about 4 pints) of fluid each day for the first week or two, to continue the flushing process and to help prevent infection. Increase fluids, if you notice the urine becoming more bloodstained. Alcohol is permitted in moderation. Try to reduce drinking after 6–8 pm so you do not have to get up during the night.

Driving

Do not drive for the first 2 weeks after the operation. This is because if you had to do an emergency stop, the sudden jerking movement could damage the healing wound. Before you come to hospital we suggest you contact your motor insurance company. Many companies will not provide full cover for patients who have had major surgery, for the first 3 months after the operation.

Work

You may return to work a month after the operation. If you have a heavy manual job, the recovery time may be longer.

On discharge, the nursing staff can give you a sick note to cover the time you have been in hospital. When this runs out, you will need to get further sick notes from your GP.

Sex

You should not have sex for 3 weeks after the operation, as this may cause the internal wound to bleed.

Possible Complications

The removal of prostate tissue usually has no effect on a man's ability to have sex. However, it can result in retrograde ejaculation, or 'dry orgasm'. This means that when the man has an orgasm, the sperm flows back into the bladder rather than out of the penis. This is not harmful and the sperm will be passed out the next time, the man urinates. This operation can therefore prevent you from fathering a child. If this concerns you, please ask the doctor for advice.

A few men have problems with potency after a TURP. These are more likely to be men over 70 years of age or those in whom erections were already reduced before the operation. If you have problems with sex, or your sex life is particularly important to you, please mention this to your doctor before the operation.

Excessive bleeding can occur during the first 24–48 hours after the operation. We have the facilities to deal with this should it occur. A small number of patients continue to bleed, requiring a further operation or blood transfusion.

Heavy bleeding or blood clots may block the flow of urine and will become very painful. However, this is uncommon. If this occurs, please call your GP or visit your local Accident and Emergency Department.

Finally, about 1 in 10 men who have a TURP will need a further operation as the prostate tissue regrows. However, this may take several years to happen.

Follow-up

We will arrange for you to see your Consultant in the Outpatient Department 6–8 weeks after your operation.

Further Information

If you have any concerns or questions about your TURP, please contact the urology department or your urologist's secretary. They will be glad to help.
(*Courtesy* of North Devon NHS Trust)

TUTORIAL 13: Fluid and Electrolyte Balance/ Parenteral Nutrition

Answer 1:

Na	135–145 mmol/L
K	3.5–5 mmol/L
Cl	98–106 mmol/L
Bicarbonate	21–28 mmol/L
Urea	2.5–6.7 mmol/L
Creatinine	70–150 umol/L or 0.05–0.12 mmol/L

Answer 2:

pH	7.35–7.45
PaO_2	10.6 kPa
$PaCO_2$	4.7–6.0 kPa
HCO_3	21–28 mmol/L
Base excess	+/– 2 mmol/L

Answer 3a:

Water 1 liter
Na 131 mmol   K 5 mmol
Cl 111 mmol (+ Ca 2 mmol and HCO_3 29 mmol)

Answer 3b:

Water 1 liter
Na 154 mmol   K 0 mmol   Cl 154 mmol

Answer 3c:

Water 1 liter
Na 0   K 0   Cl 0   Sugar 50 g

Answer 4:

1. Correct the pre-existing deficiency
2. Continue the maintenance requirements
3. Replace ongoing losses.

Answer 5:

From skin	600 mL
From respiration	400 mL
From kidneys	1500 mL
From feces	100 mL
Total	2.6 liters

Answer 6: Table 13.1

Table 13.1 Insensible loss -special situations

Fever: Add 10% for each degree above 38°C

Sweating: Add 10–15%

Hyperventilating: Add 25–50%

Hypermetabolic: Add 25–50%

Less fluid, if patient is humidified or ventilated. Replace as water.

Answer 7: Movement of fluid into the interstitial space due to tissue damage associated with major surgery/sepsis/inflammation/burns—the interstitial space (parenchymal and loose CT) is normally dry but in sequestration fluid accumulates there. It is a "physiological" compartment.

See Module 2 Tutorial 11: Third space and Third spacing.

Answer 8: 3rd space sequestration causes an increase in the ECF with depletion of the intravascular space; use balanced electrolyte solution (Hartmann's) to optimize the intravascular fluid volume. The real treatment for third spacing is to treat the underlying disease pathology.

Answer 9a: Replace with appropriate volume of 0.9N saline with added potassium as indicated. Pure gastric secretion contains a lot of Na, Cl and K ions.

Answer 9b: Hartmann's solution +/– potassium supplements.

Answer 10:

2:1:1

$\left.\begin{array}{l}\text{2 liters water} \\ \text{1 mmol/kg Na}^+ \\ \text{1 mmol/kg K}^+\end{array}\right\}$ per 24 hours

Answer 11: The metabolic response to surgery results in Na^+ and water retention and K^+ excretion. However, the latter is reversed by the K^+ released by cell injury.

Answer 12: Means that first 1–3 days give less water, less Na and less K than the 'formula'.

CASE SCENARIOS

Answer 13.1: Surgery for Crohn's disease (Figs 13.2 and 13.3).

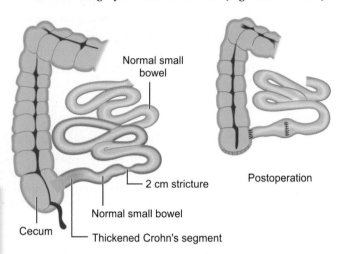

Fig. 13.2 Limited right hemicolectomy and stricturoplasty

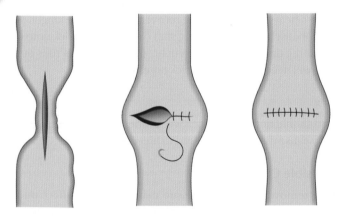

Fig. 13.3 Details of stricturoplasty.
Strictured bowel opened longitudinally and closed transversely

Answer 13.2: Device that allows hourly urine output to be measured easily by the nurses—used when you wish to monitor the urine output closely (see Fig. 13.4).

Answer 13.3:

a. Urine output during surgery and volume and type of fluids given by anesthetist during surgery
b. The estimated blood lost during surgery (and see how replaced by anesthetist)
c. IV fluids given in recovery and what urine output has been recorded
d. Pulse/BP/CVP and O_2 sats.

Answer 13.4: Chart 13.2 (page 287).

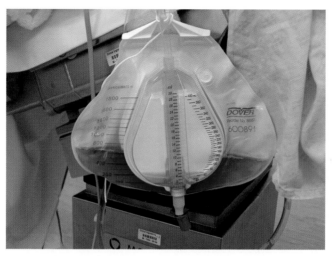

Fig. 13.4 Urimeter (Copyright RCSI with permission)

Chart 13.2 Daily intravenous fluid-order chart

Name	Miss H					
First Name						
Reg. No.						
Ward	GEN SURGERY					

Bag/Bottle Order	State infusion fluid/blood, volume to be given period of infusion and drip site, if applicable			State drug and dosage to be added	Doctor's initials	Blood bottle/bag no. infusion batch no. to be confirmed by nurse
1	HARTMANN's	500 mL	8 hours		ℛ	
2	DEXTROSE	5% 500 mL	8 hours		ℛ	
3						
4						
5						
6						
7						
8						

Answer 13.5: The total intake is 1110 mL and total output is 790 mL. She is therefore 320 mL in +ve balance. Despite this, the urine output is tailing off in the hours 3 am to 7 am—so she may be becoming fluid depleted.

Note: In line with current 'fast recovery' surgical management, she does not have a nasogastric (NG) tube and oral fluids are allowed early.

Answer 13.6: Chart 13.5 (page 288).

Prescribed 1.5 liters water in all to cover the maintenance requirements and no added electrolytes other than Hartmann's content—because of the metabolic response to surgery. (Miss H weighs 64 kg.) The patient's oral intake will also increase as she tolerates greater amounts through the day.

Note that the British Consensus Guideline recommends 1.5 to 2.5 liters of water maintenance per day. In this case, the urine output was starting to tail off—this may be an indication of dehydration but may also be a normal response in the early postoperative period.

The patient's CLINICAL STATUS and output should be reviewed routinely twice per day—in this case, to ensure there are no signs off overload or dehydration.

Chart 13.5 Daily intravenous fluid-order chart

Name	Miss H				
First Name					
Reg. No.					
Ward	GEN SURGERY				

Bag/Bottle Order	State infusion fluid/blood, volume to be given period of infusion and drip site if applicable	State drug and dosage to be added	Doctor's initials	Blood bottle/bag no. infusion batch no. to be confirmed by nurse
1	HARTMANN's 500 mL 8 hours		↙	
2	DEXTROSE 5% 500 mL 8 hours		↙	
3	DEXTROSE 5% 500 mL 8 hours		↙	
4				
5				
6				
7				
8				

5–6 May 2010

Please note the difference from the much used 1 liter 0.9 N saline and 2 liters 5% dextrose with added potassium.

Answer 13.7: To make sure she does not have any signs of a chest infection or DVT. You will do this at least once everyday.

Answer 13.8: There is no indication for transfusion with a Hb of 10 g/dL.

Answer 13.9: Look back to Module 1, Tutorial 19.

Transfusion trigger is defined as the Hb or hematocrit laboratory level at which most patients require red blood cell transfusion.

The lower limit of transfusion trigger for general medical and surgical patients is 7.0 g/dL or hematocrit of 21% (note the transfusion trigger may vary slightly from hospital to hospital).

Current data suggests that restraining transfusions favors positive outcomes except when significant underlying cardiac disease is present (may benefit from putting hematocrit up to 33).

Answer 13.10: She may have leaked from one of her anastomoses. Abdominal X-rays suggest an ileus and her electrolytes suggest she may be fluid depleted—all of which would fit with a leak.

Answer 13.11: Write her up for total of 3 liters in next 24 hours—using Hartmann's (1 liter) and dextrose 5% (2 liters).

This will give her the MAINTENANCE 2 liters and additional fluid to cover the likely dehydration.

The Hartmann's will give the necessary Na ions but you may need to add potassium to the regime depending on her electrolytes.

This regime will need to be REVIEWED depending on her CLINICAL hydration status/urine output and electrolytes (Chart 13.7).

Answer 13.12: Abdominal pain spreading over the whole of her abdomen with diffuse tenderness, guarding and rebound and absent bowel sounds. Fever, tachycardia and possibly hypotension may be present.

Answer 13.13: What he means is that the track of the fistula/abscess has walled off. The small bowel contents pass along the fistula track to the surface and do not leak into the general peritoneal cavity.

Answer 13.14: Chart 13.10.

The patient's urea and electrolytes are within normal limits—the potassium is at the lower limit of normal.

The patient has been given 1 liter of Hartmann's and 2 liters of dextrose; she has an adequate urine output (approx 1.5 liters) and the fistula output—which will be small bowel contents—is about 1 liter.

She is in positive balance of + 690 mL.

So we need to be careful not to overload her—give her 1.5 liters of Hartmann's which will provide a balanced electrolyte solution to replace the fistula loss (including K^+) and 1 liter of dextrose 5% to make up a 2.5 liter input which

Chart 13.7 Daily intravenous fluid-order chart

Name	Miss H
First Name	
Reg. No.	
Ward	GEN SURGERY

Bag/Bottle Order	State infusion fluid/blood, volume to be given period of infusion and drip site, if applicable			State drug and dosage to be added	Doctor's initials	Blood bottle/bag no. infusion batch no. to be confirmed by nurse
1	HARTMANN's	500 mL	4 hours		✓	
2	DEXTROSE	5% 500 mL	4 hours		✓	
3	HARTMANN's	500 mL	4 hours		✓	
4	DEXTROSE	5% 500 mL	4 hours		✓	
5	DEXTROSE	5% 500 mL	4 hours		✓	
6	DEXTROSE	5% 500 mL	4 hours		✓	
7						
8						10 May 2010

Chart 13.10 Daily intravenous fluid-order chart

Name	Miss H
First Name	
Reg. No.	
Ward	GEN SURGERY

Bag/Bottle Order	State infusion fluid/blood, volume to be given period of infusion and drip site, if applicable			State drug and dosage to be added	Doctor's initials	Blood bottle/bag no. infusion batch no. to be confirmed by nurse
1	HARTMANN's	500 mL	4 hours		✓	
2	DEXTROSE	5% 500 mL	6 hours		✓	
3	HARTMANN's	500 mL	4 hours		✓	
4	DEXTROSE	5% 500 mL	6 hours		✓	
5	HARTMANN's	500 mL	4 hours		✓	
6						
7						
8						13–14 May 2010

should cover the MAINTENANCE and REPLACEMENT losses (she is + 650 mL already).

Answer 13.15: TPN stands for Total Parenteral Nutrition, i.e. all the patient's nutrition is administered via a central or peripheral vein.

Answer 13.16: Can be given via:

a. A peripheral cannula—for short-term (<2 weeks)—problems with thrombophlebitis/uses up veins.

b. Peripherally inserted central cannula (longer term—4–6 weeks avoids complications of CVP but needs 'team' insertion and care).

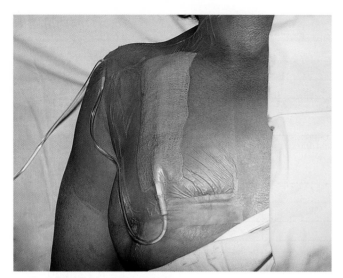

Fig. 13.5 Tunneled infraclavicular subclavian line
(From Bailey and Love. A Short Practice of Surgery. Ed. Williams N Hodder, 2008 Reproduced by permission of Taylor and Francis Books, UK)

c. Central cannula (non tunneled)—when used for nutrition need special care team.
d. Central cannula tunneled—for longer term/home care (Fig. 13.5).

Answer 13.17:
- Need about 1800 kcal/day
- If septic need about 2300 kcal/day
- Use amino acid solutions to provide nitrogen
- Use carbohydrate and fat to provide non-protein energy
- Usually mixed under sterile precautions in a 3-liter bag in pharmacy together with electrolyte and mineral contents and administered via control of a syringe pump.
  An example of typical contents is shown in Table 13.3.

Table 13.3 Typical constituents of TPN 'bag'

Constituents	Quantity
Amino acids	13.5 g
Fat/CHO	2200 kcal
Na	115 mmol
K	65 mmol
Calcium	10 mmol
Mg	9.5 mmol
Phosphate	20 mmol
Zinc	0.1 mmol
Cl	113 mmol
Acetate	135 mmol
Plus vitamins and trace elements	

Answer 13.18:

Insertion-related	Line-related	Feeding-related
• Pneumothorax • Arterial puncture • Hemothorax • Wrong position	• *Catheter-related sepsis:* • Infection at exit site • Tunnel infection • Venous thrombosis • Line occlusion	• *Metabolic:* Fluid + electrolyte imbalance hypo/hyperglycemia • Hepatobiliary disease (jaundice gallstones)

Note: Peripheral cannulae: Malposition and thrombophlebtis (after Kaushal, Surgery, 2004, 22.8.)

Answer 13.19: Monitoring of parenteral nutrition: This involves clinical, nutritional and biochemical parameters:

Clinical and nutritional (daily)	Biochemical		
Clinical condition	Daily	Weekly	Monthly
Temperature, pulse, BP, RR	Na	FBC	Selenium
Fluid balance	K, urea	LFTs	Zn
Weight	Creatinine	Phosphorus	Cu
Food chart (if on enteral feed as well)	Glucose	Ca, Mg	Urinary electrolytes
Entry site of catheter			

(after Kaushal)

Answer 13.20:
Definition: Enteral nutrition is the provision of nutritional supplements via the gastrointestinal tract.

It may be given by the oral route (i.e. sipping), if the patient is able to drink. Use flavored liquids in carton form (e.g. Ensure)—contains 250 kcal and 10 g protein—take up to 3 per day.

If patient cannot drink use enteral tube feeding; Nasogastric or nasojejunal (fine bore 'skinny' tube)—check position by either X-ray or litmus paper (stomach) or percutaneous gastrostomy/jejunostomy—either inserted at operation or by endoscopist/radiologist (see Figs 13.6 and 13.7).

Usually, use polymeric feeds containing protein, carbohydrate and fat 1 kcal/mL. Start with small (30 mL) hourly volumes and increase every 4 hours until target volume is reached. Give intermittently with rest periods 4–8 hours and sit patient up (30°).

Complications of enteral tube feeding:
Procedure related: Malposition/esophogeal ulceration/blockage (nasal)/pain/bleeding/infection (percutaneous).
Enteral feed related: Vomiting/aspiration/reflux/diarrhea/constipation/fluid imbalance.

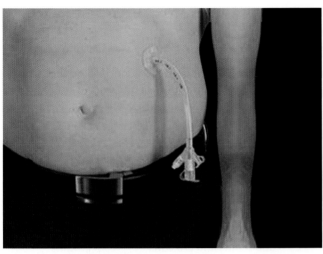

Fig. 13.6 Percutaneous gastrostomy tube
(Reproduced with permission of Kimberly-Clark Corperation, USA)

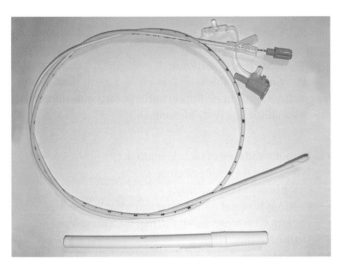

Fig. 13.7 Fine bore enteral feeding line
With permission: Corpak Med Systems, Buffalo Grove, Il, USA

Answer 13.21:

Patient's name   : Miss H
DOB   : 25/04/1986
Admitted   : 01/05/2010
Discharged   : 24/05/2010
Ward 6 university hospital
Consultant   : Mr X
Diagnosis   : Crohn's Disease
Operation   : Right hemicolectomy + stricturoplasty
Complications   : Anastomotic leak/small bowel fistula

The patient underwent surgery on 3/05/2010. She developed a fistula postoperatively and was treated conservatively with TPN and then enteral feeds.

The wound sutures have been removed and the wounds require a dry dressing only.

Drugs on discharge : Enteric-coated salazopyrin 500 mg TDS orally; 'Ensure' enteral supplements 3 × 250 mL cartons per day

OP follow up   : Mr X's clinic in 2 weeks
Histology   : Not yet available
District nurse/   : Not required
  clinic nurse

TUTORIAL 14: Gastrointestinal Bleeding

CASE SCENARIOS

Answer 1.1:

1. Very quickly assess the stability of the patient by feeling his pulse, noting his BP and checking his peripheral circulation. Unless his condition is critical.
2. Take a very quick history from the patient (or the relatives) mainly to make sure first of all that he has had a hematemesis.
3. If the nurses have not already done so put him on a monitor to measure his pulse, BP, O_2 sat and ECG.
4. Put up a large bore IV line and while doing so take off blood for FBC, U and Es, group and X-match, clotting screen.
5. Only then start and take a full history and examination (i.e. you are now in control).

Answer 1.2:

- Ask him what he has vomited and how did he know it was blood?
- How much was there and when?
- Look to see if there is blood on his face or clothing, sometimes they may have a vomit bowl or container.
- If necessary, ask the relatives or persons accompanying him.

Note: Later on, if still in doubt, passing a NG tube may help, as will rectal examination.

Answer 1.3:

Set ready the equipment.
- BP cuff or tourniquet
- Grey or green cannula 18/20 gauge
- IV giving set and Hartmann's solution
- Tubes for blood collection
- Swabs, gauze squares, etc.
Blow up BP cuff or place tourniquet.

Choose appropriate vein—usually the one on lateral side of wrist (continuation of cephalic vein, see Fig. 14.1) or the cephalic or basilic in the cubital fossa but be careful of brachial artery.

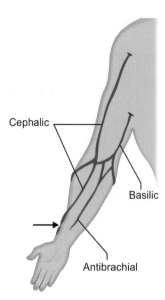

Fig. 14.1 Veins of forearm

(Arrow indicates vein to use at wrist—usually big, straight and does not move about)

Answer 1.4:
1. Put on oxygen mask (type = facemask, flow = 10 liters/min).
2. Put up 500 mL of Hartmann's on IV line and run in as fast as will go (if no improvement in pulse/BP use colloid solution next).
3. Ask nurses to send for the senior surgeon straight away.
4. Arrange for high dependency bed.
5. Put in urinary catheter while waiting.

Answer 1.5:
- He will assess the patient and the response to the fluid challenge.
- He will decide about more fluid or whether to use uncross matched blood.
- He will put in a CVP line.
- May also advise early ABGs (arterial blood gases).
- He will either arrange for immediate upper GI endoscopy/admission to high dependency ward for further monitoring or occasionally take straight to the operating room for 'in-theater' endoscopy.

Answer 1.6: Take a full 'problem-orientated' history and examine him fully.

Answer 1.7: Will tell you if he has melena/fresh blood on PR—confirms diagnosis of bleed and gives indication of severity.

Note: If there is no melena or blood: THINK AGAIN.

Answer 1.8:
- Peptic ulceration
- Gastritis/gastric or duodenal erosions

- Esophageal varices
- Gastric carcinoma
- Uncommon others, e.g. Mallory-Weiss/leiomyoma.

Answer 1.9: Mallory-Weiss syndrome is bleeding from a mucosal tear at the junction of the esophagus and the stomach which is associated with severe retching, coughing or vomiting. Also associated with alcoholism and eating disorders and there is some evidence that a hiatus hernia is a requisite predisposing condition. Diagnosis is made on history and findings at endoscopy.

Answer 1.10:

In UK		
Peptic ulcer disease		50%
Mucosal lesions including gastritis duodenitis and erosions		30%
Mallory-Weiss tear		5–10%
Esophageal varices		5–10%
Reflux esophagitis		5%
Angiodysplasia		5%
Carcinoma		Uncommon
Aortoduodenal fistula		Uncommon
Dieulafoy's syndrome		Rare
Coagulopathies		Uncommon

(Dieulafoy's syndrome = Rupture of large tortuous submucosal artery usually in the body of stomach.)

Answer 1.11:
- Amount and type of blood vomited.
- When the 1st episode occurred.
- Past history of indigestion.
- Previous hospital admissions and what happened.
- Current GI symptoms—pain, nausea, vomiting.
- Drug ingestion.
- Lifestyle—smoking, stress, alcohol.

Answer 1.12:
Differential diagnosis: Peptic ulcer
                        Gastritis.

Answer 1.13:
- History of indigestion
- History of painkiller ingestion—possibly NSAIDs
- History of traditional medicine ingestion—possibly with steroid content
- Alcohol (spirits) ingestion—approx 14 units per week.

Answer 1.14:
1. Full history and examination
2. IV line in place and running with Hartmann's
3. Bloods taken off
4. On high dependency unit on monitor, input-output chart and NBM.

Answer 1.15: Upper GI endoscopy on next routine list.

Answer 1.16:
- Wash off the clot.
- Inject the ulcer with adrenalin or a sclerosant or coagulate the vessel with heater probe or laser.

Note: There is no EBM that this affects mortality but it does reduce the incidence of rebleeding.
- Take biopsy for HP.

Answer 1.17:
1. Back to high dependency ward.
2. Routine monitoring.
3. Commence medical therapy.

Answer 1.18:
1. Start IV proton pump inhibitor, e.g. omeprazole (low dose no less effective than high dose—40 mg omperazole IV bolus and then 40 mg IV 6–12 hourly for 3 days (Wu et al. World J Gastroenterol. 2010;16(20):2558-2565).
2. Start HP eradication.
3. If settles: • Discharge on PP inhibitor orally for 6 weeks
   - Reduce spicy and oily foods
   - Stop smoking and drinking.

Answer 1.19: In UK: Omeprazole 20 mg + metronidazole 400 mg + clarithromycin 500 mg (all BD) orally for 7 days
   OR
   Omeprazole 20 mg+ clarithromycin 500 mg + amoxicillin 1g (all BD) orally for 7 days.

NB For world wide drug choice see BMJ 2015;351:h 4052

Answer 1.20:
1. Speed up his IV fluids—ask the nurses to get a packet of blood and put this up.
2. Ring the Specialist Registrar and ask him to see the patient urgently.
3. Put in urinary catheter and CVP (If you can).
4. Increase the X-match.

Answer 1.21:
1. Could rescope and reinject, or
2. Could advise surgery.

Answer 1.22:
- Using the EBM technique:
- Evidence would suggest that there is no increase in morbidity or mortality, if a second attempt at endoscopic management is made, provided the expertise is available on an emergency basis.
- *Used Google* keywords: e-medicine/duodenal ulcer/ management of rebleed/injection/surgery.
- Selected prospective randomized trial published in New England Journal of Medicine (articles in the top cited journals will already have been assessed by someone very skillful in EBM!!!).
- *Reference:* Lau JYW, et al. Endoscopic retreatment compared with surgery in patients with recurrent bleeding after initial endoscopic control of bleeding ulcers. New Eng J Med. 1999;340:751-6.

Answer 1.23:
1. Book the operating theater.
2. Send off bloods for FBC and U and Es, make sure that the patient has 4 units of packed cells available.
3. Speak to the anesthetist.
4. Explain what is happening to the patient and obtain consent.
5. Speak to the relatives.

Answer 1.24:
- The operation of choice will usually be under running of the ulcer (Figs 14.2 and 14.3).
- Because the surgeon knows the ulcer is in the 1st part of the duodenum, he makes a pylorotomy centerd on the pyloric veins of Mayo.
- He identifies the ulcer, its size and accessibility.
- Usually, it is possible to oversow the ulcer (three point ligation) and then close the pylorotomy as a pyloroplasty.
- Occasionally, the surgeon has to extend the pyloric incision to obtain access to the ulcer.
- Occasionally, the ulcer is too big to oversow and a gastrectomy has to be performed.

Answer 1.25: The vagus nerves control the acid secretion of the stomach. At the abdominal level (at the hiatus), there are usually one or two anterior trunks and a single posterior trunk. Division of these main 'trunks' is called a truncal vagotomy.

The nerves which come off the main trunk to specifically supply the acid secreting part of the stomach are called the nerves of Latarjet. Division of only these nerves is called a highly selective vagotomy (HSV) or a proximal gastric vagotomy (PGV)—it has the advantage of leaving the non-secretary (motor) functions of the vagus intact and allows a

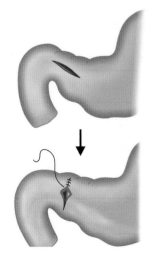

Fig. 14.2 Pylorotomy (longitudinal) closed as pyloroplasty (transverse)

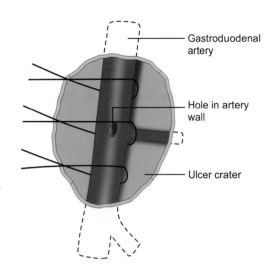

Fig. 14.3 Three point ligation of bleeding duodenal ulcer

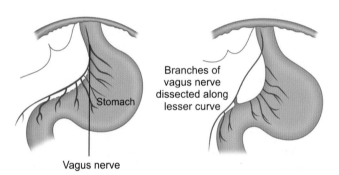

Fig. 14.4 Highly selective vagotomy (HSV) sometimes called proximal gastric vagotomy (PGV)

pyloroplasty or gastroenterostomy to be avoided (when the operation is planned or non-emergency).

The operation of HSV is illustrated in Figure 14.4.

Answer 1.26: No. With the advent of medical blockade of acid secretion by H_2 antagonists and proton-pump inhibitors, vagotomy is now rarely required. The main indication for vagotomy is failure of medical treatment to heal an ulcer—this is uncommon.

Answer 2.1:
1. Stabilize in casualty—oxygen mask, IV line, urinary catheter, continuous monitor, CVP.
2. Send-off urgent bloods for FBC, U and Es, clotting screen and X-match 4 packs of packed cells.
3. Admit to HDU for observation.
4. Inform senior and arrange urgent upper GI endoscopy.

Answer 2.2: Esophageal varices. No active bleeding.

Answer 2.3:
- Do nothing, or
- Injection of varices, or
- Banding of varices.

Answer 2.4: This is done via the endoscope using a long needle inserted through the instrument channel. Paravariceal injection is usually carried out first followed by intravariceal. Usually, use either ethanolamine oleate (5%) or sodium tetradecyl sulfate—same as is used in injection of varicose veins.

Answer 2.5: Institute medical therapy:
- Vasopressin (0.4 units/min for 24 hours or 20 units in 100 mL 5% dextrose over 20 min) usually combined with oral GTN tablets to reduce cardiac side effects.
- *IV somatostatin,* reduces the splanchnic and hepatic blood flow: loading bolus of 250 µg then 250 µg/hr IV infusion.
- Propanolol—decreases the portal pressure.
- Oral lactulose—eliminates old blood from the GI tract and helps to prevent encephalopathy.
- All patients with variceal bleeding and cirrhosis should have antibiotic prophylaxis with ciprofloxacin 1 g/day/orally/7 days.

Answer 2.6: The Sengstaken tube has three lumens—one for blowing up the esophageal balloon, one for the gastric balloon and one for gastric aspiration. The tube is better placed with the patient sedated and with throat local anesthetic spray or if the patient is stuporose or comatose, they should be intubated to protect the airway from aspiration. The Sengstaken tube has now been largely replaced by the Minnesota tube which has an additional lumen for saliva aspiration.

The problems are pressure erosion from the tube at esophageal level (the balloons have to be deflated and inflated regularly to avoid this—5 minutes every 6 hours) and aspiration of esophageal saliva.

It is generally regarded as a temporary measure to control hemorrhage prior to more definitive treatment or while the patient is transferred to a specialist center.

Procedure:
The tube is stored in a refrigerator which makes it less pliable and easier to insert. The balloons are checked for leaks and then completely deflated. The nose and throat are sprayed with local anesthetic. If the patient cooperates the tube can be put down the nose but usually it is put down the mouth with the patient on their side.

The tube is advanced 60 cm and the gastric balloon filled with 150–200 mL water or air and then drawn back until it holds at the cardia. The esophageal balloon is then inflated with air to approx 40 mm Hg (use sphygmomanometer) while an assistant holds the tube in place.

The tube is secured with tape. The stomach is aspirated hourly through the main lumen to check for continued bleeding. The esophageal balloon is deflated for 5 minutes every 6 hours. The tube is not usually left in place for more than 24 hours.

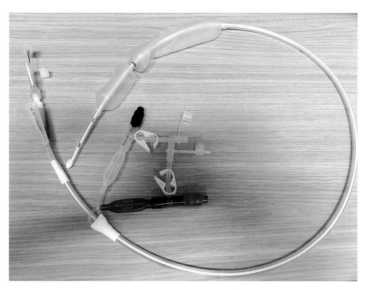

Fig. 14.6 Sengstaken Blakemore tube

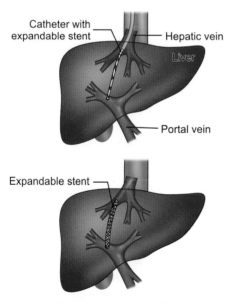

Fig. 14.7 TIPSS procedure

Flow chart 14.1 Management of bleeding esophageal varices

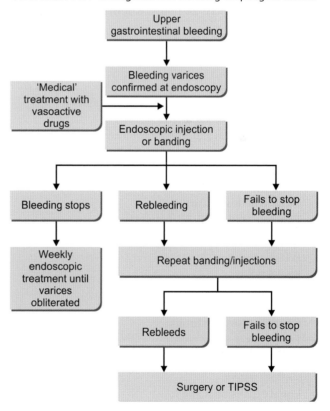

Answer 2.7:
- Portocaval shunt
- Gastric/esophageal transaction
- Devascularization of the stomach.

As an undergraduate, you do not need to know the details of these operations.

Answer 2.8: In centers where the expertise is available they have been replaced by:

Transjugular Intrahepatic Porto Systemic Shunt (TIPSS).

Answer 2.9: This is the creation of an artificial shunt between the portal vein and hepatic vein. The effect is to decrease the effective vascular resistance of the liver and lower the portal venous pressure.

TIPSS is carried out as an endovascular procedure by an interventional radiologist (see Fig. 14.7).

Answer 2.10: Flow chart 14.1

TUTORIAL 15: Irreducible Scrotal Swelling

CLINICAL SCENARIO

Answer 1.1:
- Who told you it was a heart attack?
- Were you in hospital and for how long?
- What investigations did you have done?
- Did you have coronary angiograms? (explain)
- Do you have chest pain now?
- Do you have shortness of breath, palpitations or ankle swelling?
- What medications are you on?

Answer 1.2:
- How long have you had it?
- Do you wheeze or have asthma?
- Are you short of breath?
- Do you bring up sputum or phlegm and what color is it?
- Is there any blood in the sputum?

Answer 1.3: A 68-year-old man, known hypertensive with a groin swelling for 5 years which has become painful and irreducible in the last 24 hours. Known history of MI and chronic cough.

Answer 1.4:
General:
- Conscious level
- Whether in any distress—pain or respiratory
- Query anemic or jaundiced
- Hydration status and whether well nourished
- Query cyanosed
- Any mucous membrane abnormality/intraoral pathology
- Oral hygiene and dentition
- Signs in hands and arms
- Vital signs pulse/BP/RR/temperature.

Cardiovascular system:
- JVP
- Radial pulse
- Apex beat
- Heart sounds
- Carotid pulses and bruits
- Leg pulses
- Ankle edema.

Respiratory system:
- Equal expansion R and L
- Added sounds.

Abdominal system:
- *Inspection:* Particularly distension and visible peristalsis
- Palpation
- Percussion

- *Auscultation:* Particularly obstructive bowel sounds
- Examination of groins and external genitalia
- *Rectal examination:* Particularly any prostatic abnormality.

Answer 1.5: Obstructed/irreducible right inguinal hernia.

Answer 1.6: Has had a swelling in groin for 5 years, previously reducible and now irreducible and painful. Findings of scrotal swelling extending into groin that cannot get above it.

Answer 1.7:
1. *Obstructed hernia:*
   - NBM
   - Start IV fluids
   - Take off routine bloods
   - Start on routine readings and input and output chart
   - Ask if he needs analgesia and provide
   - Write up fluid chart, medications and DVT prophylaxis
   - Arrange chest X-ray, erect and supine abdominal films
   - Check Hb and electrolytes results—query urea raised.

2. *History of MI:*
   - Arrange chest X-ray and ECG and look at results, if abnormal inform senior.

3. *Cough:*
   - Check CXR, send off sputum for culture, give spirometer and arrange physiotherapy.

4. *Hypertension:*
   - Note that it is reasonable, if elevated see, if he has taken his atenolol that day. Remember to tell anesthetist he is hypertensive and write-up antihypertensives postoperatively.

5. *Prostate:*
   - Make sure that he is passing urine postoperatively (if he is not catheterized).

6. Ring your Specialist Registrar; tell him you have a patient admitted with an obstructed hernia who is likely to need surgery. Inform him that he has hypertension, PH of MI and probably has COPD. You have done the investigations and would he/she come and look at him as soon as possible.

7. Speak to the patient and, if possible, the relatives.

Answer 1.8: Tell the anesthetist that there is a 68-year-old man who needs surgery for an obstructed hernia. He is not a very good risk because he has myocardial disease, probable COPD and hypertension. You have done the investigations and would she/he come and look at him as soon as possible.

Answer 1.9: Tell him that he has a hernia which has become 'stuck' and that he will need this to be operated on. Say that the specialist and the anesthetist will be coming to see him. Ask if he has any questions? Ask if he would like you to speak with his relatives?

Answer 1.10: I am the surgical house officer who is looking after you. Do you know what is wrong with you? You have a hernia on the right side which has become stuck and needs an operation. The specialist has asked me to explain this to you and get your consent for the operation. The operation may be done under a general anesthetic and you will be asleep the whole time and will not feel anything, or because of your chest and heart problems the anesthetist may give you what is called a spinal anesthetic and he or she will explain this to you.

The surgeon will make an incision (cut) in your right groin and the surgeon will dissect out your hernia, cut-off the sac and put in a strengthening repair (usually a mesh) to stop it coming back. This is a safe operation but because of your chest and heart problems, we will be keeping a close eye on you to make sure you do not get complications—as regards the hernia repair sometimes you can get a hemorrhage or bleed which may need further surgery, sometimes you can get problems passing urine which we will deal with for you. Occasionally, the wound may get infected. The recurrence rate of the hernia coming back after the operation is about 2–10%. After the operation, you will be able to drink almost straightaway and eat soon after. You may have some pain and we will give you pain killers. You may have a drip (IV line) for a short while. We will keep you on a cardiac monitor for a while and the physiotherapist will help you to cough and deep breathe. You should be able to go home in a day or two and may have to visit your doctor to get the stitches out. You will be seen for follow-up at the outpatient clinic in 2 weeks to make sure everything is as it should be. Do you have any questions? (NB: open repair is described, laparoscopic approach may now be used).

Answer 1.11:
1. Adjust water to comfortable temperature. Rinse your hands and arms. Pump onto hands the antimicrobial solution and wash hands for 30 seconds. Then wash arms up to and just beyond elbows.
2. Pick up the sponge/nail brush, put antimicrobial on brush and scrub nails with brush. Wash under running water.
3. Wash your arms and hands for a further 1 minute, rinse off, put on more antimicrobial and repeat for another 30 seconds and rinse off.
4. Turn off taps and walk to gowning area. Unfold the sterile gown packet. Use the towel to dry off your hands first and then arms. Discard.

5. Grasp the sterile gown by neckline, let it unfold and insert arms. Ask assistant to tie your back tapes.
6. Put on sterile gloves using no direct touch technique.
7. Hand the waist tie strip to your assistant, rotate and fasten waist tie.

Answer 1.12: Groin incision.

Answer 1.13:
1. Reduce the omentum from the sac.
2. Carry out a herniotomy.
3. Carry out a herniorraphy—usually a mesh repair.

Answer 1.14: A spinal anesthetic is when a needle is inserted into the subarachnoid space and local anesthetic introduced—this is done below L2—usually between L3 and L4. The procedure is similar to a lumbar puncture and the needle is correctly placed when there is free aspiration of CSF. A small amount of lidocaine or bupivacaine (2–4 mL) is used. A single injection usually gives 2–3 hours of surgical anesthesia.

Epidural is when the local anesthetic is injected into the epidural space. The level of injection is dictated by the level of block required and can be done from the cervical level to the sacrum (caudal block). More local anesthetic is required than for a spinal so a small catheter is introduced into the epidural space which can be 'topped up'.

Answer 1.15:
Complications of spinal anesthetic:
Common:
1. Postoperative hypotension
2. Itching
3. Urinary retention
4. Headache (postdural puncture).
Rare:
- Nerve damage
    If you want more details of the technique of spinal anesthesia, look at *www.youtube.com/watch?v = LpLlK2XmbVc*
Complications of epidural
Common:
- Hypotension
Uncommon:
    - Local anesthetic toxicity
    - Injection into intrathecal space producing high block
    - Epidural hematoma
    - Look at *https://www.youtube.com/watch?v = nWLQbewSjlg*
With epidural inadvertent intrathecal or intravascular injection of large amounts of drug is possible, producing total spinal blockade and local anesthetic toxicity.

TUTORIAL 16: Inflammatory Bowel Diseases: Ulcerative Colitis and Crohn's Disease

CASE SCENARIOS

Answer 1.1:

- How many times a day do you open your bowels?
- How long have you been opening your bowels like this?
- Do you open your bowels at night?
- Have you felt like you have not emptied your bowels fully when you finish passing stool (tenesmus) or do you ever need to rush to the toilet or have an accident when you need to open your bowels (fecal urgency)?
- What does the stool look like? What color and consistency is it?
- Is there any blood? If so, what color is it, how much is there, is it mixed in or separate to the stool, is it in the pan, is it always there?
- What is your normal bowel habit like?
- Is this the first time you have had diarrhea like this?
- Have you had anything suspicious to eat or has anyone traveling with you had similar symptoms?

Answer 1.2:

- Past history—other medical problems, previous surgery?
- Travel history—where had he been traveling, where had he stayed and what had he eaten?
- Social history:
  - Smoking history (smoking makes Crohn's disease worse. Stopping smoking may actually bring on or worsen UC).
  - Alcohol consumption.
  - Risk factors for hepatitis or HIV such as intravenous drug use, sexuality, high-risk sexual practices (Causes of immunosuppression).
- Family history of IBD (Risk of UC in first degree relative is 5–15%, stronger familial association in Crohn's).
- Systemic enquiry:
  - Any eye problems (uveitis or episcleritis)
  - Any joint problems (large joints or sacroileitis)
  - Any skin problems (erythema nodosum—painful rash on shin).

Answer 1.3:
General:

Eyes—conjunctival pallor, jaundice, red eye
Mouth—ulcers
Hands—clubbing.
Observations—pulse, BP, respiratory rate, temperature

Specific:

Abdomen—Previous scars
Distension
Tenderness/guarding
Bowel sounds.
Rectal examination—Skin tags
Fistula
Blood on glove.
Skin: Erythema nodosum (painful red raised lesion on the shin)
Pyoderma gangrenosum (ulcer with red or blue overhanging edge).

Answer 1.4:
1. Inflammatory bowel disease (UC or less likely Crohn's)
2. Infection (gastroenteritis).

An acute flare up of ulcerative colitis is the most likely cause, especially given the subacute presentation and history of stopping smoking. Crohn's tends to present with a longer history of pain and diarrhea (as we shall see in the next case!) so is less likely but this could be colonic Crohn's.

Infection is the other major differential but the 3- month history does not fit. Possible infections include *Campylobacter*, *Shigella*, *Salmonella*, *E. coli*, amebic dysentery, CMV (if immunocompromised) or schistosomiasis.

Ischemic colitis would have to be considered, if the patient was older with a cardiovascular risk profile.

Irritable bowel syndrome or a malabsorptive condition such as celiac disease would not account for the rectal bleeding or physical signs.

Answer 1.5:
1. Bloods—full blood count, renal function, inflammatory markers (ESR +/− CRP), liver function tests, coagulation profile.
2. Stool cultures X3 (including fresh stool microscopy).
3. Urgent plain abdominal X- ray.

Answer 1.6: Truelove and Witt criteria help you decide how severe the attack of UC is. Severe disease is characterized by:
- > 6 motions per day
- Large amount of rectal bleeding
- Temperature >37.8
- Pulse rate >90
- Hemoglobin <10.5 g/dL
- ESR > 30 mm/hour.

Features of a severe attack suggest a complication such as toxic dilatation (toxic megacolon) or perforation is more likely to occur and that the patient is more likely to need surgery. The plain abdominal X-ray will tell you:
- How extensive the disease is [how much of the colon is affected—affected colon has a thickened wall due to edema (thumb-printing) and does not contain feces].

- Whether there is toxic dilatation (suggested by dilated bowel greater than 6 cm in diameter).

Answer 1.7:
1. Intravenous fluids—he is tachycardic and likely to be dehydrated.
2. Intravenous hydrocortisone—100 mg IV qds.
3. Rectal steroids, e.g. prednisolone enemas twice daily.
4. Thromboprophylaxis with LMWH.
5. He will require close monitoring and observation with twice daily clinical examination and daily full blood count, electrolytes, CRP and abdominal X-ray until his clinical condition has improved.

Answer 1.8: If after 3 days of medical treatment the stool frequency is > 8/day, or if the frequency is 3–8/day with a CRP over 45, the patient has an 85% chance of requiring colectomy (Travis' rule). This is described as a failure to respond to medical therapy, so this patient is likely to need a subtotal colectomy (removal of the entire colon and formation of an ileostomy). Other medical options such as treatment with intravenous cyclosporin or a biologic anti-TNF-α agent (such as infliximab) are options with specialist gastroenterologist involvement.

If any of the following had been present, more urgent surgery would have been indicated:
- Toxic dilatation
- Perforation
- Massive hemorrhage.

Answer 1.9: Treatment of mild-to-moderate ulcerative colitis should be based on an assessment of the severity and extent of the colitis. This is done by performing a flexible sigmoidoscopy or colonoscopy. If the colitis only affects the rectum (also called proctitis) or the distal sigmoid, topical treatment with suppositories and enemata should be adequate. If the disease is more extensive, then systemic treatment will be required. Remember UC always starts at the rectum and spreads proximally to the cecum. Treatment of mild-to-moderate UC therefore consists of:
1. Controlling the current flare with oral steroids and high dose oral 5-ASA (such as mesalazine).
2. Topical application of 5-ASA preparation (or a topical steroid), if the colitis is confined to the distal colon.
3. Once the flare has subsided, gradually reduction of the steroid dose and conversion to maintenance treatment with an oral 5-ASA preparation to prevent relapse.
4. Considering assessment of the colon using colonoscopy to survey for cancer, if the patient has had pancolonic UC for more than 8–10 years (Patients with UC affecting the whole colon have an increased risk of colorectal cancer

after 10 years). The risk of colorectal cancer is even higher, if primary sclerosing cholangitis is also present.

Answer 1.10a: The whole of the colon, rectum and anal canal are removed. An endileostomy is made in the right iliac fossa (see Fig. 16.1).

Answer 1.10b: The whole of the colon and rectum are removed but the anal canal is left in place. The terminal ileum is then formed into a pouch which is attached (usually by stapling) to the top end of the anal canal. In most cases, the operation is covered by a loop ileostomy proximal to the pouch. This is closed about 3 months later and the GI tract is then back in continuity (see Fig. 16.2).

Answer 1.10c: Proctocolectomy and pouch anastomosis is now regarded as the 'gold standard' operation for patients whose UC is severe enough to warrant excision of the colon and rectum.

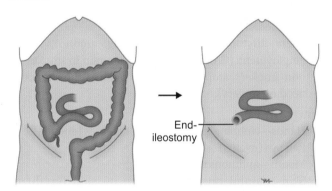

Fig. 16.1 Panproctocolectomy

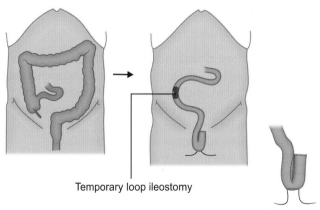

Fig. 16.2 Panproctocolectomy and ileoanal pouch

The main indications are:
1. Severe chronic disease not responsive to medical therapy.
2. Long-standing disease with dysplasia of the mucosa on colonoscopy biopsies.

3   Operable large bowel malignancy developing in the large bowel of a patient with UC.

4.   In selected patients with familial adenomatous polyposis—no connection with UC but included so you are aware this is also the operation of choice for this disease.

Note: Patients who require urgent surgery for severe extensive ulcerative colitis (e.g. toxic megacolon) usually have a subtotal colectomy performed which is converted to an ileoanal pouch when the patient is fit and well again.

Answer 2.1:

• Perianal symptom such as pain or discharge from a fistula.

• Relationship of symptoms to diet.

• Extra-GI manifestations of IBD—any eye, skin or joint problems?

• Family history (44% concordance in monozygotic twins, one affected parent has a 10–20% chance of having an affected child).

• Past medical history.

• Social history including smoking, alcohol, stress, employment. (Crohn's is twice as common in smokers as non-smokers, stopping smoking reduces the chance of needing surgery).

Answer 2.2:

• Hands—clubbing, pallor of palmar creases (anemia).

• Red eye (uveitis).

• Mouth—aphthous ulcers.

• Skin—painful raised red lesion on shin (erythema nodosum, bluish edged ulcer—pyoderma gangrenosum).

• Joints—large joint arthritis or sacroileitis.

  Extra-GI manifestations occur in up to 30% of patients with Crohn's.

Answer 2.3:

1.   Inflammatory bowel disease—Crohn's disease is a definite possibility given the presence of abdominal pain, diarrhea, and weight loss and perianal disease. Ulcerative colitis is less likely in the absence of rectal bleeding.

2.   Irritable bowel syndrome.

3.   Malabsorptive conditions such as celiac disease.

4.   Chronic GI infection such as giardiasis.

5.   Intestinal TB.

6.   *Yersinia enterocolitis*—cause an ileitis which can be confused with terminal ileal Crohn's.

Answer 2.4a: Mouth to anus, the whole of the GI tract can be affected by Crohn's disease. This is in direct contrast to UC which only affects the colon and rectum. In addition, Crohn's disease may have 'skip lesions'. These are patches of inflammation throughout the bowel with normal mucosa in between. UC is always continuous from the rectum proximally.

Answer 2.4b: The most common sites affected by Crohn's disease are:

• Small bowel—particularly, the terminal ileum. This leads to the classical symptoms of abdominal pain, diarrhea and weight loss. Chronic inflammation in the small bowel may lead to fibrosis and stricture formation. This in turn may lead to symptoms of subacute obstruction such as abdominal pain, distension and vomiting.

• Colon—Crohn's colitis tends to cause worse diarrhea than small bowel disease. Rectal bleeding is less common than in UC. The rectum is sometimes spared.

• Perianal disease—fistulae and recurrent abscesses may be features of perianal Crohn's. Perianal disease is more likely, if both the colon and the ileum are affected as well.

  Roughly 1/3rd of patients with Crohn's have disease only affecting the terminal ileum, 1/3rd have disease confined to the colon and 1/3rd have ileocolonic disease. Perianal disease may occur in any group or in isolation but is more common in ileocolonic disease.

Answer 2.5:

• Bloods—full blood count, urea and electrolytes, liver function tests, inflammatory markers (CRP or ESR).

• Stool culture and microscopy.

• Colonoscopy with terminal ileum intubation and biopsy (to look for evidence of colonic or terminal ileal involvement and provide a biopsy for confirmation of the diagnosis).

• Small bowel follow through (an NG tube is passed to 4th part of duodenum and barium instilled via the tube to image the small bowel with a series of X-rays). Ulceration in the small bowel may be described as 'cobblestoning' and 'rose-thorn ulcers'. Strictures and fistulae may also be demonstrated by this method. Increasingly small bowel MRI studies may replace barium imaging.

• CT scan—Indicated, if an inflammatory mass or intra-abdominal abscess is suspected.

  Investigations are aimed at assessing the extent and the severity of the affected GI tract.

Answer 2.6: Table 16.1

Table 16.1 Histological changes of ulcerative colitis and Crohn's disease		
	Ulcerative colitis	*Crohn's disease*
Distribution	Mucosal only	Transmural
Granuloma	Absent	Diagnostic
Crypts	Distorted	Not distorted
Goblet cell depletion	Common in active disease	No distortion
Cellular infiltrate	Polymorphs	Lymphocytes

(This table is part of the larger table comparing UC and Crohn's Table 16.2).

Answer 2.7: You could ask her about her:

Ideas, Concerns and Expectations (ICE)

It may well be that she has some pre-conceived ideas about Crohn's disease based on what she has read about, seen on the TV or looked up on the internet. It can be a very 'scary' disease. She may be concerned she will need an operation or need a stoma bag. Body image issues can be a major concern. She may be worried about how it will affect her relationships and her chances of having children. She may have a friend or a family member who has had a bad experience with Crohn's disease. She may be worried how it will affect her ability to work or to socialize or play sport.

On the other hand, she may be relieved that the cause of her symptoms has finally been found and she may be able to begin treatment to get better.

You should explore her ideas and concerns with empathy and try to reassure her when possible. It may help to tell her that medications are usually enough to keep the disease under control. Surgery may be required but may improve her quality of life. It is more than likely that she will be able to work, socialize and have children as normal. It is helpful to tell her not to believe all she reads on the internet. Point her in the direction of reputable websites and give her information about patient support groups if possible.

There may be a specialist IBD nurse available to put her in touch with. Specialist nurses are very good at managing chronic diseases such as IBD and particularly in providing support to patients. She is at the beginning of a lifelong journey with a chronic disease. The doctor-patient relationship is crucial to effective management of her condition so it is important to develop a trusting, open and honest relationship with the patient at this point.

Finally, if she asks any questions you do not know the answer to, offer to talk to your Consultant to find out.

Answer 2.8:

Medical Treatment

- Steroids—oral prednisolone is used to bring a flare up under control. The dose is then gradually reduced. IV steroids may be needed for a severe flare.
- Once the flare is under control, 5-ASA medications (e.g. mesalazine) may help to keep colonic disease under control but does not prevent small bowel disease relapsing.
- If a patient has a second flare requiring steroids within a year, it may be necessary to start an immunosuppressive medication. The options are:

  Azathioprine: The most commonly used immuno-suppressant in Crohn's. Side effects include pancreatitis, abnormal LFTs, neutropenia and a possible risk of lymphoma with long-term use. Regular monitoring of FBC and LFTs are therefore mandatory.

  Methotrexate: Less frequently used but may help, if relapse occurs despite azathioprine. Side effects include liver toxicity, neutropenia and it is teratogenic so contraception is an important consideration.

- Smoking cessation is very important.
- Increasingly, biologic agents such as Infliximab (an anti-TNF-α agent) are being used in Crohn's, both to induce and maintain remission. It is important to exclude active infection and TB before using an anti-TNFα agent. Side effects include immunosuppression and overwhelming infection. There is no long-term safety data (over 10 years) for these medications.

Surgical Treatment

Surgical intervention is indicated, if:

- The flare of Crohn's is not settling with medical therapy. A limited ileal resection or limited right hemicolectomy for terminal ileal disease can be very effective.
- Fistulae and abscesses and small bowel strictures often require surgical intervention.

Answer 2.9:

- Small bowel Crohn's disease.
- Figure 16.3 shows the typical 'cobblestone' appearance of Crohn's disease.

  Figure 16.4 shows, at laparotomy, the thickened, inflamed, 'hosepipe' like appearance of small bowel Crohn's disease which occurs together with mesenteric fat enhancement and lymph node enlargement (not shown).

Answer 2.10:

Figure 16.5A shows large, hypertrophied, edematous perianal skin tags.

Figure 16.5B shows edematous skin tags and an external fistula opening at 1 o'clock.

Figure 16.5C shows peri-anal scaring and multiple fistulae. The red rubber band is called a seton and is sometimes used in the management of complex fistulae.

The above are all features of perianal Crohn's disease. Remember that fissure and ulcers also occur in the Crohn's perineum—sometimes these are relatively painless and may have a blue coloration.

Be careful about the diagnosis as HIV disease can present with perianal ulcers and fissures.

Answer 2.11: These are the colonoscopic changes of colitis—loss of normal vessel pattern of the mucosa; contact bleeding from the colonoscope indicating mucosal inflammation; reddening of the mucosa with multiple superficial ulcerations.

In the Western world, these would almost certainly represent ulcerative colitis or less likely Crohn's disease. Remember in the Far East and Africa, these changes can occur in infective/protozoan colitides, e.g amebiasis/schistosomiasis/giardiasis.

TUTORIAL 17: Multiple Trauma

CASE SCENARIO

Answer 1.1:

1. Decide with the triage nurses who will be responsible for which patient.
2. Check with the triage nurses that the "bays" are allocated and all equipment and staff ready.
3. Send a message to trauma team and A and E Consultant informing them about imminent patient arrivals and requesting their presence as soon as possible.

Answer 1.2:

1. Speak to the patient; ask him his name and where he has pain, i.e. quick assessment of mental status.
2. Perform a quick primary survey.
3. As you do this, listen to the paramedics telling you what has happened and what action they have taken.

Answer 1.3: From your primary survey (ABCDE), you prioritize

1. The hypovolemia—probably due to blood loss from his limb fracture and possibly the chest injury
   - Insert a second IV line
   - Blood to be sent for FBC/U and Es/group and X-match
   - 500 mL gelofusine to be run in down the as quickly as possible.
2. The chest injury is the next most immediate problem and you proceed to examine his chest in detail.

Answer 1.4: Surgical emphysema is air in the subcutaneous tissues usually of the chest or abdominal wall.

Its presence is detected by running the fingers over the area and feeling a 'crackling' like crushing eggshells.

Answer 1.5: Fractured ribs with either a pneumothorax or hemothorax on the left side.

Answer 1.6: Insert a chest drain into the left side 'safe triangle'.

5th intercostal space, anterior auxiliary line, immediately above the rib below.

Answer 1.7:

Signs: Hyper-resonance of chest wall on affected side
Diminished breath sounds on affected side
Tracheal deviation towards contralateral side
Cyanosis
Hypotension.

This is a life-threatening condition. Put patient on 100% oxygen and perform immediate needle decompression. Then reassess the patient and prepare to inset a formal chest drain.

Needle decompression:

- Insert a large bore (14 or 16 gauge) IV needle into the second intercostal space just superior to the 3rd rib in the mid-clavicular line (1–2 cm lateral to sternal edge).

- Remove stylet. Listen for the hissing sound of escaping gas.
- Tape needle in place and put a flutter valve over the end.

Answer 1.8:

1. The Anesthetist and the Orthopedic Surgeon agree that the patient is stable enough for a SECONDARY SURVEY.
2. The Anesthetist arranges for blood gases and a chest X-ray.

Answer 1.9: Detailed examination of the limb including assessment of the vascularity and neurological status (sensory and motor).

Answer 1.10:

1. Intravenous antibiotics—cephalosporin and metronidazole.
2. Tetanus prophylaxis.
3. Irrigation of wound in A and E: Sterile dressing; leg splint.
4. *X-ray:* 2 views 2 legs.

Answer 1.11:

1. Wound debridement under general anesthesia should be carried out within 6 hours.
2. Fractures treated by either internal fixation or external fixation depending on type of fracture.

Answer 1.12: The primary survey should be preceded by a quick history from the patient, if possible, but if not from the paramedics or witnesses.

You need to know:

1. When the accident occurred.
2. Type of accident (e.g. head on car crash, seat belts).
3. Conscious level of the patient when ambulance crew arrived and any changes.
4. Blood loss at accident scene.
5. Any drugs, fluids, treatment given at scene of accident.
6. If available, previous past medical history/drugs/allergies of patient.

Some of this information will already have been phoned in by the ambulance crew. In a major trauma situation, the other information can be listened to as you go about your primary survey.

The primary survey is designed to assess and institute treatment for the IMMEDIATE life-threatening problems. It is based on the well known mnemonic ABCDE:

A: Is the AIRWAY obstructed?
   - Remove any oropharyngeal obstructions—dentures/blood/vomit.
B: Is the patient BREATHING spontaneously and adequately ventilated?
   - If no—needs immediate intubation
   - If severe facial/jaw injuries may need immediate cricothyroidotomy

- Open chest wounds need covering
- Tension pneumothorax immediate chest needle/drain
- Neck collar.

C: State of CIRCULATION is assessed by pulse/BP/cyanosis/peripheral circulation:

- Control any obvious external hemorrhage by pressure dressing
- Large bore IV lines (X2, if deemed necessary) + immediate fluid replacement—crystalloid/colloid/unmatched O negative blood
- Rarely aspiration cardiac tamponade
- Cardiac massage in case of arrest.

(If circulation compromised will need urinary catheter once primary survey and immediate treatment instituted.)

D: DISABILITY of central nervous system—assess level of consciousness by quick Glasgow coma score.
Use Glasgow Coma Scale (score) (Table 17.1).

Table 17.1 Glasgow coma score					
Eye opening		*Verbal response*		*Motor response*	
Spontaneous	4	Orientated	5	Obeys command	6
To speech	3	Confused	4	Localizes pain	5
To pain	2	Inappropriate words	3	Flexion to pain	4
None	1	Incomprehensible words	2	Extension to pain	2
		None	1	None	1
Total Score = 15					
Minor head injury score = 13–15; Moderate HI = 9–12; Severe <8					

What you actually do:

1. Eyes: *Look at patient's eyes:* are they spontaneously open? If not ask him to open and close his eyes (shout), if does not, rub his sternum (pain). See if opens his eyes.
2. Verbal response: Shout at him, and ask him if he knows where he is and his name. Note his response—answers correctly/answers but in confused manner/answers in a confused manner wrongly/answers in "gobble de gook".
3. Motor response:
   - Shout at him and ask him to move arms or legs.
   - See, if responds appropriately.
   - If not, pinch his arm or leg, ask if this hurts him and see if he responds to this by either flexing it (withdraws leg) or extending it.

E: EXPOSURE: Remove all of clothing and examine quickly from 'head-to-toe' for other life-threatening injuries.
With nursing help turn the patient with head supported to EXAMINE THE BACK.

Answer 1.13: The major problem seems to be likely intra-abdominal bleeding (because of the hypotension and evidence of blunt trauma to abdomen with abdominal tenderness).

1. You ask the nurse to put a gauze pad on the bleeding scalp laceration and keep pressure on it.
2. Ask nurse to put a neck collar on (if not done by paramedics) and put on facemask with 100% oxygen.
3. You put a large bore cannula into the cubital fossa and start 500 mL Hartmann's running in. You ask the nurse to put a line in the other arm.
4. As you put the line in take off bloods for FBC/bioprofile/group and X-match 4 pints/clotting screen.

Answer 1.14: The secondary survey is carried out after the IMMEDIATE life-threatening injuries have received initial management. Sometimes, progression of the primary survey injuries will take precedence over the secondary survey

e.g. Deteriorating head injury
Uncontrollable intrathoracic bleeding
Non-responsive (to fluid) suspected intra-abdominal injury

The secondary survey is a more detailed head-to-toe examination to identify and assess signs of serious head/spine/chest/abdominal/pelvic/limb injuries.
Systematic examination is carried out to identify:

Head and Neck:
- Lacerations
- Depressed fractures
- Facial and jaw injuries
- Otorrhea/rhinorrhea
- Pupil size and responsiveness
- Assessment of neck injury

Chest:
- Penetrating injuries (back + front)
- Abrasions/bruising
- Crepitus/tenderness ?fracture ribs
- Rate and pattern of respiration/cyanosis
- Symmetry of chest movements
- Mediastinal shift
- Percussion and auscultation of chest (differences)

Abdomen:
- External injuries
- Distension by gas or fluid
- Increase in abdominal girth
- Tenderness
- Palpable bladder
- Pelvic fracture
- Bleeding from the urethral meatus

Limbs:
- Neurovascular status of both limbs
- Lacerations
- Deformities
- Soft tissue swellings
- Fractures and dislocations.

(After *Burkitt and Quick:* Preliminary Hospital Management of the Multiple and Serious Injuries in Essential Surgery, 3rd edn, Harcourt Health Sciences)

Answer 1.15: The surgeon thinks the lady has intra-abdominal bleeding from blunt trauma.

Answer 1.16: He tells the nurse to start a bag of haemaccel and run it in fast and to tell him if it increases her blood pressure.

He tells another nurse to catheterize the patient and make sure the input and output charts are being completed (IV fluid in/urine out).

He tells the nurses to get the Anesthetist and Neurosurgical Registrar to look at the patient as soon as possible and to warn the emergency theater she may be coming down for a laparotomy soon.

Answer 1.17: In the HDU, the patient is connected to a 'dinamap' so has continuous measurement of pulse/BP/CVP/ECG and Oxygen saturation.

The Anesthetist decides an arterial line is not necessary.

The nurses start an input-output chart and put a urimeter on the bladder catheter.

The Anesthetist writes up the fluid chart.

Answer 1.18: Following splenectomy the patient has a lifelong susceptibility to overwhelming postsplenectomy sepsis and should receive immediately postoperatively the following prophylaxis:

1. Pneumococcal vaccine (boost 5 yearly).
2. *Haemophilus* type B vaccine.
3. Meningococcal group C conjugate vaccine unless previously immunized.
4. Phenoxymethyl penicillin IM and then orally (lifelong) penicillin V 250–500 mg daily.
5. The patient should be given written information about the effects of splenectomy and carry a card or wear a bracelet to alert health professionals.
6. The patient should be educated about the risks of overseas travel (malaria risk).
7. The patient should keep a course of broad-spectrum antibiotics available and start immediately, if have fever or infection.
8. The patient should be advised to have yearly influenza vaccination.
9. Vaccination and revaccination status should be clearly explained to patient and documented with GP.

Note: These are the 2002 updates of the NHS Clinical Guidelines.

Do not forget anti-DVT prophylaxis with LMWH and stockings.

Answer 1.19:
1. Routine ward round questions and examination of the patient to ensure, they are not developing a complication. *General:*
   Chest infection/UTI/DVT/wound infection.
   Examine the routine charts; pulse/BP/RR/temperature
   Examine chest daily/examine legs daily/look at wound when dressing changed. Check wound drain, if present.
2. Check the input and output charts to make sure these are balanced.
3. Check the blood results (FBC/bioprofile). *Specific to splenectomy:*
4. Check platelet count on alternate days—a small percentage of postsplenectomy patients develop thrombocytosis.
5. Check drain, if present—may damage tail of pancreas during splenectomy and develop pancreatic fistula.

Answer 1.20: There is a linear fracture of the parietal bone.

Answer 1.21: His Glasgow Coma Score and pupillary responses are recorded hourly.

Answer 1.22: The CT suggests R extradural hematoma.

Answer 1.23: (see Module 1, Tutorial 16)
a. Most commonly due to middle meningeal artery laceration due to a fracture of parietal or temporal bone (MVA/Fall/sporting injury).
b. Usually following head injury with or without loss of consciousness or drowsiness. Only 30% have the classic lucid interval (hours to days) followed by progressive headache, vomiting, confusion, fits.
   Signs: Hemiparesis, brisk reflexes and upgoing plantars
   Deepening coma, spastic paresis, irregular breathing
   Hypertension, bradycardia
   Ipsilateral pupil dilatation = late
c. *The management:*
   1. Immediate surgical evacuation or
   2. If the lesion is small and patient in good neurosurgical condition may manage conservatively with frequent neurological examinations.

Two attributes are essential in an outstanding doctor. First you must be knowledgeable, skilled and up-to-date and secondly you must be able to talk to patients and inspire trust and confidence. Remember, medicine is not really about money, self esteem or privilege, it is about caring and, in particular, caring about patients.

– Peter Lee

Useful Protocols

- *Surgical History*
- *Gastrointestinal/Abdominal Examination*
- *Problem-based History and Examination*
- *Thyroid/Neck Examination*
- *Inguinal Hernia Examination*

- *Male Genitalia/Scrotal Examination*
- *Breast Examination*
- *Lump or Bump Examination*
- *Examination of a Skin Ulcer*
- *Physical Examination of a Vascular Patient*

SURGICAL HISTORY

The central theme of Module 1 is History Taking and Physical Examination. Early in your course, you will have been introduced into the 'art' of taking history and examining a patient (be this with actors, simulation or 'real' patients). This book is not intended to replace the many excellent texts on the techniques of the subject. However, an accurate history and complete physical examination are the basis of all clinical medicine. To do this you must have a defined protocol on which to base your routine approach to the patient. This protocol must be short, complete, succinct and easily learned. At Penang Medical College, the surgical students were obliged to learn the protocols by heart (rote learning !!—so frowned upon by the medical educationalist) and stand up and repeat them out loud! Brain washing, but many students continued to use the 'surgical protocols' as the basis for their history and examination in all branches of their medical training and afterwards into their medical career.

So, as the first 'task' of this course write down the protocols you have been taught, i.e. the questions, you will routinely ask and the physical examination steps, you will routinely perform to elicit a general surgical history and examination of the gastrointestinal tract/abdomen.

You may find this difficult to do—do not worry, just learn the ones provided below—they work—and will enable you to approach even your first patient with some confidence.

As you become more experienced do not stop using the protocols, they mean

- You can perform an adequate history and examination in a short time (e.g. when you are a house officer with 7 acute admissions to see or a consultant with 15 new patients to see at the OP clinic.
- You will not omit a vital piece of information important to the patient's surgical management, even at times of severe stress.

SURGICAL HISTORY: SUGGESTED PROTOCOL

Name:		Age:	Occupation:

Presenting complaint(s): Duration of each

History of presenting complaints:

Past medical history: Serious illnesses/operations/ever been in hospital/had anesthetic, if so any problems—diabetes/jaundice/heart attack/high BP/stroke/Rh-Fever/TB

Family history: Mother died of, father died of ? brothers/sisters; Any family illness

Social history: Married?, children?, smoke, drink, home/financial circumstances diet, travel

Review of systems:

CVS:	Chest pain	**RS:**	SOB/asthma
	SOB		Cough
	Palpitations		Sputum +/– blood
	Ankle swelling		Fever/night cough

Abdominal:	Difficulty in swallowing	**GUS:**	Frequency
	Nausea/vomiting +/- blood		Dysuria
	Heartburn/acid reflux		Nocturia
	Indigestion/abdo pain/abdo distention		Hematuria
	Change in bowel habit +/– blood		Periods/pregnancies
	Appetite		Postmenopausal bleeding
	Weight loss		(+ if indicated: History of sexual contact)
CNS:	Headaches	***MS:**	Painful//stiff/swollen joints
	Fits/blackouts/dizziness		Neck/back pain
	Weakness/numbness/tingling		Fingers white/blue in cold
	Stroke/sleep well/depressed		
Hemo:	Bruise easily	**Endocrine:**	Swelling in neck
	Difficulty stopping bleeding		Hands tremble
	Lumps under arms, in neck, groins		Prefer hot/cold weather
	Clots in legs/lungs: DVT/PE		Increased sweating/fatigue
			Change in appearance/voice
?Drugs?Medications		**Allergies**	

*Musculoskeletal system

GASTROINTESTINAL/ABDOMINAL EXAMINATION—SUGGESTED PROTOCOL

GENERAL: Write or say (if presenting). The patient is or has:

Face:	• Alert, conscious and orientated	(or otherwise)
	• Not in obvious distress	(or in pain, sweating, tachypneic)
	• Well nourished	(or cachexic/malnourished)
	• Well hydrated	(dehydrated—sunken eyes)
	• Not obviously clinically anemic	(pallor of conjunctivae)
	• Not obviously jaundiced	(sclera)
Mouth:	• No abnormality of mouth	(or otherwise, e.g. angular stomatitis)
	• No abnormality of lips	(or otherwise, e.g. central cyanosis)
	• No intraoral pathology	(or otherwise: poor hygiene)
	• Dentition is good	(teeth decay)
Hands/Arms:	• No obvious abnormality of fingernails	(or otherwise: clubbing, koilonychia)
	• No palmar crease pallor	
	• No palmar erythema	
	• Palms are moist	
	• No abnormality of arms	(scratch marks, muscle wasting)
	• No other signs of liver failure	(liver flap)
Vital signs:	Pulse, BP, RR, temperature/peripheral perfusion	
Neck:	No visible or palpable neck swellings or lymph nodes	
Chest:	No obvious abnormality of chest wall	(spider nevi, gynecomastia)
SPECIFIC: Abdomen:	Write or say (if presenting)	
Inspection:	Moving normally with respiration	(or otherwise-held rigid)
	Not distended	(or otherwise)
	No visible skin changes or scars	(jaundiced/bruising/midline scar)
	No visible mass/veins/pulsations	(or otherwise; mass present/caput medusa)
	Normal umbilicus	(everted umbilicus/hernia)
Palpation:	Presence or absence of tenderness/guarding/rebound organomegaly	
Percussion:	Presence or absence of dullness/ascites	

Auscultation:	Bowel sounds—normal/abnormal; absent/high-pitched
Groins and hernia orifices:	Normal
External genitalia:	Normal
Rectal examination, if indicated	**Vaginal examination, if indicated**

Legs: Normal (or otherwise: pitting edema)

Then examination of any other specific system, the history may indicate in the presenting symptoms, e.g. neurological/musculoskeletal

Followed by basic routine examination of the other systems:

- Cardiovascular system
- Respiratory system
- Musculoskeletal system
- Neurological system

PROTOCOL FOR PROBLEM-BASED HISTORY AND EXAMINATION

Once you have gained the necessary knowledge, all your histories and examinations should be problem based, i.e. once you have made your diagnosis or differential diagnosis you should make a list of the patient's problems you have elicited from the history and examination. Equally important is to write opposite each problem what you propose to do about it (and then do it!). Usually, 'Problem 1' will be to attempt to confirm your diagnosis.

So, the complete scheme will be:

History (as per protocol + added questions as you formulate a diagnosis)	THINK
Summary (key points only-2 lines maximum)	THINK
Examination (protocol led but looking specifically for signs, which fit with your evolving diagnosis)	THINK
Differential diagnosis (obeying Lee's law)**	THINK
Investigations (appropriate and justifiable)	THINK
Diagnosis	THINK
List of problems and action	THINK

e.g.

1. Confirm diagnosis, e.g. of intestinal obstruction
2. Chest pain—organize CXR/ECG/?cardiac referral
3. Diabetic—controlled or not? Blood glucose, U and Es need diabetologist/anesthetist advice
4. Patient does not know names of drugs: Ask for bottles
                                        Ask relatives
                                        Ring GP

The word *think* has been appended to each step. This is to emphasize that, although you have been taught to use basic protocols, the history and examination is a *dynamic* process evolving as the patient provides you with information. You must think as you go along, ask additional relevant questions and not just write down a set of cyclostyled questions and answers.

** No differential diagnosis must be entered, unless the patients symptoms and signs are suggestive of that diagnosis (and you must be able to justify)

THYROID/NECK EXAMINATION: INSPECT/PALPATE/PERCUSS/AUSCULTATE

INSPECT from in front	• Any obvious generalized or localized swelling?
	• State anatomical location of swelling
	• If swelling present does it move on swallowing?
	• On putting out tongue?
	• Any visible scars/skin discoloration
	• Any dilated veins
	• Any arterial palpations

PALPATE from behind	• Size/Shape/Consistency/Tenderness/Temperature of swelling
	• Mobility of swelling—is it fixed to skin/deeper structures
	• Palpable thrill?
	• Ask to swallow again—does it move?
	• Identify carotid pulses
	• Feel for lymph nodes: Submental/submandibular/tonsillar cervical chain/posterior triangle
	(Tricks for feeling swelling: Put head down push swelling to one side)
PALPATE from in front	Is trachea central?
PERCUSS	Over manubrium for retrosternal extension
	Pemberton's sign, if indicated
AUSCULTATE	For bruit

Description of Multinodular Goiter Based on Protocol

On examination: Inspection shows a large irregular swelling involving the right and left anterior triangles and the midline. There are no obvious scars; the overlying skin is normal. There are no obvious arterial or venous pulsations. The swelling moves up and down when she swallows and does not move when she puts out her tongue. On palpation from behind, the swelling measures about 14 cm × 10 cm, it moves on swallowing and appears to involve both the left and right lobes of the thyroid gland and the isthmus. It is irregular. There are several separate nodules which vary in size between 2 and 4 cm diameter. The swellings are firm in consistency, smooth-surfaced and have well-demarcated edges. The swelling is non-tender, does not pulsate and none of the nodules transilluminate. The carotid pulses are palpable, the skin moves freely over the swelling but it appears to be 'fixed' deeply. There are no palpable neck nodes. The trachea is not palpable, auscultation is negative but Pemberton's sign appears to be positive, in that she is a little plethoric and breathless when asked to elevate her arms.

INGUINAL HERNIA EXAMINATION

Patient lying supine

Look

1. Any visible swelling? Note position and size.
2. Any other relevant signs, e.g. scars, change in color of skin.
3. If swelling is present ask patient if they can reduce it for you and then proceed as follows. If they are unable to reduce—see instructions below.
4. Ask patient to cough: Look to see if a swelling appears—if so look very carefully, and see if the swelling comes down lateral to medial (indirect) or posteroanterior (direct). This is probably the most 'accurate' test of all—so do it carefully.

Palpate

1. If swelling present, then ask the patient to reduce again.
2. Place hand flat on the line of the inguinal canal and ask patient to cough—note, if there is a cough impulse or a swelling appears and in which direction the impulse or swelling travels.
3. Identify the anatomical landmarks of the inguinal ligament. Anterior Superior Iliac Spine (ASIS) and the pubic tubercle. Note the latter lies in the crease at the bottom of the abdomen and not in the groin crease.
   Ascertain if the swelling is above and medial to pubic tubercle—inguinal hernia or below and lateral—femoral hernia.
4. Identify the mid point of the inguinal ligament (half-way between the ASIS and the pubic tubercle)—one cm above this is the position of the deep inguinal ring.
   With the swelling reduced place one or two fingers of your right hand over the deep ring and press firmly. Ask the patient to cough. If the swelling is controlled the hernia is indirect; if the swelling appears medial to the fingers it is direct. This is called the *deep ring occlusion test*.
5. *Scrotal invagination test:* 'Free the scrotum'. Invaginate the little finger (gently) into the neck of the scrotum and pass it upwards to the position of the external ring to enter the inguinal canal. Ask the patient to cough. Can you feel a swelling coming into the canal? If so does the swelling hit the tip of your finger (indirect) or back of your finger (direct)?
6. Complete the examination by examining the scrotum and testis.
7. Examine the other groin and scrotum in exactly same way.

Ask the Patient to Stand
- If no swelling visible ask the patient to cough.
- Look for cough impulse or swelling.
- Note the size and position of swelling in relation to pubic tubercle.

If a swelling is seen, ask the patient to reduce it and hold it reduced for you. Identify your landmarks, occlude the deep ring and ask the patient to cough again—does it remain controlled (indirect).

Note: If on standing, a swelling is seen that is painful or difficult to reduce by the patient, do not progress with the standing examination any further—just do the examination with the patient lying down.

Hint: When the patient is standing probably the best way of feeling a swelling or cough impulse is to stand at the side of the patient or behind him and put your left hand on his inguinal canal for the patient's left side and right hand on the inguinal canal for right side.

If you are examining a patient with a large scrotal swelling—visible on standing or lying down you are best to examine him lying down first. Ask him to reduce the swelling. If he can reduced it proceed with the 'hernia protocol'. If he cannot, you have to decide one thing—can you get above the swelling—if so it is a 'scrotal problem' and you examine accordingly. If you cannot get above the swelling, then it is an inguinoscrotal swelling and is an indirect inguinal hernia until proven otherwise.

MALE GENITALIA/SCROTUM EXAMINATION

- Patient supine to start with.
- Examiner preferably wearing gloves (nonsterile).

Inspection
- **Inspect the penis**—including the glans and meatus-dorsal and ventral surface look for size, shape, skin color, discharge, any discrete abnormality, e.g. ulcer/lump—use appropriate protocol to describe (e.g. Size, Shape, Surface, etc. or for an ulcer Base Edge Depth Discharge: BEDDS mnemonic). Retract prepuce if indicated.
- **Inspect—the scrotum** from front and then lift up and look underneath; looking for any difference in size or shape (Left versus Right), any skin abnormality, any lumps, ulcer.

Palpation
- **Palpate**—the contents of the scrotum starting with the normal side first. Compare Right to Left side.
  Identify and palpate:
  – Testis
  – Epididymis
  – Cord (feel vas deferens and vessels)
- If swelling is felt: determine four facts:
  1. Is the swelling confined to the scrotum? (i.e. can you get above it?)
  2. Can the testis and epididymis be defined?
  3. Is the swelling transilluminable?
  4. Is the swelling tender?
- Define the characteristics of any swelling using the standard protocol for lump/bump (SSS, etc.).
- Finally; stand the patient up: Is the swelling still palpable or is a new one present? (e.g. varicocele).

BREAST EXAMINATION

Inspect, palpate—breast first then axilla
First examine, the patient sitting on the edge of examination couch facing you with arms at sides.
Inspect: Sequence: Breast Areola Nipple
   Inspect the breasts for swellings, size, R and L disparity, skin tethering, color change, distended veins
   Then inspect aerola—both sides—size, shape, ulcer
   Then inspect nipple—both sides—size, shape, ulcer, discharge.
   Ask patient to put arms above head—any change in skin contour (tethering), does lump become visible or more obvious.
   Ask patient to put arms on hip and press in—any change?—any skin tethering
Palpation: • Same sequence: Breast Areolar Nipple
   • With patient sitting comfortably arms at side
   • Palpate normal breast first

- Palpate four quadrants in systematic manner: identify swelling/thickening/tenderness
- If lump identified assess size, margin, consistancy, temperature, fixity
- ? Skin mobile over it locally: move swelling, raise arms test fixity to chest wall by tensing pectoralis major
- Palpate nipple—gentle squeeze ? discharge
- Palpate areola
- Then palpate abnormal breast—exactly same sequence
- Then palpate both axillae with patient still sitting:
- Rest patient's arm on yours
- Examine medial chest wall, apex of axilla, anterior wall over pectoralis, posterior wall over subscapularis
- If lymph nodes felt: note number, site, consistency, fixity
- Feel supraclavicular area for nodes
- Go behind patient and feel anterior and posterior triangles for nodes
- Then lie the patient on the examination couch, supine with 1 or 2 pillows under her head and her hand behind her head

Then repeat the same sequence of examination, you have performed above: Breast/Areola/Nipple, and then palpate both axillae. Finally, examine the abdomen, for evidence of enlarged liver or presence of ascites

---

Remember: LOOK, FEEL, MOVE BREAST, AREOLA, NIPPLE

Look: R and L disparity in size/lumps/skin tethering abnormal skin changes, distended veins then areola changes, then nipple changes or differences

Raise arms—look for tethering/mass

Feel: By quadrants, systematically, describe lump by set criteria (site, size, shape, surface, etc.)

Do not forget

Move: (i.e. fixity to skin and pectoralis muscle), then examine areola and nipple

- Examine normal breast first and then the other
- Feel axillae CORRECT WAY: ant/post/medial walls and apex
- Feel supraclavicular areas
- Then lie paient down on 1 pillow, hand behind head and repeat whole sequence
- Check for ascites and liver enlargement

LUMP OR BUMP EXAMINATION

LOOK   FEEL   MOVE: (4 S 1C 1E 3T 1P)

4 × S	Size
	Site
	Shape
	Surface
1 × C	Consistency (fluctuates)
1 × E	Edge
3 × T	Tenderness
	Temperature
	Transilluminates
1 × P	Pulsatile
MOVE	Superficial fixation
	Deep fixation

SURROUNDINGS + lymph nodes

PERCUSSION

AUSCULATE   bruit

EXAMINATION OF A SKIN ULCER

LOOK   FEEL   MOVE

Look   Position

Size

Shape

Number

BEDDS

Base: Healthy granulations, dead slough, tendon, bone

Edge: Sloping, punched out, undermined, rolled, everted

Depth: mm's and anatomical structures reached

Discharge: Serous, serosanguinous, blood, pus

Surroundings: Color

VV's

Wasting

Feel
- Temperature/Tenderness
- Peripheral pulses
- Sensation
- Lymph nodes

Move
- Loss of muscle power
- Fixed deformities
- Wasting of muscle groups

PHYSICAL EXAMINATION OF A VASCULAR PATIENT

GENERAL:

Face:
- Alert, conscious and orientated?
- In pain or distressed?
- Pale or jaundiced?
- Well nourished?
- Well hydrated?
- Lips/Mouth: Cyanosed/plethoric/intraoral pathology and dentition?

Hands: Fingernail changes, palmar crease pallor, palmar erythema, moist palms

ARMS

Vital signs: Pulse/BP/RR/temp/peripheries

CVS: Cardio: Lips
        JVP
        Inspection of chest
        Apex beat
        Auscultation
        Leg edema

Remember this is a 'vascular case' so you have to examine the upper limbs/neck/face for evidence of vascular disease:

COMPARE BOTH UPPER LIMBS:

Inspection	Color	• Normal
		• Pale
		• Congested
		• Blotchy
		• Ischemic changes – Thinning of skin
		– Hair loss
		– Ulceration

Palpation	Temperature
	Capillary refilling
	Pulses Distal to proximal comparing both sides
	Radial
	Ulnar
	Brachial
	Axillary
	+/– Thrills

Auscultation for bruits

Palpate and ausculate carotid arteries in neck

Face: Cyanosis/plethoric
        Arcus/xanthelasma
        Fundi

Appropriate neurological assessment, if relevant history or local signs, e.g. weakness

RS: • Inspection
       • Auscultation
       • Percussion

Abdomen: Pulsatile mass
           Bruit

Specfic: Lower limbs (including full vascular assessment)

Look: Compare both limbs – Any swelling/deformity/muscle wasting
                            – Any bruising
         Change in color, e.g. pale/blue
         Varicose veins

Then **Look** at right leg
         Any signs of ischemia – Thickened, dystrophic toenails, ulcers, gangrene
                                – Look at pressure points

Feel: • Temperature/tenderness (especially calf)
         • Pulses (dorsalis pedis, posterior tibial, popliteal, femoral)
         • Capillary refill
         • Sensation

Move: Limitation on movements
         Muscle wasting
         Fixed deformities
         Burgers angle/test

Then Look, Feel/Move for other leg.

Neurological Examination: Back and legs.

How to Read Plain Chest and Abdominal Radiographs

In many parts of the world, plain abdominal X-rays in the acute abdomen have been replaced by CT abdomen, which include 'plain' scout films of the abdomen. However, this facility is not available in all hospitals and throughout the world, hence the continued inclusion of abdominal X-rays in this book.

Suggested Protocols for interpretation of chest and abdominal X-rays *(by kind permission of the editor, Penang Hospital Journal).*

How to Read Plain Chest and Abdominal Radiographs: A Systematic and Standardized Approach

Kok Hong Kuan, Gooi Boon Hui, Dennis Tan Gan Pin, Salwah Hashim, Peter Lee
Department of Surgery, Penang Medical College
Departments of Surgery and Radiology, Penang General Hospital

INTRODUCTION

Chest and abdominal X-rays are the two most frequently requested imaging modalities in the clinical setting and play a pivotal role in the management of cardiorespiratory and abdominal diseases. Although the interpretation of these X-rays is often left to the junior doctors, there may be a lack of formal instruction on the approach to these radiographs in medical schools. Thus, junior doctors often have to learn the techniques through clinical experience.

In order not to miss important findings on a radiograph, a systematic and standardized approach must be applied. There are numerous guidelines available in textbooks and the web, however, they are often technically detailed and few are targeted at students or junior doctors.

We recommend a structured approach (or protocol) for reading these radiographs which is simple, systematic and easily remembered. This approach is routinely adopted in clinical teaching at Penang Medical College. We find that students are now more confident and are better able to read and elicit the essential radiographic findings.

PLAIN CHEST X-RAYS (Fig. 1)

Plain chest radiographs (CXR) are the most common radiographs that junior doctors or medical students will be expected to interpret on the ward. However, it is important to note that the chest radiograph should be used as an adjunct

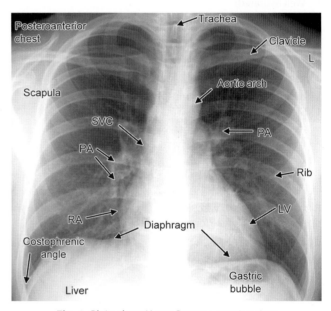

Fig. 1 Plain chest X-ray: Posteroanterior view
Abbreviations: LV, left ventricle; PA, pulmonary artery; RA, right atrium; SVC, superior vena cava

to diagnosis and should be interpreted in the light of the patient's clinical history and physical findings. The reading of the plain chest X-ray should begin with the following introductory sequence:

State: Patient's name and date of X-ray taken.
(If the patient is present, make sure the X-rays match the patient's name).

State: Type of X-ray (Erect PA/Supine AP/Semi-erect/ Sitting) and the extent of the field of the film (e.g. cervical spine to upper abdomen).
- *CXR are routinely taken in the erect PA view. Unlabeled films are generally considered to be erect and PA.*
- *Supine AP films are normally taken when patients are not able to stand erect. The AP film magnifies the heart and is generally of poorer quality.*

State: Whether the X-ray is orientated correctly right to left.
- *Most films will be marked with a R or L radiological marker. The heart shadow and*

gastric bubble are on the left. Be aware that dextrocardia and situs inversus do occur.

State: The adequacy of exposure, i.e. is it overexposed (dark) or underexposed (white)?
- *Generally, only the first 4 thoracic vertebrae will be visible in a well-exposed film.*
- *>4, if overexposed and low density lesions may be missed.*
- *<4, if underexposed and the lung may appear falsely white.*

State: The alignment of the X-ray, i.e. is the patient straight on or rotated?
- *Well centered film, if the medial ends of both clavicles are equidistant from the central spinous process of the vertebrae.*
- *A rotated film can cause distortion of the heart size and shape, altered prominence of the hilum, spurious displacement of the trachea, altered size of the aortic arch and altered relative densities of the hemithoraces.*

State: The degree of inspiration
- *A well-inspired film exposes the 6th rib anteriorly or the 10th rib posteriorly in the middle of the right hemidiaphragm.*
- *Poor inspiration will make the heart appear larger and give the appearance of basal shadowing.*

Your introduction may be presented as follows:

This is an erect PA chest X-ray of Mr Smith taken on the 2nd May 2009 extending from the lower neck to the upper abdomen, including the diaphragms. The film is correctly orientated right to left, is well penetrated, not rotated and has been taken in full inspiration.

The X-ray is then examined on a protocoled basis (i.e. the same every time).

If you are presenting the findings, you can state them as you go along.

The protocol we are going to use is to look in sequence at:

1. The trachea — Central or not
2. The mediastinum — Any widening / Any mass / Position (shifted or not)
3. Cardiac shadow — Estimate the cardiothoracic ratio / Identify single/multiple chamber enlargement / Any displacement of cardiac shadow
4. Hilar shadows — Look for increased density/irregularity/enlargement/abnormal vessels (left hilum is usually above the right)
5. Lung fields — Compare both sides as a whole divide into upper, middle and lower zones; look at each and compare with other side (concentrate on looking for homogeneous shadowing or mass lesions)
6. Diaphragms — Right hemidiaphragm usually above the left / Check the costophrenic angles
7. Visualized abdomen — Stomach bubble / Air under diaphragm / Calcified lesions, e.g. gallstone / Hepatosplenomegaly
8. The bony structures — Go through all the bony structures—the ribs and visualized portion of spine first
9. Soft tissues — Breast shadows / Soft tissue neck swelling and alignment of trachea / Soft tissue swelling over thoracic cage / Abnormal calcifications, e.g. in thyroid
10. Additions — NG tube, chest drains, ET tube, artificial valve, sternotomy wires, pacemaker, ECG leads, central line

Please note that this is an orderly progression and is easy to remember (Fig. 2).

Reminder!
Places where things are often missed on a chest X-ray:
- Look at the lung apices
- Look behind the heart
- Look at the bones

Sample chest X-ray Report for Figure 3.

This is an erect PA chest X-ray of Mr Smith taken on (date), extending from the lower neck to the upper abdomen. The film is correctly orientated right to left, well penetrated, not rotated and has been taken in full inspiration. The trachea is central. No mediastinal widening. The heart is enlarged with a cardiothoracic ratio of 0.7. The right and left heart borders are visible. The left ventricle is dilated. The right hilum appears normal. The left hilum is not visualized. Sternotomy wires in upper mediastinum and a radiopaque ring shadow in the left cardiac chamber, suggestive of a metallic mitral valve replacement. Normal lungs but the left lower zone is obscured by the enlarged cardiac shadow. The stomach bubble is noted on the left upper abdomen. No abnormality detected in upper abdomen. No soft tissue or bony abnormalities.

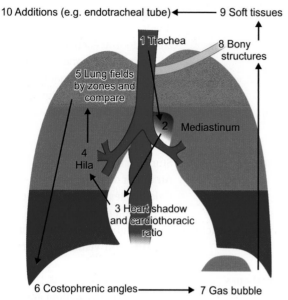

Fig. 2 Suggested approach to the chest X-ray

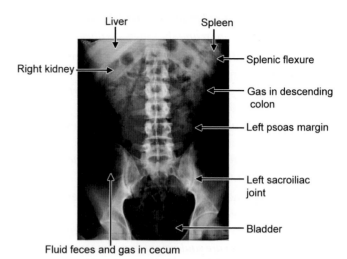

Fig. 4 Normal plain abdominal X-ray: anteroposterior view

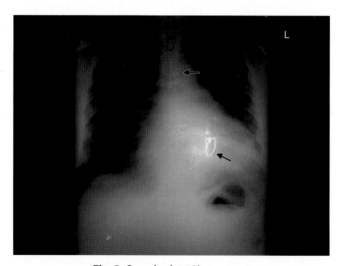

Fig. 3 Sample chest X-ray report

PLAIN ABDOMINAL X-RAYS (AXR) (Fig. 4)

- Plain abdominal X-rays are frequently ordered in the assessment of patients with an acute abdomen.
- Usually an erect chest X-ray (to visualize air under the diaphragm) together with an erect and supine abdominal X-ray are requested.
- Occasionally, if the patient cannot take up the erect position then a lateral decubitus film with the patient lying on his/her side is taken. This view is particularly useful for demonstrating small amounts of free air.
- The KUB film (kidneys, ureters and bladder) ordered by the urologists may differ from plain abdominal X-rays

only in the extent of the radiograph—by necessity, it must include the area from the diaphragms to the lower border of the bony pelvis.

- The reading of a standard plain abdominal X-ray should begin with the following introduction:

State: Patient's name and date of X-ray

(If the patient is present, make sure that the X-rays match the patient's name)

State: Type of X-ray (supine/erect/decubitus) and the extent of the field of the film

- *Erect films are decided by annotation, i.e. it is marked erect or by presence of air fluid level in stomach or bowel.*
- *Supine films are also decided by annotation, i.e. it is marked supine or by gaseous bowel distension with no fluid levels.*
- *Lateral decubitus films are recognized by fluid levels lying parallel to the long axis of the body.*
- *The extent of field is important: Are the diaphragms included? (free air)*
  Is the entire pelvic area included? (hernia shown)

State: Is the X-ray orientated correctly right to left?

- *Remember most films should be marked with an R or L, but these are not always correct! Look for the liver outline on the R or the gastric bubble on the L (or a nasogastric tube).*

State: The adequacy of exposure, i.e. is it overexposed (dark) or underexposed (white)

- *A well-penetrated film will show some or all of the lumbar vertebrae, the psoas shadows and the preperitoneal fat line.*

State: The alignment of the X-ray, i.e. is the patient straight or rotated?

Your introduction may be presented as follows:

This is an erect abdominal film of Mr Smith taken on the 24th February 2009 and includes the area from above the diaphragms down to the pelvis. It is correctly orientated right to left, well penetrated and the patient is not rotated.

The X-ray is then examined on a protocoled basis (i.e. the same every time). If you are presenting the findings you can state them as you go along.

The protocol we are going to use is to look in sequence for:

- The hollow organs (stomach, small bowel, large bowel including rectum and bladder).
- The solid organs (liver, spleen, kidneys, pancreas, prostate in male, uterus in female).
- Calcifications within abdominal organs (e.g. gallstones in gallbladder, calcifications in liver, spleen, pancreas, kidneys, ureters, uterus, ovaries, prostate and bladder).
- Calcifications within blood vessels (e.g. abdominal aorta, iliac vessels, phleboliths in veins).
- The bony structures.
- Soft tissue structures.
- Additions (e.g. drains, foreign bodies, catheters, staples).

Proceed as follows:

Hollow Viscera

Work your way down from the stomach to the rectum:

Stomach	• Gas outlining the body and antrum of the stomach with air fluid level in erect film, presence of NG tube
Small bowel	• Presence of valvulae conniventes encircling the jejunum • Lumen caliber, abnormal, if dilated more than 3 cm diameter. Often, only visualized clearly when abnormal air distension seen in supine film or air-fluid levels in erect film • Edema of the wall shown by increased radiolucency (white) and fuzziness of outline • Free gas can be seen 'outlining' the bowel wall, as free bubbles or under the diaphragms in the erect film or under the abdominal wall in a decubitus film
Large bowel	• Located in the periphery (i.e. frames the abdomen) • Presence of haustra (incomplete folds) are characteristic • May contain air on supine film, air fluid levels on erect films or fluid only • Dilated, if the transverse colon diameter is >5.5 cm or the cecal diameter at its base is >8 cm • Look for any cut off point—air proximal, none seen distally suggesting point of obstruction, check if air is seen in the rectum • Fecal material is speckled and granular (particularly seen in cecum)
Bladder	• Soft-tissue density emerging from pelvis only seen, if distended with urine

Solid Viscera

Liver	• Large soft tissue density in the right upper quadrant • More easily seen, if enlarged
Kidneys	• Not always visible • Smooth outline visible at level of upper border of T12 to L2, normally 10–12 cm long or 3.5 vertebrae in longitudinal length • Left higher than right • Enlarged or small • One kidney may be absent, horse-shoe kidney may be seen
Spleen	• Usually only seen, if enlarged • Enlarges inferomedially and may displace bowel
Pancreas	• Usually only seen if calcified, crosses the midline in an oblique axis
Psoas muscles	• Lateral border not always seen
Uterus	• May be seen if enlarged or calcified

Calcifications in Abdominal Organs

Gallstones	• Usually RUQ, solid or layered, 10–20% are radiopaque • In gallstone ileus, may be seen outside of the gallbladder
Hepatic calcifications	• Cysts, granuloma
Splenic calcifications	• Cysts, granuloma
Pancreatic calcifications	• Chronic pancreatitis
Renal calcifications	• 90% of kidney stones are radiopaque, one kidney or both, small or large or classical staghorn • Medullary nephrocalcinosis in hyperparathyroidism, renal tubular acidosis
Calcifications in line of ureter	• Ureters run down tips of lumbar transverse processes, crosses pelvic brim at sacroiliac joint, passes downwards to enter the bladder opposite the ischial spines (trace down this line)
Uterine calcifications	• Fibroids
Ovarian calcifications	• Dermoid cyst—teeth, bone
Bladder calcifications	• Bladder calculi are classically laminated
Calcification in prostate	• Stones
Calcification in appendix	• Appendicolith

Calcifications in Blood Vessels

Abdominal aorta in abdominal aortic aneurysm, iliac phleboliths in pelvic veins, rarely splenic artery aneurysm. Phleboliths are oval, smooth and have a small internal lucency.

Soft Tissues

- Abdominal wall swellings
- Irreducible hernia as scrotal swelling
- Breast shadows may be seen.

Bones

- Lower ribs, lumbar spine, sacrum, pelvis and hips
- Look carefully at each
- Abnormalities may include cortical thinning in osteoporosis, osteolytic or sclerotic lesions in metastasis, and Paget's, myeloma
- Sacroiliitis in Crohn's disease and ankylosing spondylitis.

Additions

- Drains, tubes (e.g. nasogastric, nephrostomy) catheters, foreign bodies and caval filter.

To finish: Once you have worked through the above protocol and noted your abnormal findings, it is helpful to conclude by once more looking at the X-ray as a 'whole' and then dividing it into four quadrants and checking each for the abnormalities, you have already identified or may have missed (Fig. 5).

Sample abdominal X-ray report is shown in Figure 6.

This is a supine abdominal X-ray of Mr Smith taken on (date) extending from the T11 vertebrae down to the bony pelvis. It is correctly orientated right to left, well penetrated and the patient is not rotated. The liver and kidney shadows are visualized with a large radiopaque staghorn calculi seen in the pelvicalyceal system of the right kidney. Both psoas shadows are normal. A large calcified lymph node in front of the sacral promontory with smaller calcified lymph nodes above and below it. No other soft tissue or skeletal abnormalities in this film.

CONCLUSION

- When asked to present your interpretation of a chest or abdominal X-ray, always start with the introduction, we have recommended. This approach indicates you know what you are talking about, prevents errors and sounds impressive.

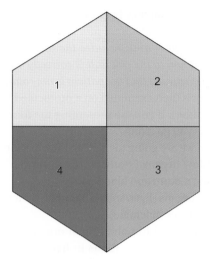

Fig. 5 Conclude by evaluating the film as a whole, looking through each quadrant

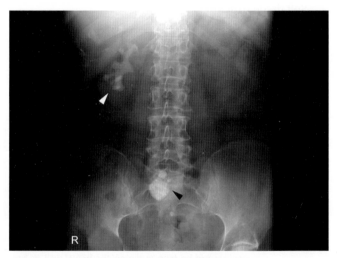

Fig. 6 Sample abdominal X-ray report

- You may not always be afforded the time or space to present the whole of the protocol as described above but always work through it in this standardized manner even, if you only present the abnormal findings.
- If you practice in this protocoled, standardized manner everytime, it will soon become second nature. You will not miss important findings, even if you do not know the correct diagnosis.
- Students may find it helpful to copy out just the 'protocol' parts of this article on to a card and carry it as an 'aide memoire' on the wards.

FURTHER READING

1. Armstrong P, Wastie M. Diagnostic Imaging, 4th edn. London: Blackwell Scientific, 1998.
2. Begg JD. Abdominal X-rays Made Easy, 2nd edn. Edinburgh: Churchill Livingstone, 2006.
3. Corne J, Carroll M, Brown I, Delany D. Chest X-ray Made Easy, 2nd edn. Edinburgh: Churchill Livingstone, 2002.
4. Erect Chest X-ray. Radiology Picture of the Day, 22 July 2008. *http://radpod.org/wp-content/uploads/2007/05/erect_chest.jpg*.
5. Hogan B, Looby S. Thoracic and Abdominal Radiology Manual, Department of Radiology, Beaumont Hospital.
6. Lee PWR. The plain X-ray in the acute abdomen: A surgeon's evaluation. Br J Surg. 1976; 63(10):763-6.

INDEX

Page numbers followed by *f* refer to figure and *t* refer to table.